D0916636

THE GREAT AMERICAN NUTRITION HASSLE

Edited by
LIESELOTTE HOFMANN

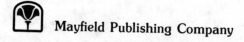

Mayfield Publishing Company

Library of Congress Catalog Card Number: 78-51947
International Standard Book Number: 0-87484-446-0

Manufactured in the United States of America
Mayfield Publishing Company
285 Hamilton Avenue, Palo Alto, California 94301

This book was set in Souvenir Light by Typesetting Services and
was printed and bound by the George Banta Company.
Sponsoring editor was C. Lansing Hays, Carole Norton supervised
editing, and Meryl Lanning was manuscript editor. Michelle Hogan
supervised production, the book and cover were designed by
Nancy Sears.

Contents

Preface

"Some people," said Samuel Johnson in 1763, "have a foolish way of not minding, or of pretending not to mind, what they eat. For my part, I mind my belly very studiously and very carefully; for I look upon it that he who does not mind his belly will hardly mind anything else." About a century later, Mark Twain countered this wise Englishman's observation with the revelation that "part of the secret of success in life is to eat what you like and let the food fight it out inside."

Today, in a land of cooking crazes and diet crazes, some Americans veer toward Johnson's view, but probably more go along with Mark Twain. In any case, Americans are becoming increasingly obsessed with food, and some of them are even worrying about nutrition. Many, of course, don't give a damn; others are so confused that they give up, and still others are so concerned that they become nutritional neurotics. The growing number of citizens who have become suspicious of their standard fare and of the programming that has led them to eat the way they do are frustrated by the contradictory advice of nutritionists and by the paucity of conclusive data on diet.

This book of readings reflects the main currents of thought and contention regarding nutrition in America. As both a nutrition handbook and a forum for diverse views, it includes topics that basic nutrition texts do not discuss at length or at all. Commingling here are biochemistry, behavioral science, sociology, medicine, politics, and economics. Nutritionists, biochemists, physicians, psychologists, food technologists, consumer groups, lawyers, and biomedical writers have their say in these pages and frequently disagree. Some of the authors are moderates, some are mavericks; many are eminent in their field. Their articles, whether sober, humorous, vitriolic, or salty, are never too technical. Extricated from a torrent of words in a wide variety of sources, the forty selections here have been chosen for their readability, currency, diversity of views, and potential appeal to even the frantic and the blasé.

ix

Although science is a dispassionate, impartial body of knowledge, scientists are not necessarily a dispassionate, impartial lot. Like the rest of us, scientists, as well as nutritionists and physicians, sometimes wear blinders, harbor biases, and have axes to grind. They are capable of, as Ralph Nader once put it in another context, slipping on their premises and sprawling to their conclusions. They may cling to a beloved hypothesis when evidence proves it to be flawed; they may pick their cases and ignore those that undermine their position.

These readings may cement your biases, unglue them, or cause you simply to rearrange them. But they invite you to consider the issues from more than one angle. They are meant to spur discussion in or out of the classroom.

When used along with other sources, the readings and the introductory comments may help nurture an understanding of the forces that shape nutrition in this country and of what you can do to meet your unique needs, without qualms and without complicated formulas. Perhaps this book will also help you see what nutritionist Jean Mayer meant when, serving as nutrition adviser to the President a few years ago, he lamented, "All the medical advances in the past 25 years have been wiped out by the decline in nutrition." Aided by this book it is hoped that you—either as a student of nutrition or as a general consumer—may come to realize that optimum rather than adequate nutrition is within your reach; that you will become more aware of your right and your obligation to be in charge of your own health; and that you will be encouraged and enabled to make reasoned judgments and to forge a personal course that avoids the Scylla of apathy and the Charybdis of fanaticism.

Because nutrition is a young science, the student of nutrition today must struggle through a maelstrom of theories, opinions, facts, fetishes, and new findings. If the readings seem to pose more questions than they answer, you can always fall back on these words of Alfred Korzybski: "There are two ways to slice easily through life; to believe everything or to doubt everything. Both ways save us from thinking."

To the dozens of authors and publishers who granted permission to reproduce the selections in this volume, I offer my deep gratitude.

I am indebted to C. Lansing Hays, not only because he commissioned me to prepare this book but because he remained so enthusiastic and forbearing during its genesis. And my thanks are extended to the nutrition educators who reviewed drafts of the manuscript and offered valuable suggestions and cautionary advice: Richard A. Ahrens, University of Maryland; Stanley G. Miguel,

Arizona State University; Rose Tseng, San Jose State University; Jack D. Osman, Towson State University; and Nancy Hufstetler, El Camino College. In addition, I wish to thank Professor George M. Briggs of the University of California, Berkeley, for so graciously taking the time to go over the manuscript, and for his kindness, encouragement, and gentle admonitions.

My thanks go also to Dr. Sumner Kalman of the Stanford School of Medicine for genially giving me access to a wealth of material; and to Meryl Lanning for her fine editorial advice.

Special gratitude is reserved for Carole Norton—for prodding my dream into reality, for her stalwart support and peerless counsel, and for giving this book its title.

Part I
Nutrition Attitudes, Needs, and Hazards

*Food is the first
enjoyment of life.*

—LIN YUTANG

Introduction to

Part I

Why do we eat the way we do? Why do we relish certain edible materials and shun others? If Americans were to dub grasshoppers "brushwood shrimps" and rats "household deer," as the Chinese once did,[1] would it give them gustatory appeal? Why have we long enjoyed eating cheese, while the Chinese have been persuaded by neither Mongols nor Europeans to eat it?*

During a famine, humans will eat *anything* edible. But when extreme hunger is not at issue, "food with man is not just food; it is the crossroads of emotion, religion, tradition, and habit."[2] With a flawed understanding of why people eat as they do, it is difficult, perhaps impossible, to fully apply knowledge of nutrition.

For many persons, the range of familiarity with foods is quite limited. Food acceptability hinges not only on an individual's past experience and on social, economic, and environmental conditions, but also on the biochemical state of the body and the response of sense organs. For instance, as we grow older, our taste buds gradually disappear. Most or all of the taste buds that abound in the cheeks and throat during early childhood make their exit, leaving only those of the tongue; and by later adulthood the structure and function of these, too, decline.[3]

Yet, as the French gourmet Brillat-Savarin wrote over 150 years ago, taste remains a delight because

> the pleasure of eating . . . is of all times, all ages, all conditions. . . . Because it may be enjoyed with other enjoyments, and even console us for their absence. . . . Because its impressions are more durable and more dependent on our will. . . . Because in eating we experience a certain indescribably keen sensation of pleasure, by what we eat we repair the losses we have sustained, and prolong life.[4]

Scientific logic may incite that small minority of Americans who have a deep concern with nutrition and health to change their eating practices. But the food intake of

---

*For one thing, some Chinese say, it smells like unwashed feet.

3

most people is ruled by learned and habituated preferences, by the senses, by external influences, and by the emotions; and those who most sorely need their nutrition improved know and care the least about the subject. Those nutritionists who are both sensitive and sophisticated realize that it is nonnutritional factors that for the most part determine food choices; they try to address themselves to those, instead of relying simply on concepts and terminology as in the past.[5]

Although food advertisers make much ado about the taste of their products, there is sturdy evidence that they have helped bring about a decline in America's food tastes. A few years ago Jacques Pépin (whose credentials include having been Charles de Gaulle's personal chef and a saucier at Maxim's in Paris) tried an experiment at the Campbell Soup Company, where he worked as chief of research. He prepared cream of tomato soup in the manner of Maxim's, with fresh tomatoes and real cream. Ninety-seven percent of the people who tasted it against Campbell's—not knowing which was which—preferred Campbell's. The real, the basic soup didn't taste "right"; Campbell's did, because the tasters were accustomed to thinking of it as "cream of tomato soup." Similarly, a taste panel recently chose canned pineapple juice over fresh. Why? Because the fresh juice didn't taste tinny, and that's what their palates were used to.[6,*]

In *Selection 1*, Jack Star offers a diverting analysis of the psychology and physiology of eating. He describes how our changing tastes and eating habits have eroded traditional food preferences and narrowed our choices. Particularly awry are family eating patterns: the sit-down dinner is now more a theory than a reality. To some, this alone is cause for concern. As John Keats puts it,

> When we make our conscientious selection of foodstuffs, when we go to work in our kitchens and dress our dinner tables, we are celebrants of an immemorial mystery. . . . The ultimate and principal ritual in our celebration is the evening communion around the dinner table. This is our daily statement of faith, our daily thanksgiving, and the way we celebrate it reveals what we believe to be true about ourselves. . . . The entire circumstances of the evening meal combine to state what family life means to us and what we actually think of one another.[7]

---

*It is true that, for some segments of the population, Lucullan repasts and exorbitant expenditures for elegant and exotic foodstuffs are "in" (see, for instance, "Love in the Kitchen," *Time*, December 19, 1977, pp. 54–58, 60–61). But the bulk of the nation's annual $215 billion food budget is not earmarked for such gourmet fare.

The decline in tastes and the desultory eating patterns of Americans probably have much to do with government findings that about half our population—rich, poor, and in-between—is not getting adequate nutrition from "the average American diet." But nutritional science, too, may be at fault. Says one critic:

> Nutritional science is not significantly advanced beyond the stage of the Ten Commandments. We have a science of nutrition based on the avoidance of deficiencies, of ill health. What we lack, and sorely need, is a science of well-being, of nutritional sufficiency. We have some idea of what deficiencies are most dangerous, particularly in the area of vitamins. We have very little scientific knowledge of the nutritional qualities of a diet that will maximize well-being and healthy growth.[8]

As Nevin Scrimshaw and Vernon Young demonstrate in *Selection 2,* dietary, physiological, and environmental factors interact to determine the nutritional needs of individuals and populations. For this reason, recommended energy and nutrient allowances can be but statistical approximations. The authors show why estimates of caloric requirements and recommended dietary allowances (RDAs) must, in spite of their limitations, serve as a guide for both individuals and populations; but they emphasize the urgent need for research in this realm. They might well agree with Garrett Hardin's dictum: "Blessed are the statistical tables, for they delay the day of our thinking."[9]

So different are the quantitative and qualitative needs of individuals that it has been suggested that the abbreviation RDA stands for "ridiculous, dangerous, and arbitrary." (Curiously, the National Academy of Sciences reportedly recommends 4 to 13 times the RDA of some nutrients for the optimum health of monkeys used in research work.[10]) The 1968 RDA list underwent 55 changes in values from the 1964 list, with variations from 20 to 700 percent; the 1974 list involved similar seesawing. This instability has aroused the suspicions of Senator William Proxmire of Wisconsin, who states that the Food and Nutrition Board of the National Research Council, which sets the RDA standard, "is both the creature of the food industry and heavily financed by the food industry." The lower the RDAs, Proxmire contends, the more nutritious the products of the food industry will appear: "At best the RDAs are only a 'recommended' allowance at antediluvian levels designed to prevent some terrible disease. At worst they are based on the conflicts of interest and self-serving views of certain portions of the food industry. Almost never are they provided at levels to provide for optimum health and nutrition."[11]

In *Selection 3,* D. Mark Hegsted, like the authors of Selection 2, takes a different (and apolitical) view; he states that the RDAs are deliberately set well *above* the estimated average requirement. Hegsted elaborates on the difficulties of using the RDA standard as a guide for specific situations, of explaining to people how they should eat, and of evaluating what they have been eating. What do you think—that the many changes in the RDA list are the result of food-industry clout, or research findings, or both?

Michael Jacobson takes a discouraging look at changes in the American diet, offering in *Selection 4* an overview of matters that are the core of several later selections. From infancy through old age, we eat more sugar, salt, and fat, but less fiber, than did our grandparents, he points out; and many of us end up paying the penalty.

Contributing to our dietary indiscretions are fast-food meals. Fast-food outlets receive an estimated 40 cents of every dollar spent on food eaten away from home; they are expected to take in $20 billion in 1977, the year McDonald's will sell its 23 billionth hamburger. Because they alleviate hunger (real or imagined) quickly in familiar, casual surroundings, fast-food outlets have become a ubiquitous lure. The massive number of Americans who want food and want it fast are undaunted by the dismay of nutritionists, the contempt of gourmets, the twinges of their own consciences.[12] Facing up to the real world, *Mademoiselle* recently persuaded a highly reluctant nutritionist to put together, as a stop-gap procedure only, a "junk-food" reducing diet based on fast-food meals.[13]

A couple of years ago Consumers Union tested the typical meals purveyed by eight of the largest fast-food chains. *Selection 5* describes the findings which, if you are a fast-food aficionado, may or may not ease your conscience.

Thanks mainly to the plethora of high-protein diets and the pushing of protein products by the livestock, dairy, and meat-packing industries, Americans have been led to believe that they need far more protein than in fact they do. Although some Americans are actually protein-starved, recent studies reveal that many, if not most of us consume considerably more protein (largely in the form of animal products) than our bodies can use.[14]

Were we to reduce our livestock population by half, the grains released for human consumption would add up to roughly 100 million tons. We stuff our livestock annually with as much grain as all the people in India and China consume in one year. Nutritionist Jean Mayer comments that "the same amount of food that is feeding 210 million Americans would feed 1.5 billion Chinese on an average Chinese diet."[15] The Chinese diet is regarded as one of the healthiest in the world, which means that we could manage very well on about a seventh of the food we now consume.

In *Selection 6*, D. Mark Hegsted examines the question of protein needs from several angles and ponders the ramifications of modifying the American diet. He shows that "the protein mystique" stems from acceptance of the belief that supply is the world's major nutritional problem, and he asks whether this is a valid concept on which to base major policy decisions.

Today, for the first time in history, Americans are buying more processed than fresh food. This increase is accompanied by a rapidly growing number of additives (their use went up by 50 percent in the decade 1965–1975). Fears about the side effects of additives have mounted apace; so worried are some people that their motto is: "If I can't pronounce it, I don't buy it." If, for instance, a product were labeled as containing para-hydroxylphenylbutanone-2, they would dismiss it out of hand. Yet, ominous as this chemical may sound, it is one that occurs naturally in raspberries, giving them their unique flavor.[16] Laypersons, including some self-appointed nutritionists, often do not realize that foods are themselves chemicals (the term "chemicalized foods" translates into "chemicalized chemicals").

Indeed, the trump card played by some proponents of additives is that certain naturally occurring chemicals are toxic.[17] What they fail to stress is that during the course of history, human beings have managed by trial and sometimes tragic error to separate the poisonous from the nonpoisonous; that natural toxic substances are rarely ingested in massive doses; and that there will always be some persons sensitive to certain natural ingredients in foods. The present uproar over additives is a reaction to thousands of substances concocted by technologists who are engaged in a possibly dangerous game of one-upmanship with nature. The question is whether augmenting the chemicals apportioned by nature is sensible, especially if, as the proponents of additives are fond of emphasizing, so many natural hazards already exist.

Each day the average American consumes several hundred food additives. A single food may contain well over a dozen unnatural, chemically modified substances. The human body, which has no antidotes for them, is expected to cope with them by its normal processes. If there are ill effects, now or 20 years from now, which chemical or chemicals can be blamed? Of the 3,800 to 4,000 additives now used, none has undergone pharmacological studies such as those required for licensing drugs—though additives can act like drugs.

Enter the "single rat" argument. Under the Delaney Amendment (1958) to the Food and Drug Law, if any substance is found to induce cancer in laboratory animals it must be banned from food. Opponents of the law maintain that it nullifies scientific judgment about safety: if a single rat gets one tumor, "even when fed in massive doses and by an unusual route (such as implantation), then the chemical must be banned, and maybe a whole industry wiped out."[18] Biochemist Magnus Pyke notes, however, that "even when toxic effects are found for the test animals, it does not necessarily follow that human beings would be affected, although it is prudent to assume that they would be. On the other hand, one could argue that even when a test substance has no effect on animals it may still harm people."[19]

"Americans," one gourmet laments, "will eat anything if you can manage to color it orange."[20] Food dyes, which have been used so extravagantly, have recently come under heavy fire, and the Food and Drug Administration has begun to take action. But the FDA still lets the food industry decide which of the more than 1,500 food flavorings and flavoring adjuncts in use are to be considered "Generally Recognized As Safe" (GRAS). Data on adverse effects have commonly remained unpublished. The government also tolerates package labels that reveal little about the contents, use misleading or cryptic terms, and deliberately leave out the names of some ingredients.[21] For instance, although monosodium glutamate must be listed on soup labels, it need not appear on labels for mayonnaise or salad dressing; and more than 30 nondairy additives permitted in processed cheeses do not have to be listed. On the occasion of his forced retirement as Commissioner of the FDA in 1969, Dr. Herbert Ley noted: "The thing that bugs me is that the people think the FDA is protecting them—it isn't. What the FDA is doing and what the public thinks it's doing are as different as night and day."[22]

Because many food shoppers are now wary, and claim that they have legitimate concerns, government food controllers and public-relations personnel in the food industry can no longer brush off as quacks or mental cases those who question the rampant use of additives. It is ceaseless political and industrial pressures on the FDA that are largely responsible for the agency's inconsistencies, tardiness, and laxity in warnings and inspections. When the FDA does take a stand against additives, it can count on attacks from a diversity of protesters, including members of Congress, food-industry lobbyists, the American Medical Association, financial journals, and even—as in the case of the proposed ban on saccharin—the general public.

Because science is presently unable to give a straight answer on additives, some laypersons and nutritionists consider the dangers negligible and greatly exaggerated. Harvard nutritionist Fredrick Stare, for example, insists that additives are not "badditives": you should eat them because they're good for you.

Less than 1 percent of our total diet, he points out, is made up of additives; and "our current food laws are such that an additive—especially one from a synthetic source—doesn't have a chance if it is found to pose even a slight health hazard to man or animals."[23]

Nevertheless, with additives entering the American diet at the rate of a billion pounds a year, the FDA recently announced plans for a far-reaching review of them. But perhaps most promising is the development of a new family of additives composed of chemicals bonded to special polymers. Called hitchhikers, they literally go along just for the ride. Once foods are eaten, these substances quit work; they cannot be absorbed by the body, supply no calories, and, according to their developers, cannot cause health problems. They will probably be on the market by 1980.[24]

In *Selection 7*, Joan Majtenyi presents a dispassionate, informative survey of additives: the various types and their uses, benefits, and potential hazards. Spokespersons for the food industry have suggested that the benefits to a consumer from additives make their "calculated risk" worthwhile. To which one skeptic has responded: "It looks to me as if industry is doing all the calculating, and the consumer public is taking all the risks."[25] Do you think the risks are minimal and exaggerated? Or do you think they are sufficient to warrant more careful food selection and more constructive criticism of regulatory agencies?

References

1 Reay Tannahill, *Food in History* (New York: Stein and Day, 1973), p. 152.

2 Ercel S. Eppright, "Factors Influencing Food Acceptance," *Journal of The American Dietetic Association* 23 (July 1947), p. 579.

3 Ibid., pp. 580–581.

4 Anthelme Brillat-Savarin, *Handbook of Dining,* quoted in Ann Seranne and John Tebbel, eds., *The Epicure's Companion* (New York: David McKay Co., 1962), pp. 431–432.

5 Godfrey M. Hochbaum, "Human Behavior and Nutrition Education," *Nutrition News* 40 (February 1977), pp. 1, 4; and Howard E. Bauman and Dudley Ruch, "Problems of Researching and Marketing Fortified Foods and Their Implications for Consumption Trends," in American Medical Association, *Nutrients in Processed Foods: Vitamins, Minerals* (Acton, Mass.: Publishing Sciences Group, 1974), p. 148.

6 Harvey Steiman, "Culinary Madness—Imitating the Imitators," *San Francisco Examiner,* July 27, 1977, p. 19.

7 John Keats, *What Ever Happened to Mom's Apple Pie? The American Food Industry and How to Cope with It* (Boston: Houghton Mifflin Co., 1976), pp. 231–232.

8   Larry P. Gross, "Can We Influence Behavior to Promote Good Nutrition?" *Bulletin of the New York Academy of Medicine* 47 (June 1971), p. 616.

9   Garrett Hardin, *Stalking the Wild Taboo* (Los Altos, Calif.: William Kaufmann, 1973), p. 96.

10 Carlton Fredericks, "Hotline to Health," *Prevention,* May 1977, p. 48.

11 William Proxmire, quoted in Richard A. Passwater, *Supernutrition* (New York: Pocket Books, 1976), pp. 185, 188.

12 Paul Gray, "Want Food Fast? Here's Fast Food," *Time,* July 4, 1977, p. 46.

13 "The Junk-Food Diet," *Mademoiselle,* August 1977, p. 178.

14 See, for instance, Ronald M. Deutsch, *Realities of Nutrition* (Palo Alto, Calif.: Bull Publishing Co., 1976) pp. 2–3, 195–197.

15 Jean Mayer, quoted in Allan Cott, with Jerome Agel and Eugene Boe, *Fasting: The Ultimate Diet* (New York: Bantam Books, 1975), p. 38.

16 James Trager, *The Bellybook* (New York: Grossman Publishers, 1972), p. 372.

17 See, for instance, Alfred H. Wertheim, *The Natural Poisons in Natural Foods* (Secaucus, N.J.: Lyle Stuart, 1974); Elizabeth M. Whelan and Fredrick Stare, *Panic in the Pantry: Food Facts, Fads and Fallacies* (New York: Atheneum, 1975), pp. 82–105; and Vernal S. Packard, Jr., *Processed Foods and the Consumer: Additives, Labeling, Standards and Nutrition* (Minneapolis: University of Minnesota Press, 1976), pp. 145–168.

18 Nicholas Wade, "Delaney Anti-Cancer Clause: Scientists Debate an Article of Faith," *Science 177* (August 1972), p. 589.

19 Magnus Pyke, quoted in Beatrice Trum Hunter, *Food Additives and Federal Policy: The Mirage of Safety* (New York: Charles Scribner's Sons, 1975), p. 51. See also Julie Miller, "Testing for Seeds of Destruction," *The Progressive,* December 1976, pp. 37–40.

20 Waverley Root, quoted in "What's in This Stuff?" *Esquire,* June 1974, p. 92.

21 "Food and Nutrition," *Consumers' Research Magazine,* October 1976, p. 56. See also Jacqueline Verrett and Jean Carper, *Eating May Be Hazardous to Your Health* (New York: Simon and Schuster, 1974); Michael F. Jacobson, *Eater's Digest: The Consumer's Factbook of Food Additives* (Garden City, N.Y.: Doubleday and Co., 1972); and William Longgood, *The Poisons in Your Food,* new rev. ed. (New York: Pyramid Books, 1969).

22 R. D. Lyons, "Ousted FDA Chief Charges 'Pressure' from Drug Industry," *New York Times,* December 31, 1969.

23 Whelan and Stare, *Panic in the Pantry,* p. 129.

24 Alton Blakeslee, "'Hitchhiking' Food Additives Are Coming," *San Francisco Examiner,* July 20, 1977, p. 24. (Dynapol, a firm in Palo Alto, Calif., is developing these additives.)

25 Wertheim, *Natural Poisons,* p. 48.

1 | The Psychology and Physiology of Eating

JACK STAR

Jack Star, a magazine writer, was a *Look* reporter for 20 years.

From *Today's Health,* February 1973, pp. 32–37. Reprinted by permission of the author.

Last night, in a Mexican restaurant, my 14-year-old son watched with astonishment as I devoured a half dozen red hot peppers. My eyes streamed, my nose ran, and fires raged in my mouth and throat. "Oh, this is so good!" I said, extinguishing the flames with scalding coffee—the way I like it.

It seems that my love of hot Mexican food may be related to a love of pain. My authority for this is a book called *Principles of Sensory Evaluation of Food,* which is considerably more interesting than its title would seem to indicate. Its authors, Maynard A. Amerine, Rose Marie Pangborn, and Edward B. Roessler, all of the University of California in Davis, point out: "Some people apparently derive pleasure from a certain degree of pain, as in the eating of excessively 'hot' curries or chilies, drinking very hot coffee or distilled beverages 'straight.' " With the dry wit of the scientist, the authors suggest that "a certain degree of adaptation to these foods is involved."

But why do people like me go through the suffering required to "adapt" to spicy food, while other people never try it more than once ("How can you stand to eat that stuff?")? Are such preferences really "a matter of taste" in the *physical* sense, or are they *social* and *cultural* preferences, determined by our parents, friends, social class, and need for status?

As is often the case with scientific questions, the answers are complicated and always incomplete. Thanks to the labors of sociology, anthropology, and even psychology, much is known about the role of status in food selection, about food taboos and superstitions, about the function of more obvious factors, such as memory and the attraction of familiar foods.

But when it comes to describing exactly how we taste foods, the explanations are less clear and more problematical. Only during the last decade or two have scientists focused their attention on the chemistry of taste, and each year scientific journals publish scores of articles on "the chemical senses."

One reminder: The word *taste*, referring to the physical faculty (as opposed to flavor, as in the taste of butter), has two common meanings. The first is the sense of taste that resides in the taste buds on the tongue, which distinguish only sweet, sour, salty, and bitter "tastes." The second, more inclusive meaning is the sense of taste that comes from the tongue working in combination with the sense of smell. It is from this more complicated sense of taste that we are able to distinguish, often with the help of other senses as well, hundreds of different flavors.

Look at your tongue in a mirror—or without a mirror, if you're agile enough—and you will see many tiny dots, bumps, and craters. These are the papillae. In each papilla there are from 33 to 508 taste buds—an average of about 250. Each taste bud has from 5 to 18 taste cells, each of which may respond to all four basic tastes identified by the tongue—sweet, sour, salty, and bitter—or just some of them. A bitter taste is best sensed at the back of the tongue; the sour taste is most sensitive at the edges of the tongue; sweet and salty tastes are most easily detected at the tip of the tongue—one reason that candies like gum drops are made so that the tip of the tongue is used most. Where there are no papillae, there is no taste. Most of the tongue's sensitivity is at the tips and edges—there is little in the middle.

The nose is just as important to the tasting process as the tongue—and probably more so—because man's nose is far more acute and versatile at identifying substances than his tongue. By smelling, a man can detect dilutions of alcohol, for example, that are 24,000 times greater than those that can be detected by the tongue. Smelling is an infinitely more sophisticated process: A person can be trained to distinguish among several thousand different odors, while the tongue has to make do with sweet, sour, salty, and bitter and their combinations.

How does the sense of smell, so important to identifying—and enjoying—the flavors of foods, really work? The exact mechanism is yet to be discovered, but it is a chemical process: The nose and nasal passages have chemical receptors that identify molecules that are given off by food and many other objects in our environment. The molecules of a particular substance—popcorn, say—enter the nose and cling to mucosal linings, where they are picked up by the chemo-receptors in the nose, which chemically analyze the molecules and send the information that this particular chemical combination (or smell) belongs to popcorn.

Whatever the precise workings of our complicated sense of smell, there is no doubting its importance to our enjoyment of eating. We all know that when we come down with colds the joy of eating becomes a sad ghost of its former self. (Interestingly, in the very early stages of a cold, the inflamed, swelling nasal tissues are *more* sensitive, for a short while, so this would be the ideal time to enjoy a gourmet meal.)

In general, the sense of smell is more acute in the morning hours and decreases after eating. Sipping a martini or popping a sugar cube in the mouth helps accelerate this decrease, while bitter tonics and dry white wines help prevent the decrease.

Besides taste and smell, the nerves around the mouth and even inside the dental pulp and gums help make a meal pleasurable by telling the eater about the texture and temperature of the food.

The color of food, of course, is an important key to food selection and enjoyment. White oleomargarine, for example, tastes and smells exactly the same as yellow oleomargarine—but just try to make the average housewife buy white margarine. She won't. It doesn't taste like margarine to her.

Most shoppers, in fact, associate the color of fruits and vegetables with ripeness, juiciness, or flavor. Changing colors also serve as a guide to poor flavor in too-old cheese, fish, and meat. But even when a color has little to do with flavor, the consumer has his preferences. Experiments have shown that orange orange juice is vastly preferred to yellow orange juice—even when the taste is the same. And poorer-tasting orange juice tastes better to people when coloring is added.

One diabolical scientist badly confused a test panel by serving its members six flavors of sherbet (lemon, lime, orange, grape, pineapple, and almond) in their uncolored, natural form. Then he baffled them even more by tinting the lemon sherbet an orange color, the pineapple a grape color, and the almond a lemon color.

That is why butter has been artificially colored when the natural carotene was low. That is why artificial green color has been added to mint-flavored ice cream, which is naturally white. And that is why oranges have been tinted a deeper orange, and coloring added to maraschino cherries, candy, jelly, and syrup.

In one famous experiment a number of shoppers wearing tinted goggles were turned loose in a supermarket. When they took off the goggles at the check-out counter, the shoppers were astonished at their strange selection of brands and at their unusual choices of meats, cheeses, fruits, and vegetables. And they were noticeably slower than usual in doing their shopping.

I recently received a powerful lesson in the importance of sight to the enjoyment of eating. I attended a banquet sponsored by the American Foundation for the Blind. At each of 12 tables a sighted person wearing a blindfold had to struggle through a meal with the aid of a blind person. This was an experiment in role reversal—to see what it was like to be blind. I was one of the dozen persons wearing a blindfold. I was amazed to find that much of the flavor of my food had simply vanished. I was told by my blind helper at the meal that if I were to actually become blind, I would in time adjust to the missing visual stimuli. But for now, there was no question that I lost much of my eating pleasure because of the blindfold, lack of my sight of food. But as important as our senses are to eating, a moment's reflection should tell us that social influences are probably just as important. Why does the sugar content of the same brand of soft drink vary, because of the customers' preferences, from region to region? Why do people in New Orleans like so much chicory in their coffee? Why do people in Hawaii and the Carolinas prefer wieners with an orange casing, and people in Kansas and Georgia a red casing—and Milwaukee residents a casing with no color at all? Why does a Boston housewife usually prefer brown eggs and a Chicago shopper white ones?

One of the most important determinants is simply what you're used to. "What people eat is what food is available and what they've been taught to eat by their mothers," says Minneapolis biochemist Arthur D. Odell, Ph.D., a pioneer in developing a whole line of synthetic meats from soy beans. "Europeans are in a meat culture, but 60 percent of the world lives on cereal grains, because that's all they have to eat."

Taboos also are significant, he says. "A Hindu would no more eat a cow than he would eat a cat. In some parts of the world taboos affect diet enormously—take the prohibition in some primitive societies against pregnant women eating meat or drinking milk, the very foods they need most."

When the biochemist told me that most Europeans regard sweet corn as swine food, I remembered the time I invited the captain of a Swedish ship to my home for dinner. He enjoyed the steak but despite his natural politeness had trouble disguising his revulsion for the ear of corn as he poked it gingerly with his fork.

A food consultant for the U.N. and for the U.S. State Department, Dr. Odell travels to every part of the world. "Do you know what the universal food is?" he asks. "Coca-Cola, that's what. Why? The bubbles in the mouth are pleasant. You get a feeling of both sweetness and tartness. The aroma is pleasant. And you unconsciously realize you are getting an energy lift from the sugar, particularly between meals when your sugar level has dropped down."

Dr. Odell notes that exotic food tastes are often acquired through necessity. The Greeks like a white wine called *retsina* that is heavily flavored with resin—a most unusual taste—because the wine was originally shipped in pine casks that exuded the substance. The Scandinavians acquired a taste for heavily salted fish—heavily salted originally so that it would not spoil, and now salted through preference. British sailors got to like pickled and dried meats—prepared that way out of necessity and later out of choice.

James L. Breeling, director of the section on food science in the American Medical Association's Department of Foods and Nutrition, explains how a food can attain almost a mystical significance for a people.

"On the Western Amazon River," he says, "the staple food is yucca, sometimes called manioc—a high-carbohydrate root. When the river is steady or falling, the people catch fish, both to eat and to sell. They also plant and harvest yucca. Fish, chicken, wild game, and fruits can all be sold for cash in the towns and villages. Manioc is what the people live on. Yet, manioc is highly regarded by these people. It is not consumed only for the economic reason. Belief in its value is beyond anything that can be substantiated by chemical analysis."

Manioc falls within the group of foods which Derrick Jelliffe, M.D., professor and head of the department of population, family health, and international health at UCLA and a nutritional anthropologist who studied infant feeding in many parts of the world, has named "cultural superfoods." Such a food is not only a community's main source of calories, "but one that has a tremendous emotional, historical, mystical, and religious hold on the community." In Ireland and Russia the superfood is the potato. In Central America it is corn.

The superfoods are often bound up with rites and used in a variety of ceremonies, says Breeling, adding: "As Jelliffe points out, all of us base our food preferences upon *irrational* factors. We eat for the symbolic value of the food as much as, or even more than, for the nutritive value. Food advertisers give practical recognition to the symbolic foods . . . in the advertising of products as giving status, sexual attractiveness, upward social mobility."

In *The Status Seekers,* Vance Packard vividly describes a typical example of the role of food preferences during one American's climb up the social ladder: "As a lad, this man had grown up in a poor family of Italian origin. He was raised on blood sausages, pizza, spaghetti, and red wine. After completing high school, he went to Minnesota and began working in logging camps, where—anxious to be accepted—he soon learned to prefer beef, beer, and beans, and he shunned 'Italian' food. Later, he went to a Detroit industrial plant, and eventually became a promising young executive. This was in the days when it was still fairly easy for a non-college man to rise in industry. In his executive role he found himself cultivating the favorite foods and beverages of other executives: Steak, whiskey, and seafood. Ultimately, he gained acceptance in the city's upper class. Now he began winning admi-

~~~~~~

ARMY MEN PREFER ALL-AMERICAN FOOD

With all the jokes about Army food, it may surprise some to learn that the Army has spent a lot of time and money to find out which foods soldiers prefer. Why? Believe it or not, it's so that their preferences could be taken into account when planning mess hall menus.

Among the findings of the latest such study were these:

- The more educated the soldier, the more he liked such foods as mushrooms, hot tea, and grapefruit, and the less he liked ham salad and mashed potatoes.
- The younger the soldier, the fewer foods he liked.
- More intelligent soldiers preferred crisp relishes, relish trays, and maple syrup, among other foods—and had significantly less interest in cherry drink, corn flakes, and instant coffee.

The findings also confirmed what has already been known for some time and can be demonstrated by almost anyone's experience: As one grows older, the general trend in food preference is away from the sweet foods beloved in childhood, and toward tart, bitter, or more subtly flavored foods.

The results of the survey, which was conducted by Joseph M. Kamen, Ph.D., now professor of marketing at Indiana University Northwest in Gary, were published in 1963 as a 400–page technical report titled *Analysis of U.S. Army Food Preference Survey*.

The study was carried out by means of questionnaires filled out by more than 2,000 soldiers, and evaluated their attitudes toward 263 foods—everything from Knickerbocker soup to cabbage, apple, and raisin salad. Preferences also were compared to the size of hometown, marital status, education, intelligence, and a number of other factors.

Although the survey was limited to a

~~~~~~

ration from people in his elite social set by going back to his knowledge of Italian cooking, and serving them, with the aid of his manservant, authentic Italian treats such as blood sausage, spaghetti, and red wine!"

Breeling also calls attention to the heavy symbolic meaning that the so-called organic and macrobiotic foods have for their users—a meaning that is not backed up by scientific evidence. George Christakis, M.D., of the Mt. Sinai Hospital and Medical School in New York City, learned this when working on a drug rehabilitation program with children who "frequently had

~~~~~~

restricted range of men, the relationships found should apply to people generally. "According to psychometric theory," Dr. Kamen says, "the relationships should be even stronger among the general population."

With this likelihood in mind, we used Dr. Kamen's study to put together the average soldier's—and perhaps the average American's—favorite and least-favorite dinner menus. The favorite menu reads like a list of foods straight out of the American Dream:

Grilled Steak
Mashed Potatoes
Tossed Vegetable Salad
or
Fresh Sliced Tomatoes
Hot Cross Buns and Butter
Apple Pie
Fresh Milk and Coffee

The least favorite menu shows a democratic abhorrence of the unusual bordering on the obsessive:

Baked Liver
Fried Rice
Spinach with Cheese Sauce
or
Cabbage and Cottage Cheese Salad
Whole Wheat Bread and Margarine
Rhubarb Pie
Buttermilk and Iced Coffee

In light of this research, is it any wonder that parents often have such trouble getting their children to eat nutritious, well-balanced meals? Children usually don't get to choose their own menus; they prefer sweet foods; and they like relatively few foods.

Knowing all this may not solve any problems, but it may make you less annoyed the next time your family is headed for a fine restaurant and a child asks you, "Do they have hamburgers?"

~~~~~~

been led into drugs through some ideological or religious commitment, which included acceptance of macrobiotic foods for their symbolic value." Even after the children had been cured of their drug habit they were "unable to reject the nutritionally unsatisfactory foods and eating patterns which continued to hold symbolic values important to them."

The French anthropologist Claude Lévi-Strauss also writes of such food myths in *The Raw and the Cooked,* saying that the conventions of society decree what is food and what is not food, and what kind of food shall be eaten on what occasions. The surprising thing is how alike the American housewife and the Amazon Indian matron are in their view of food. Breeling offers some examples: "Wherever the menu includes a dish of roast meat, it is accorded pride of place. Steamed and boiled foods are considered especially appropriate to men. Fatter cuts of meat are given to women and strong-tasting foods are often forbidden to children.

"Lévi-Strauss has even claimed that the high status given roasting is highly regarded only in very democratic societies. Boiling provides a means of conserving meat and its juices, whereas roasting is accompanied by destruction and loss. Thus boiling denotes economy, roasting prodigality; boiling is plebian, roasting aristocratic."

In New York, I visit with a psychologist-sociologist, Paul A. Fine, Ph.D., who had made over 100 food studies and come up with some stunning conclusions about our changing food habits. A white-bearded man with a black mustache, Dr. Fine talked to me with the aid of a blackboard, on which he sketched a circle, like a clock face, with 10 arrows like clock hands. Each "hand," arrowing toward the center, is labeled "German," "Swedish," "Hungarian," "Southern," "Jewish," etc.—symbolizing the food preferences of America's ethnic groups which, he says, are blending together in one big mish-mash.

"The old idea of meat and potatoes hangs on," he says, "but in a different form—including steak and baked potato, 'Salisbury' steak and mashed potatoes, sliced beef with mashed potatoes and gravy. Certain Italian foods have been 'discovered' by the average man, 'flattened out' to an acceptable blandness and incorporated into mainstream eating—most notably, spaghetti and meatballs, and, of course, the pizza (which would go unrecognized in Italy)."

It is Dr. Fine's conclusion, based on extensive research, that the American woman's feelings about her family's eating habits are one thing, and the reality another. A "sit-down" breakfast has great symbolic significance, for example, but in actuality no more than 25 percent of American households engage in this ritual.

It seems that most households are like mine. My son eats a bowl of cereal, alone at the kitchen table, before leaving for high school. My daughter munches on a piece of raisin bread while walking to school. My wife breakfasts standing up, having only a cup of Sanka. I sit in solitary splendor in the living room, digesting the morning paper along with fresh orange juice, coffee, and perhaps a poached egg—the closest thing to a "sit-down" breakfast.

"At work Dad has coffee and some kind of cake or roll for his real breakfast," says Dr. Fine. "The kids at school, the secretary at her desk may get so hungry by mid-morning that they steal from or eat up their lunch. In the summer, kids swarm in and out of the kitchen and the 'fridge' all morning. Pre-schoolers beg for this and that or take this and that all morning."

Lunch is simple if the kids come home—maybe soup, sandwich, milk, and a couple of cookies. At school "they trade sandwiches, spend their lunch money on a Coke and hot dog at a corner store instead of at the school cafeteria. Dad may be having the biggest meal of his day at a fancy restaurant with clients. The canteen machines get big play."

Mid-afternoon is an important eating time when the kids burst in the door from school—starving. They eat steadily until dinner time—a big peanut butter and pickle sandwich, some cake, whatever is in the refrigerator.

In her shopping habits, the housewife is actually an order-filler with the inventory in her head, visualizing the normal eating habits of her family. She knows perfectly well, says Dr. Fine, that there will be an enormous amount of snacking and she prepares for it. She stakes out only a tiny portion of the refrigerator or freezer as sacred from the family members' attacks.

Sit-down dinners are the theory seven days a week. In reality, Dr. Fine has found, the whole family sits down together as seldom as three days a week or less! The whole meal time may last only 20 minutes. "And no sooner is the table cleared and dishes washed, than the eating starts again. Someone makes a sandwich. Older kids go out for a while, come back with friends, fix food and do homework together, or sit in front of the TV and snack." A bedtime snack is the rule, not the exception, says Dr. Fine, and even then it doesn't end—"people can't sleep, they are restless, they are hungry. They get up and raid the 'fridge,' the pantry for cereal, eat apples and cheese, raid the leftovers they would not eat at dinner."

The changing tastes and eating habits, says Dr. Fine, have been brought about by a changing society. Menus are extraordinarily limited, with some women serving as few as seven basic meals rotated through the calendar week. "Most seem to use 10 to 14 basic meals," he says, "with the rare 'experiment' thrown in. If the experiment is successful, it tends to *replace* a less popular meal, rather than be added to the repertoire."

The reason for this state of culinary affairs, Dr. Fine says, is that many women now in their 20s and 30s did not learn to cook at home, as did older women, because of the breakdown of the "authoritarian" home that followed the Depression and World War II. Instead, young women now learn to cook after marriage, from friends, neighbors, and cookbooks, as well as mothers and mothers-in-law, but the learning process takes years and the family becomes accustomed to her first few basic dishes.

The mainstream Americans, as Dr. Fine characterizes the majority in the middle of the eating diagram he sketches on his blackboard, have moved, with the aid of massive advertising, to what he calls "common denominator" foods that fit the new eating habits: "Oreos, peanut butter, Crisco, TV dinners, cake mix, macaroni and cheese, Pepsi and Coke, pizza, Jello, hamburgers, Rice-a-Roni, Spaghetti-O's, pork and beans, Heinz ketchup, and instant coffee. It is the world of General Motors, Kleenex, Ford, television, and processed foods. It is the world of 'the Joneses' next door: doing what others do, keeping up rather than reaching up, following the advice of the mass media."

Dr. Fine's sketch also shows groups with different eating habits. At the left are the first-generation "ethnics," like those who stil prefer the unique foods their geography and culture conditioned them to like. The "ethnics," says Dr. Fine, are destined to join the mainstream as they become Americanized.

At the right of Dr. Fine's groupings are "the gourmets, the experimenters, the seekers after the new and different." These are "mostly upwardly-mobile, educated and self-reliant Americans, usually at least one generation removed from their ethnic origins. They are deeply concerned with naturalness and nutrition, and tend to reject food packaging, and especially processing in any form. Though most are using processed foods out of necessity, they are doing so increasingly 'under protest,' and always seeking alternatives."

Dr. Fine's conclusions seem to mesh with those of Dr. Odell, with the biochemist foreseeing even more erosion of traditionally conservative food preferences. When he was developing his synthetic soybean "meat," Dr.

Odell says, he recognized the essential food conservative in all of us by trying to mimic nature as much as possible with textures and flavors.

"Still, I see the time coming," he predicts, "when we can get kids to eat red 'mashed potatoes' and blue 'hamburger patties.' We're going to have food in shapes and with flavors we don't even have a name for now. But it will take a new generation to accept all this—one with no food hangups."

| 2 |

The Requirements of
Human Nutrition

NEVIN S. SCRIMSHAW and VERNON R. YOUNG

Nevin S. Scrimshaw holds the rank of Institute Professor at the Massachusetts Institute of Technology and has been head of the Department of Nutrition and Food Science at M.I.T. since 1961; before that he served for 12 years as director of the Institute of Nutrition of Central America and Panama (INCAP). A physiologist and M.D., he continues to serve as a consultant to INCAP and travels frequently to Asia to advise on nutrition and health problems there. In addition he is a member of numerous advisory committes to government departments, international agencies, and private foundations. Vernon R. Young is associate professor of nutritional biochemistry in the Department of Nutrition and Food Science at M.I.T. His research has tended to concentrate on the relations between aging and nutrition.

From Scientific American 235 (September 1976), pp. 51–64.

Human beings lack the biochemical machinery to manufacture a variety of carbon compounds required for the formation and maintenance of tissues and for the metabolic reactions that sustain life. These compounds, which all animal cells and organisms must obtain preformed from the environment, together with a number of mineral elements, are termed the essential nutrients. Over the past few million years of evolutionary time the competitive struggle to obtain them in sufficient amounts has favored the emergence and dominance of the human species and has profoundly influenced man's social and cultural ascent. At the same time man's inability to manufacture the essential nutrient compounds has exposed him to deficiency diseases that continue to threaten hundreds of millions of people in today's world.

How did the diverse nutritional requirements of animals, including man, evolve? A significant clue was provided some 30 years ago when the pioneering studies of George W. Beadle and Edward L. Tatum of Stanford University with the red mold *Neurospora* demonstrated that gene mutation can bring about alterations in the needs of cells and organisms for an external supply of compounds. Like all other plants, *Neurospora* normally requires no vitamins or amino acids for its metabolism and growth; it makes them itself. When Beadle and Tatum exposed the mold cells to X rays, however, the resulting mutations caused a loss in the cells' ability to synthesize vitamins such as thiamine, pyridoxine and para-aminobenzoic acid and the amino acids histidine, lysine and tryptophan.

Evolutionary biologists now believe a similar series of mutations occurred in the remote past to give rise to the nutrient-synthesizing deficiencies of animals. The earliest forms of life appear to have been simple bacteriumlike organisms that were capable of manufacturing all the compounds they needed from mineral salts, nitrogen, simple compounds of carbon and of course water. This ability entailed the storage of an enormous amount of genetic information, and cells that could reduce the metabolic costs of replicating and maintaining genes gained a selective advantage. With natural selection favoring mutations that eliminated the "unnecessary" enzymatic synthesis of readily available nutrients, primitive forms of life evolved and ultimately developed into animal cells.

When the first single-cell animals appeared about a billion years ago, they lacked a number of the biosynthetic pathways found in plant cells, notably the photosynthetic pathway that enables a plant to convert the energy of sunlight into the energy-rich compounds that drive the metabolism of cells. All the animal species that subsequently emerged from these ancestral beginnings had similar deficiencies, but they survived by obtaining the energy and nutrients they needed from external sources. For example, plants have retained the ability to make all the 20 amino acids found in their proteins from simple carbon and nitrogen compounds, whereas animals depend on their diet to supply about half of these amino acids.

An interesting and quite recent evolutionary development of nutritional significance is the inability of certain animals to synthesize ascorbic acid (vitamin C). I. B. Chatterjee of the University College of Science in India has
estimated that some 350 million years ago the capacity for synthesizing this
vitamin arose in amphibians, but that a gene mutation about 25 million
years ago in a common ancestor of man and other primates led to a loss of
the enzyme L-gulono oxidase, which catalyzed the terminal step in the conversion of glucose to ascorbic acid. Linus Pauling has suggested that the
loss of this pathway was selectively advantageous in that it freed glucose for
energy use by the body. In any case the mutation was not lethal because
the missing compound was present in the food of the mutant animals. Their
evolution could thus continue.

Man's need to obtain an adequate supply of essential nutrients through
his diet not only is a part of his biological evolution but also has shaped his
social evolution. It has suggested that the migration of human groups to the
northern regions of the earth was slowed by the limited amounts of ascorbic
acid in the foods available in those areas during the long winter months.
Moreover, man's dependence on an adequate supply of nutrients meant
that he initially had to be a hunter and gatherer, which circumscribed his
cultural development. With the domestication of the cereal grains and other
plants, along with a limited number of animal species, he was able to organize a stable way of life and secure the essential nutrients without foraging
over substantial areas. This freed his energies for new kinds of social,
economic and artistic activities.

At least 45 and possibly as many as 50 dietary compounds and elements
are now recognized as essential for a human being to live a full, healthy life.
Plant and animal foods cannot, however, be directly utilized by the cells of
human tissues. The nutrients contained in foods are released by digestion,
absorbed in the intestine and transported to the cells by the blood. As long
as the overall diet supplies all the essential nutrients, the cells and tissues of
the body are capable of synthesizing the many thousands of additional
compounds required for life.

Since the body is dependent on a regular supply of nutrients, intricate
biochemical mechanisms have evolved to regulate the availability of the nutrients to the cells so that the organism can adjust to a wide range of intakes.
Those nutrients that have been acquired in excess of cellular needs are han-
dled by catabolic pathways that bring about their breakdown. The break-

down products are then eliminated in the urine, bile, sweat and other body secretions so that they do not accumulate and reach toxic levels.

The importance of regulating nutrient levels is dramatically illustrated in certain human diseases. In the genetic disorder known as maple-syrup-urine disease infants cannot adequately metabolize the branched-chain amino acids (leucine, isoleucine and valine). In another genetic disorder, phenyl-ketonuria, the enzyme for breaking down the amino acid phenylalanine is lacking. Both conditions cause a buildup of amino acids in the blood and the tissues, particularly the brain, leading to cell death and mental retardation. The management of patients with these diseases consists of special diets containing a low level of the offending nutrient.

Another example of the accumulation of nutrients to toxic levels is hemochromatosis, a severe form of liver disease usually resulting from a combination of high iron and alcohol intakes that give rise to an excessive accumulation of iron in the liver. Vitamins A, D and K are also toxic in high concentrations. Hypervitaminosis from an excessive dietary intake of vitamin A, usually from the misguided use of high-potency vitamin pills, results in thickening of the skin, headaches and increased susceptibility to disease.

On the other hand, if the nutrient intake is so low that it is sufficient to meet the normal needs of cells, changes occur within the cells and tissues that act to conserve the limited supply. These changes may involve a more effective absorption of nutrients from the intestine and the activation of biochemical mechanisms that enhance the retention of the nutrient once it is inside the body. If the dietary intake continues to be inadequate, these metabolic adaptations break down and deficiency disease rises above the "clinical horizon," with characteristic symptoms that can lead to disability and death.

In addition to essential nutrients the body needs a supply of energy, that is, energy-rich compounds whose energy content is measured in calories. The assessment of the quantitative requirements for calories and the essential nutrients is clearly of great practical importance in human nutrition. The task is far more difficult than is generally realized. In animal husbandry the minimum needs of the animal for individual nutrients can be judged in relation to certain productive functions, such as rapid growth in meat-producing animals, high milk yield in dairy cows and maximum fleece production in sheep. The nutrient requirements of the human organism cannot be defined as readily because its well-being is more difficult to measure. What are the appropriate yardsticks? Maximum physical fitness and disease resistance would seem to be logical criteria for assessing the requirements for individual nutrients, but because we cannot quantify physical well-being as precisely as we can the growth of experimental animals, we must seek more objective measures.

Some nutrients or their breakdown products are excreted daily in the urine, feces and sweat and are lost through the shedding of small amounts of skin and hair. For the body to remain in metabolic equilibrium the total gain of nutrient in food must equal the total loss. Therefore by measuring the intake required to balance the amount lost daily by the body it is possible to estimate the minimum metabolic need for a given nutrient. For example, nitrogen, a characteristic and relatively constant component of protein, is measured to determine protein needs. The metabolic-balance approach has also been followed in measuring the requirements for calcium, zinc and magnesium, but it is not suited to nutrients that are oxidized and whose carbon is eliminated in the respired air, such as fats and vitamins. For those nutrients the requirements can be estimated by determining the minimum amount of the nutrient that prevents the onset of subclinical deficiency disease, although the technique has its methodological and ethical restrictions.

Even when the metabolic-balance method is applicable, it does not provide information on where in the body the nutrient is being retained or utilized; overall nutrient balance might be achieved with a given intake of the nutrient being examined, but this does not prove that the tissues are functioning optimally and that health will be maintained. In addition it is difficult to carry out balance studies for prolonged dietary periods; such studies call for sophisticated facilities and a team of trained workers. The need to carefully control nutrient-intake levels requires that the daily menu be monotonous. Losses in the urine and feces (and ideally in sweat, skin and hair as well) must be assayed quantitatively, which means additional inconvenience for the subjects and technical problems for the investigators, particularly when the subjects are infants, young children or elderly people. For these reasons metabolic-balance studies are usually of short duration: a week or less in children and two or three weeks in adults. The long-term nutritional and health significance of these brief study periods has not been critically determined, so that the adequacy of our current estimates of nutrient requirements, which have been based on short-term studies, is uncertain. This is not a satisfactory state of affairs.

In the Department of Nutrition and Food Science at the Massachusetts Institute of Technology, working with Edwina E. Murray as research nutritionist and several physician graduate students, we have been able to complete a series of long-term metabolic-balance studies with highly motivated and cooperative students. These subjects have adhered to monotonous diets and have followed strict regimens for the complete daily collection of urine and feces for periods lasting up to 100 days, a significant increase over the usual 14- to 21-day balance period.

In one study six volunteer subjects lived on a diet providing protein at a level equal to the safe practical intake recommended by the 1973 Joint Food and Agriculture Organization–World Health Organization Expert Committee on Energy and Protein Requirements. By the end of three months metabolic measurements on these subjects indicated that there were decreases in lean body and muscle mass and/or changes in liver metabolism. These results strongly suggest that short-term metabolic balance studies are not sufficient as the sole criterion for assessing human protein requirements and that the current recommendations for dietary protein intake for large population groups are inadequate. Although our own balance studies have involved experimental diet periods significantly longer than those employed for the FAO–WHO estimates, the fact remains that the experimental subjects are few in number and are confined to privileged American males, and that the duration of the study is still limited.

For some of the essential nutrients none of these approaches has been followed, and only vague epidemiological data are available. Here we must depend mainly on data obtained in animal experiments and extrapolate the results cautiously to humans, or attempt to assess how much well-nourished groups consume and consider that as an adequate intake level.

The many difficulties faced in determining the amounts of nutrients required by an individual are compounded by the problem of determining the variation in the requirements of that individual over a period of time, and with the variation encountered among individuals. It is easy to establish that physiological states such as growth, pregnancy and lactation call for greater amounts of most nutrients than those needed by healthy adults for maintenance alone. It is harder to measure the subtle changes in requirements that occur in the aging adult, a problem often complicated by the cumulative effects of both acute and chronic diseases that can affect requirements for nutrients by interfering with their absorption or utilization.

Knowledge of nutrient requirements in infants and in young children is also on uncertain ground. There is a tendency for investigators to regard such individuals as little adults and, with a small allowance for their growth, to extrapolate their requirements proportionately by weight from studies of older individuals. This approach does not take into account changes in the metabolic activities of cells and in the rates of nutrient turnover with age. For body protein, studies in our laboratory demonstrate high rates of turnover in newborn infants that diminish rapidly during the early weeks and months of infancy. Thereafter the decline is less rapid, but on a whole-body basis it probably continues with the passage of time during the adult years. Although protein requirements are not determined entirely by metabolic-turnover rate, the direction of change in the requirements for total dietary protein is the same as that for body protein turnover.

There is also variation in nutrient requirements among individuals of the same age, sex and physiological state because of the interaction of genetic and environmental factors. The important variation in nutritional requirements is the one that is due to the actual expression of genes in the individual, rather than the potential expression of genes under ideal circumstances. For example, in Japan there has been an increase in height of adults over the past 30 years, when a progressively greater proportion of the full genetic potential was expressed as dietary and environmental conditions improved.

One problem in knowing the appropriate variation to assign to nutrient requirements in normal individuals is the lack of data on the populations of different countries. In a study at M.I.T. we have given students a protein-free but otherwise adequate diet for 12 days in order to estimate the minimum level of nitrogen excretion, known as the obligatory loss. The statistical means of this urinary nitrogen value were significantly higher than those found subsequently for university students in Taiwan, who were studied under comparable conditions by P.-C. Huang of the National Taiwan University College of Medicine. Whether this disparity is due to genetic differences or to environmental and experimental factors is currently undetermined, but the fact of the difference appears to be indisputable. The nutritional significance of this observation is not fully known, but it emphasizes the great need for a large number of comparative studies on nutrient metabolism and requirements in populations of differing geographic, cultural and genetic backgrounds.

Nutrient requirements also depend on a variety of environmental factors that may be physical (for example, average ambient temperature), biological (the presence of infectious organisms and other parasites) or social (physical activity, the type of clothing worn, sanitary conditions and personal hygiene and other patterns of behavior). Environmental factors can influence nutritional status by directly modifying dietary requirements or by their effects on the production and availability of food and on its consumption.

The major dietary factors influencing nutrient requirements are threefold. The first is that the form of a nutrient in food may have a significant effect on its degree of absorption and utilization. For example, the relatively low efficiency of the absorption of iron from vegetable foods is a major factor in the total iron intake required by human beings. Ferrous iron (reduced iron, as in ferrous sulfate or finely divided elemental iron) is more effectively absorbed than ferric iron (as in ferric chloride or iron pyrophosphate). Even ferrous iron, however, is absorbed less efficiently when it is ingested in combination with phytates and oxalates, which are found in leafy green vegetables and the whole-grain, unleavened bread of North Africa and the Middle East. The iron found in meat (heme iron) is much better absorbed than iron of vegetable origin, and small amounts of red meat markedly improve overall iron absorption.

The second major factor affecting nutrient requirements is that the presence or absence of one nutrient frequently affects the utilization of another. For example, when dietary protein intake is deficient, the two proteins that play a role in the transport of vitamin A (retinol-binding protein and prealbumin) are not made by the liver in adequate amounts. The esterified form of the vitamin remains stored in the liver, unavailable to the other body tissues. Signs of vitamin-A deficiency may then appear, in spite of the fact that the intake of the vitamin (or of its precusor, beta-carotene, which is present in plant foods) would be sufficient if protein nutrition were adequate.

The third factor is the presence in the human large intestine of bacteria that live on organic molecules not absorbed in the small intestine. In the course of their metabolic activities these bacteria manufacture vitamins that their human host absorbs; it is a symbiotic, or mutually beneficial, relationship. Vitamin K, a deficiency of which causes failure of blood clotting, is synthesized in this way, as are small quantities of some of the B vitamins.

The factors influencing the adequacy of dietary protein for an individual may be even more complex. In the first place, the normal requirement is not for protein per se but, depending on the individual's age, for some nine or ten essential amino acids in adequate amounts and appropriate proportions. Whether an amino acid is utilized for the synthesis of new protein or is degraded for its energy content (a wasteful process) depends on a number of factors. First, each of the essential amino acids must be present simultaneously in the intracellular pool for protein synthesis to proceed. If a given amino acid is present only in a limited amount, the protein can be formed only as long as the supply of that amino acid (called the limiting amino acid) lasts. If one essential amino acid is missing from the pool, the remaining ones cannot be stored for later synthesis and will be catabolized for energy.

The level of nonprotein calories in the diet is also important. If it is high with respect to need, the ingested protein is spared from breakdown to meet energy requirements, but the individual tends to become obese. If it is low, some of the protein will be preempted to meet energy requirements and will not be available to fulfill the actual protein needs of the body. It is sometimes mistakenly believed that it is not worth improving the protein content of a diet if caloric intake is deficient. Our studies of young adults indicate that some improvement in protein retention is achieved even under circumstances of deficient energy intake. Adequate nonspecific sources of nitrogen are also needed so that the nonessential amino acids and other metabolically important nitrogenous compounds can be synthesized in the body.

Various proteins differ in their essential amino acid concentration and balance. A nutritionally "complete" protein source such as meat, eggs or milk supplies enough of all the essential amino acids needed to meet the body's requirements for maintenance and growth. A low-quality or nutritionally "incomplete" protein such as the zein of corn, which lacks the amino acids tryptophan and lysine, cannot support either maintenance or growth. A somewhat less inferior protein such as the gliadin of wheat provides enough lysine for maintenance but not enough for growth. Plant proteins usually contain inadequate amounts of one essential amino acid or more. Lysine and threonine levels in cereals are generally low, and corn is also deficient in tryptophan. Legumes are good sources of lysine but are low in the sulfur-containing amino acids methionine and cystine; leafy green vegetables are well balanced in all the essential amino acids except methionine.

In spite of these shortcomings of individual foods it is possible to devise meals containing acceptable proportions of essential amino acids by combining proteins from several sources. In general, cereals that are deficient in lysine are complemented by legumes that are deficient in methionine. Every culture has evolved its own mixtures of complementary proteins. In the Middle East wheat bread, which lacks adequate levels of lysine, is eaten with

Essential amino acids	RDA for healthy adult male (milligrams)	Dietary sources	Major body functions	Deficiency	Excess
AROMATIC					
Phenylalanine	1,100				
Tyrosine					
BASIC		From proteins	Precursors of structural protein, enzymes, antibodies, hormones, metabolically active compounds		
Lysine	800	Good sources			
Histidine	Not known	Legume grains			
BRANCHED CHAIN		Dairy products			
		Meat	Certain amino acids have specific functions:	Deficient protein intake leads to development of kwashiorkor and, coupled with low energy intake, to marasmus	Excess protein intake possibly aggravates or potentiates chronic disease states
Isoleucine	700	Fish	(a) Tyrosine is a precursor of epinephrine and thyroxine		
Leucine	1,000	Adequate sources	(b) Arginine is a precursor of		
Valine	800	Rice			
		Corn			

SULFUR-CONTAINING		Poor sources Cassava Sweet potato	(c) Methionine is required for methyl group metabolism		
Methionine	1,100				
Cystine					
OTHER			(d) Tryptophan is a precursor of serotonin		
Tryptophan	250				
Threonine	500				
ESSENTIAL FATTY ACIDS		Vegetable fats (corn, cottonseed, soy oils) Wheat germ Vegetable shortenings	Involved in cell membrane structure and function. Precursors of prostaglandins (regulation of gastric function, release of hormones, smooth-muscle activity)		
Arachidonic	6,000			Poor growth Skin lesions	
Linoleic					
Linolenic					Not known

Essential amino acids and fatty acids cannot be synthesized in the body and must be present in food. Amino acids are the building blocks of body proteins; essential fatty acids are involved in the maintenance of cell membrane structure and function and serve as precursors of the prostaglandins, a family of hormone-like compounds that have diverse physiological actions in the body.

cheese, which has a high lysine content. Mexicans eat beans and rice, Jamaicans eat rice and peas, Indians eat wheat and pulses, and Americans eat breakfast cereals with milk. This kind of supplementation, particularly in infants and growing children, only works, however, when the deficient and complementary proteins are ingested together or are ingested separately within a few hours.

Acute or chronic infections or other disease processes that cause decreased gastrointestinal function increase the need for dietary protein, because less of it will be absorbed. Trauma, anxiety, fear and other causes of stress have an even more pronounced effect in altering protein requirements. Stress results in an increase in the catabolism of muscle protein with respect to synthesis, leading to the transport of amino acids away from muscle and peripheral tissues to the liver, where they are converted to glucose for energy purposes. This process creates a deficit in the protein content of the body, which must be compensated for by increased protein retention during the recovery period.

With any infection, even immunization with live-virus vaccines, there is a loss of appetite that leads to a decrease in food intake. The metabolic consequences of acute infections have been most extensively documented by William R. Beisel and his collaborators at the Army Medical Research Institute of Infectious Diseases. The first changes are increased synthesis of antibodies and other proteins characteristic of acute illness, followed by catabolic responses that result in increased losses of nitrogen (from body protein), vitamin A, vitamin C, iron and zinc, and probably other nutrients as well.

Disease may also directly upset the mechanisms controlling the metabolism of essential nutrients, thereby altering dietary nutrient requirements. The conversion of vitamin D into its metabolically active form, for example, depends on the activities of the liver and the kidneys. If the kidneys are diseased, the normal utilization of the vitamin is compromised. It is for this reason that many individuals suffering from kidney disease show skeletal abnormalities similar to these seen in rickets, a disease of vitamin D deficiency. When these patients are given a synthetic form of the active derivative of the vitamin, they show a marked improvement in health.

The absorption of nutrients is reduced whenever the gastrointestinal tract is significantly affected by acute or chronic infections, by a high concentration of intestinal parasites or by malaria (which interferes with the mesenteric circulation). Chronic infections and parasitic infestations are also capable of increasing nutrient requirements in other ways. Even with a diet that would otherwise be adequate, iron-deficiency anemia can develop as a result of the intestinal blood loss associated with hookworm, schistosomiasis and certain protozoal infections. In northern European countries where the eating of raw fish commonly leads to heavy infestations of fish tapeworm, vitamin B-12 deficiency disease (anemia and neurological damage) often develops in affected individuals because the parasite has a particularly large requirement for the vitamin.

For these reasons young children in developing countries who are subject to intestinal, respiratory and other infections that increase nutrient requirements, and who at the same time have a poor diet, are particularly likely to develop acute nutritional disease. The ideal public-health approach would be to eliminate the infections rather than to provide the extra amounts of nutrients these conditions require, but that is frequently not possible because of a lack of resources or for social reasons.

All these sources of variation in nutrient requirements make it impossible to generate precise values for nutrient requirements in either individuals or population groups. Instead nutrient allowances must be viewed statistically, on the assumption that individual variation in a nutrient requirement is distributed in a bell-shaped curve above and below the mean requirement for that population group.

It is not practical to attempt to arrive at nutritional recommendations sufficient to cover 100 percent of a population, because this would require far more nutrition than is necessary for most people. There will always be a few normal individuals in a population, two or three per 100, who need more of a nutrient than can be recommended in a practical dietary allowance, and a smaller number at the extreme tail of the bell curve, two or three per 1,000, whose metabolic abnormalities significantly increase their requirements. Finally, recommended daily allowances (RDA's) are intended only to cover healthy individuals and are often not adequate for people suffering from acute or chronic diseases.

The major limitation to the practical use of RDA's is that they are based on data from small and possibly unrepresentative samples that have been extrapolated to populations of all types. In developing countries, where a large fraction of the population is likely to be suffering from disease, children have a greatly reduced weight and height for their age because of the combined effects of repeated infections and malnutrition. As a result the body

Vitamin	RDA for healthy adult male (milligrams)	Dietary sources	Major body functions	Deficiency	Excess
WATER-SOLUBLE					
Vitamin B-1 (thiamine)	1.5	Pork, organ meats, whole grains, legumes	Coenzyme (thiamine pyrophosphate) in reactions involving the removal of carbon dioxide	Beriberi (peripheral nerve changes, edema, heart failure)	None reported
Vitamin B-2 (riboflavin)	1.8	Widely distributed in foods	Constituent of two flavin nucleotide coenzymes involved in energy metabolism (FAD and FMN)	Reddened lips, cracks at corner of mouth (cheilosis), lesions of eye	None reported
Niacin	20	Liver, lean meats, grains, legumes (can be formed from tryptophan)	Constituent of two coenzymes involved in oxidation-reduction reactions (NAD and NADP)	Pellagra (skin and gastro-intestinal lesions, nervous, mental disorders)	Flushing, burning and tingling around neck, face, and hands
Vitamin B-6 (Pyridoxine)	2	Meats, vegetables, whole-grain cereals	Coenzyme (pyridoxal phosphate) involved in amino acid metabolism	Irritability, convulsions, muscular twitching, dermatitis near eyes, kidney stones	None reported
Pantothenic acid	5-10	Widely distributed in foods	Constituent of coenzyme A, which plays a central role in energy metabolism	Fatigue, sleep disturbances, impaired coordination, nausea (rare in man)	None reported
Folacin	.4	Legumes, green vegetables, whole-wheat products	Coenzyme (reduced form) involved in transfer of single-carbon units in nucleic acid and amino acid metabolism	Anemia, gastrointestinal disturbances, diarrhea, red tongue	None reported
Vitamin B-12	.003	Muscle meats, eggs, dairy products, (not present in plant foods)	Coenzyme involved in transfer of single-carbon units in nucleic acid metabolism	Pernicious anemia, neurological disorders	None reported
Biotin	Not established. Usual diet provides .15-.3	Legumes, vegetables, meats	Coenzyme required for fat synthesis, amino acid metabolism and glycogen (animal-starch) formation	Fatigue, depression, nausea, dermatitis, muscular pains	Not reported

Choline	Not established. Usual diet provides 500-900	All foods containing phospholipids (egg yolk, liver, grains, legumes)	Constituent of phospholipids. Precursor of putative neurotransmitter acetylcholine	Not reported in man	None reported
Vitamin C (ascorbic acid)	45	Citrus fruits, tomatoes, green peppers, salad greens	Maintains intercellular matrix of cartilage, bone and dentine. Important in collagen synthesis.	Scurvy (degeneration of skin, teeth, blood vessels, epithelial hemorrhages)	Relatively nontoxic. Possibility of kidney stones
FAT-SOLUBLE					
Vitamin A (retinol)	1	Provitamin A (beta-carotene) widely distributed in green vegetables. Retinol present in milk, butter, cheese, fortified margarine	Constituent of rhodopsin (visual pigment). Maintenance of epithelial tissues. Role in mucopolysaccharide synthesis	Xerophthalmia (keratinization of ocular tissue), night blindness, permanent blindness	Headache, vomiting, peeling of skin, anorexia, swelling of long bones
Vitamin D	.01	Cod-liver oil, eggs, dairy products, fortified milk and margarine	Promotes growth and mineralization of bones. Increases absorption of calcium	Rickets (bone deformities) in children. Osteomalacia in adults	Vomiting, diarrhea, loss of weight, kidney damage
Vitamin E (tocopherol)	15	Seeds, green leafy vegetables, margarines, shortenings	Functions as an antioxidant to prevent cell-membrane damage	Possibly anemia	Relatively nontoxic
Vitamin K (phylloquinone)	.03	Green leafy vegetables. Small amount in cereals, fruits and meats	Important in blood clotting (involved in formation of active prothrombin)	Conditioned deficiencies associated with severe bleeding, internal hemorrhages	Relatively nontoxic. Synthetic forms at high doses may cause jaundice

Vitamins are organic molecules needed in very small amounts in the diet of higher animals. Most of the water-soluble (B complex) vitamins act as coenzymes, or organic catalysts; the four fat-soluble vitamins (A, D, E and K) have more diverse functions. Although low vitamin intake can result in deficiency disease, the misguided use of high-potency vitamin pills can also have undesirable effects.

Mineral	Amount in adult body (grams)	RDA for healthy adult male (milligrams)	Dietary sources	Major body functions	Deficiency	Excess
Calcium	1,500	800	Milk, cheese, dark green vegetables, dried legumes	Bone and tooth formation. Blood clotting. Nerve transmission	Stunted growth. Rickets, osteoporosis. Convulsions	Not reported in man
Phosphorus	860	800	Milk, cheese, meat, poultry, grains	Bone and tooth formation. Acid-base balance	Weakness, demineralization of bone. Loss of calcium	Erosion of jaw (fossy jaw)
Sulfur	300	(Provided by sulfur amino acids)	Sulfur amino acids (methionine and cystine) in dietary proteins	Constituent of active tissue compounds, cartilage and tendon	Related to intake and deficiency of sulfur amino acids	Excess sulfur amino acid intake leads to poor growth
Potassium	180	2,500	Meats, milk, many fruits	Acid-base balance. Body water balance. Nerve function	Muscular weakness. Paralysis	Muscular weakness. Death
Chlorine	74	2,000	Common salt	Formation of gastric juice. Acid-base balance	Muscle cramps. Mental apathy. Reduced appetite	Vomiting
Sodium	64	2,500	Common salt	Acid-base balance. Body water balance. Nerve function	Muscle cramps. Mental apathy. Reduced appetite	High blood pressure
Magnesium	25	350	Whole grains, green leafy vegetables	Activates enzymes. Involved in protein synthesis	Growth failure. Behavioral disturbances. Weakness, spasms	Diarrhea
Iron	4.5	10	Eggs, lean meats, legumes, whole grains, green leafy vegetables	Constituent of hemoglobin and enzymes involved in energy metabolism	Iron-deficiency anemia (weakness, reduced resistance to infection)	Siderosis Cirrhosis of liver
Fluorine	2.6	2	Drinking water, tea, seafood	May be important in maintenance of bone structure	Higher frequency of tooth decay	Mottling of teeth. Increased bone density. Neurological disturbances
Zinc	2	15	Widely distributed in foods	Constituent of enzymes involved in digestion	Growth failure. Small sex glands	Fever, nausea, vomiting, diarrhea
Copper	.1	2	Meats, drinking water	Constituent of enzymes associated with iron metabolism	Anemia, bone changes (rare in man)	Rare metabolic condition (Wilson's disease)

		Not estab-lished	Widely distributed in foods	Function unknown (essential for animals)	Not reported in man	Industrial exposures.
Silicon Vanadium Tin Nickel	.024 .018 .017 .010	Not established				Silicon - silicosis Vanadium - lung irritation Tin - vomiting Nickel - acute pneumonitis
Selenium	.013	Not established (diet provides .05-.1 per day)	Seafood, meat, grains	Functions in close association with vitamin E	Anemia (rare)	Gastrointestinal disorders, lung irritation
Manganese	.012	Not established (diet provides 6-8 per day)	Widely distributed in foods	Constituent of enzymes involved in fat synthesis	In animals: poor growth, disturbances of nervous system, reproductive abnormalities	Poisoning in manganese mines: generalized disease of nervous system
Iodine	.011	.14	Marine fish and shellfish, dairy products, many vegetables	Constituent of thyroid hormones	Goiter (enlarged thyroid)	Very high intakes depress thyroid activity
Molybdenum	.009	Not established (diet provides .4 per day)	Legumes, cereals, organ meats	Constituent of some enzymes	Not reported in man	Inhibition of enzymes
Chromium	.006	Not established (diet provides .05-.12 per day)	Fats, vegetable oils, meats	Involved in glucose and energy metabolism	Impaired ability to metabolize glucose	Occupational exposures: skin and kidney damage
Cobalt	.0015	(Required as vitamin B-12)	Organ and muscle meats, milk	Constituent of vitamin B-12	Not reported in man	Industrial exposure: dermatitis and diseases of red blood cells
Water	40,000 (60 percent of body weight)	1.5 liters per day	Solid foods, liquids, drinking water	Transport of nutrients. Temperature regulation. Participates in metabolic reactions	Thirst, dehydration	Headaches, nausea. Edema. High blood pressure

Essential Mineral Elements are involved in the electrochemical functions of nerve and muscle, the formation of bones and teeth, the activation of enzymes and, in the case of iron, the transport of oxygen. The trace minerals nickel, tin, vanadium and silicon, previously considered to be health hazards, are now known to be essential for animals. Although they are so widely distributed in nature that primary dietary deficiencies are unlikely, changes in the balance among them may have important consequences for health.

size of adults is also small. For them the age-specific nutritional figures derived from well-nourished populations may be unnecessarily high and estimated caloric requirements may be excessive. It is therefore preferable to calculate allowances for adults in developing countries on the basis of kilograms of body weight.

Per-kilogram allowances are not sufficient, however, for children whose growth has been stunted by malnutrition and disease. Such allowances will be too low for maximum catch-up growth and will perpetuate the existing poor nutritional state of the children. A compromise in countries where nutritional dwarfism among children is common is to estimate the specific requirements of children on a per-kilogram basis and add a modest extra allowance for catch-up growth.

When acute infections are prevalent in a population, extra allowance must be made for the individual during recovery, although because of reduced food intake during the acute phase of the illness and increased retention of some nutrients in depleted individuals, the overall food requirements of the group suffering from infections may be little affected. Increased dietary allowances may nonetheless be needed to compensate for continuing high nutrient losses or for the impaired absorption associated with intestinal-parasite load and chronic disease.

In sum, recommended allowances cannot serve as an absolute indicator of the adequacy of a given intake for a given individual. They can justifiably be applied only to a reasonably healthy population. In spite of their limitations, however, estimates of caloric requirements and recommended allowances for essential nutrients must be supplied. They guide the design of diets for individuals, the evaluation of the relative adequacy of diets for populations, the content of nutrition-education programs and the planning by government of nutrition-intervention programs.

There is no area of human health in which research is more urgently needed than the nutritional requirements of representative human populations over the full range of both health and disease. Clearly an adequate knowledge of the amount and kinds of food required by man is essential for food and nutrition policy planning and will be of major importance for the generation ahead.

|3| Dietary Standards

D. MARK HEGSTED

D. Mark Hegsted is professor of nutrition at the School of Public Health, Harvard University. He is the editor of *Nutrition Reviews,* and since 1960 has been a member of various committees of the World Health Organization and of the Food and Agriculture Organization.

Reprinted, by permission, from *The New England Journal of Medicine* 292 (April 24, 1975), pp. 915–917. © Copyright, 1975, by the Massachusetts Medical Society.

Dietary standards, such as the Recommended Dietary Allowances (RDA),[1] are used for two primary purposes—to plan diets for individuals or groups of people, and to evaluate the nutritional adequacy of the foods eaten. Although much has been written about what the standards represent and how they should be used, a variety of questions remain unanswered.

Nutritional standards represent a judgment based upon practical experience with individuals or groups of individuals consuming diets of differing nutrient content, studies specifically designed to evaluate nutrient requirements of human subjects, and similar studies on the nutrient requirements of animals. The fact that different expert groups arrive at different recommendations reflects differences in judgment of the implications of the data available as well as differing opinions on the purpose and function of dietary standards.

It is generally accepted that since individuals differ in many ways, individuals of similar size, age, sex, and activity may have different nutrient needs. Unfortunately, very little evidence is available to indicate the degree of variability that may be expected. Most experimental studies on nutrient requirements yield only an estimate of the mean requirement of the group studied. Assuming that the estimate is valid, it will obviously be an inadequate amount for half the population. Thus, dietary recommendations must exceed the estimated average requirement. Judgments on the validity of estimated requirements, the spread in requirements that might be expected in the population, and the possible benefits of high intakes vary, however.

It is well to point out that other practical considerations may influence dietary standards. In an affluent country with a relatively abundant food supply, it can be assumed that errors on the high side are preferable to underestimates of the true need. The situation may be quite different in a country with a limited food supply. Dietary recommendations that call for nutrient intakes substantially above those provided by the usual food supply imply the need for extensive changes—modification of agricultural policy, importation of certain kinds of foods, or fortification of foods with nutrients. Such programs are expensive and are probably not desirable unless there is clear evidence of a beneficial effect. There is also increasing evidence of interactions between nutrients and other constituents of the diet that modify requirements—factors that modify the availability of iron or zinc are examples. Thus, even though there is little evidence of racial differences in nutrient requirements, there are rational reasons for differing dietary recommendations in different parts of the world.

There is abundant evidence that nutrient needs are modified by physiologic function, especially growth, pregnancy and lactation, sex, and physical activity, and separate standards are developed for many different groups. Infants, for example, are estimated to require approximately 2 g of protein per kilogram of body weight per day, whereas the estimated need for adults is of the order of 0.5 g per kilogram per day. This conventional method of expressing requirements seems logically to lead to the assumption that infants require high protein diets and an explanation of the high prevalence of malnutrition in infants and young children in many parts of the world. However, infants receive adequate amounts of protein from breast milk, which supplies only 6 to 7 percent of the calories as protein—a level below that of many high cereal diets. Ordinary diets in the United States supply something of the order of 12 percent or more of the calories as protein even in underprivileged groups. The energy needs of infants and young children per unit weight are high. If these needs are met, they can obtain sufficient protein even from a diet relatively low in protein. They do not require diets high in protein.

This conventional method of expressing nutrient standards has other disadvantages. Such standards imply that a homemaker feeding a family of a young child, an adolescent, her husband, a grandmother, and herself should really plan and purchase five different diets. Obviously, her job is to plan a diet that will be consumed in differing amounts and still adequately nourish each member of the family. The conventional dietary standards do not provide her with much help. One can reasonably argue that dietary standards based upon calories, which ultimately determine the amount of food eaten, and devised to provide adequate nourishment for anyone in the family would be a more useful approach.

A similar problem is apparent in the current procedures for labeling foods with their nutrient content. Current procedures call for expressing nutrient content in "a serving" as a percentage of the U.S. RDA. The U.S. RDA represents, more or less, the highest daily nutrient need expected in any age or sex group. The need for a single standard is clear. However, since the nutrient needs of young children may be adequately met by 50 percent or less of the U.S. RDA, calculating the adequacy of the diet on the basis of the U.S. RDA will be misleading or confusing. The recommendation that nutrient labeling be provided in relation to calories has obvious merit.

In contrast to the problems encountered in providing dietary instruction concerning what food should be eaten, it would seem that an evaluation of the nutritional adequacy of the food that has been or is being consumed must be based upon estimates of actual nutrient need. A number of problems arise that have not been adequately explained or investigated.

The Food and Nutrition Board[1] has repeatedly stated that the standards should serve "as guides for the interpretation of food consumption data of groups of people." It is often useful to compare nutrient intakes of Group A with Group B or the change in intake within a group over time. Yet the primary question asked in dietary surveys is not how much the group on the average consumes but rather how many, or which individuals, within the group are not adequately fed. Just how this information should be obtained is not clear, and there has been much argument over the interpretation of dietary surveys.

The Food and Nutrition Board also has repeatedly stated that an intake less than the RDA does not mean the person is malnourished, a conclusion that seems to be self-evident since the RDA's are deliberately set well above the estimated average requirement. If the nutrient needs of similar persons do vary substantially, as must be assumed, it is unlikely that dietary evaluation will ever be an effective diagnostic tool. A good dietary history, however, ought to be useful in establishing a "degree of risk." If one assumes that the dietary standard might be set at 2 standard deviations above the estimated mean requirements, only 2 or 3 per cent of the population would have requirements higher than that amount, and it would represent varying degrees of excess for most of the population. However, since one never or very rarely knows anything about the nutrient requirements of a specific person, the risk of inadequacy would increase as intakes fell below this level. This seems to be the only reasonable way to interpret dietary survey data, and a standard set at 2 standard deviations above the estimated mean requirement would be a reasonable standard. Communities might, of course, decide to accept other degrees of risk.

The other major problem in interpreting dietary surveys is the accuracy of the information obtained. In all surveys a choice must be made between a substantial amount of information obtained on few subjects or less information on a larger and presumably more representative group. Questions of cost and subject participation are involved. Most surveys opt for the so-called "24-hour recall"—an estimate of the previous day's intake. Apart from the errors involved in estimating the amount of different foods eaten and their nutrient content, it is perfectly clear that the diet on any one day or even in one week does not necessarily characterize a person's usual pattern of food consumption. Low intakes of all nutrients in such surveys are often associated with a low total food intake on that day—often so low that it is obvious that it is not typical. The vitamin A intake may vary from almost nil to many times the RDA, depending upon whether or not carrots, liver, or green leafy vegetables were consumed during that day. It is not surprising, therefore, that dietary surveys traditionally show rather large numbers with diets low in vitamin A, riboflavin, vitamin C, and calcium. The concentration of these nutrients in the diet depends upon a relatively few specific foods or classes of foods, and an adequate diet is usually obtained on the average within large daily fluctuations.

An adequate interpretation of dietary surveys to define the proportion of individuals at risk must include some estimates of the errors involved—error in the true sense as well as the variability in intake from day to day. The usual intake is the only meaningful index. To some degree each individual nutrient represents a different problem. Some suggestions have been made about how this problem might be approached,[2] but it requires additional thought and discussion.

Planning of diets or dietary instruction must consider factors other than the requirements of essential nutrients. A current example demonstrates the difficulties in standards designed for several purposes. The estimated protein requirements are substantially less than most Americans consume. Should one therefore "recommend" intakes that will approximate the requirements of protein but may be unacceptable to most people? If not, how does one use the recommended intakes to evaluate the adequacy of diets in protein? This problem epitomizes the conflict between telling people how to eat and how to evaluate what they have been eating. An attempt to fulfill both functions results in compromises that are not entirely satisfactory for either purpose.

References

1   Committee on Dietary Allowances, Food and Nutrition Board: Recommended Dietary Allowances. Eighth revised edition. Washington, DC, National Academy of Sciences, 1974.
2   Hegsted DM: Dietary standards. J Am Diet Assoc 66:13–21, 1975.

| 4 |

Our Diets Have Changed, but Not for the Best

MICHAEL JACOBSON

Michael Jacobson, a biochemist, is a director of the Center for Science in the Public Interest, Washington, D.C. He is the author of *Eater's Digest* and *Nutrition Scoreboard*.

If the bromide "You are what you eat" is true, we could all end up being very different people from our ancestors. Modern science and agriculture have freed the United States and many other nations from traditional diets based largely on natural farm products. New varieties of crops, transcontinental shipping, a wide spectrum of food additives, and new food-processing techniques have led, for better or worse, to diets different from any previously consumed by human populations. But these dietary changes reflect the decisions of business executives and investors rather than nutritionists and public health officials.

The United States, not surprisingly, has been the leader in the genetic engineering of food crops and in the laboratory creation of new foods. Benjamin Franklin and Abraham Lincoln, if they could visit us, would probably have some difficulty distinguishing between a toy store and a supermarket. They would not even recognize as foods such products as artificial whipped cream in its pressurized can, or some of the breakfast "cereals" that are almost half sugar and bear little resemblance to cereal grains. Franklin and Lincoln would probably feel much more at home in the homey "natural foods" stores that are popping up everywhere than they would in the 10,000-item supermarkets. Many of the new foods do save us time and trouble, but they are often costly, in terms of both dollars and, ultimately, health.

"Modern" eating practices start young, often with the tiny infant. Most pediatricians agree that good old-fashioned breast-feeding is the best way to feed a baby, but all too often mothers are persuaded by cultural and commerical pressures—or because of their work schedules—to bottle-feed with canned baby formula. Only about one in four infants enjoys the nutritional (and psychological) benefits of breast-feeding.

Until the 1930s solid baby food was prepared at home by the mother. Now, however, commercially prepared strained baby foods are the rule and are being introduced into a baby's diet at an increasingly early age. Mothers often compete with one another on the basis of how early little Johnny or Susie starts to eat solid food. Many researchers believe that feeding a baby solid foods too early can lead to both overfeeding and allergic reactions.

Some pediatricians and researchers worry about the health consequences of commerical baby foods. In the past 20 years canned formula has become the most popular food for infants. Although this is probably superior to the old-fashioned formulas based on evaporated milk and corn syrup, it is still a pale imitation of human breast milk. For instance, it lacks the antibodies and enzymes that help ward off disease and the "bifidus factor" that promotes the growth of favorable intestinal bacteria. Because it is based on cow's milk, infants may have allergic reactions. Differences include higher levels of sodium and unsaturated fats and lower levels of cholesterol as compared to breast milk.

A researcher at the University of Iowa, Dr. Samuel J. Fomon, suggests that formula-feeding may be more likely than breast-feeding to lead to obesity in later life. He reasons that the formula-fed infant is expected to finish the last drop in the bottle, while the breast-fed baby stops when he has had enough. Fomon and his colleague, Dr. Thomas A. Anderson (who once worked for Heinz, a major baby food manufacturer), have also suggested that early introduction of solid foods may lead to overfeeding—the infant often is expected to finish the last spoonful in the dish.

Pediatricians also wonder about strained baby foods. Although as yet they have little solid evidence, some fear that the salt and sugar used so freely as flavorings establish taste patterns that remain with a person throughout life.

In 1969 a Congressional committee held hearings that focused on the high salt content of baby food. This attention led the manufacturers to reduce voluntarily the salt levels in baby foods, but many products still contain up to ten times as much sodium (mainly from added salt) as does breast milk. Salt is of great concern to doctors and nutritionists because too much of it in the diet of adults contributes to high blood pressure (hypertension), which is the primary cause of about 20,000 deaths a year, and is the major underlying factor in some 900,000 deaths a year from stroke and cardiovascular disease. Dr. Jean Mayer, . . . probably the most influential nutritionist in the country, has said that "preventing hypertension would be much better than finding it and treating it—and a critical step in prevention is so easy: Just eat less salt."

For a child whose taste buds were initiated on blueberry buckle, raspberry cobbler, and other sweetened and salted baby foods, the step to artificially colored and flavored sugar-coated breakfast "cereals" is a small and natural one. Many of these products, which could be called candies, are 30 to 50 percent sugar. One widely known children's cereal, for instance, contains a higher percentage of sugar (approximately 50 percent) than a chocolate bar (40 percent).

Highly sweetened foods encourage young children to develop a taste for sugar, of which the average American consumes approximately 100 pounds per year. Dental researchers have proved that sugar is a major cause of tooth decay. In addition, sugar's "empty calories" displace nutritious foods and contribute to obesity, diabetes, and heart disease.

While the Food and Drug Administration has not taken any action on the higher sugar content of some cereals, Dr. Lloyd Tepper, Associate Commissioner for Science at FDA, said this at a 1973 Senate hearing on nutrition:

"I don't think you have to be a great scientist to appreciate the fact that a highly sweetened, sucrose-containing material, which is naturally tacky when it gets wet, is going to be a troublemaker. And I would not prescribe this

~~~~~~

SUCROSE CONTENT OF COMMERCIALLY AVAILABLE BREAKFAST CEREALS

Cereal Product	Sucrose Content %		
Shredded Wheat (large)	1.2	Rice Chex	10.3
Shredded Wheat (spoon size)	1.6	Special K	10.8
Cheerios	2.7	Crisp Rice	10.9
Puffed Rice	2.8	Concentrate	12.3
Wheat Chex	3.5	Rice Crispies (Kellogg)	12.9
Uncle Sam Cereal	3.6	Corn Flakes (Kellogg)	14.2
Grape Nut Flakes	3.9	Buck Wheat	15.1
Puffed Wheat	4.2	Brown Sugar-Cinnamon	
Post Toasties	5.8	Frosted Mini Wheats	16.3
Product 19	5.8	Life	17.0
Corn Total	5.8	Team	17.0
Peanut Butter	6.3	Granola	17.2
Corn Flakes (Kroger)	6.6	Sugar Frosted Corn Flakes	17.4
Grape Nuts	7.7	Granola (with dates)	17.7
Corn Chex	8.4	Granola (with raisins)	18.3
Crispy Rice	8.8	40% Bran Flakes (Kellogg)	18.3
Alpen	8.5	40% Bran Flakes (Post)	18.8
Wheaties	8.9	Raisin Bran (Skinner)	18.9
Corn Flakes (Food Club)	9.1	Heartland (with raisins)	19.1
Total	9.4	100% Bran	19.2

~~~~~~

particular food component for my own children, not on the basis of scientific studies, but because I do not believe that prolonged exposure of tooth surfaces to a sucrose-containing material is beneficial."

While tooth decay is certainly not a deadly disease, it can be both painful and costly. Army surveys indicate that, on the average, every 100 inductees require 600 fillings, 112 extractions, 40 bridges, 21 crowns, 18 partial den-

~~~~~~

All Bran	21.6	Cocoa Puffs	46.5
Granola (with almonds and filberts)	22.6	Vanilly Crunch	46.5
		Frankenberry	46.6
Fortified Oat Flakes	23.4	Cocoa Krispies	46.7
Raisin Bran (Kellogg)	24.7	Kaboom	46.8
Super Sugar Chex	25.3	Frosted Flakes	46.9
Heartland	26.3	Baron Von Redberry	47.3
Sugar Frosted Flakes	30.8	Count Chocula	47.9
Bran Buds	32.3	Froot Loops	47.9
Sugar Sparkled Corn Flakes	34.0	Boo Berry	48.5
Frosted Mini Wheats	34.0	Pink Panther	50.5
Sugar Pops	40.7	Honeycomb	51.6
Alpha Bits	40.9	Cinnamon Crunch	53.5
Sir Grapefellow	43.8	Cocoa Pebbles	54.1
Cap'n Crunch	44.1	Apple Jacks	55.5
Crunch Berries	44.4	Fruity Pebbles	56.2
Super Sugar Crisp	45.2	King Vitaman	61.6
Orange Quangaroos	45.3	Sugar Smacks	63.7
Quisp	45.5	Super Orange Crisp	70.8

From Ira L. Shannon, "Sucrose and Glucose in Dry Breakfast Cereals," *Journal of Dentistry for Children*, September-October 1974, p. 18. Copyright © 1974 by the American Society of Dentistry for Children. Reprinted by permission.

~~~~~~

tures, and one full denture. Although Americans currently pay dentists about $2 billion a year for treating decayed teeth, Dr. Abraham E. Nizel, of the Tufts University School of Dental Medicine, has estimated that we would be paying $8 billion a year if everyone went to the dentist and had all his dental needs taken care of. It is Dr. Nizel's impression that tooth decay is so rampant that even "if all the 100,000 dentists in the United States restored decayed teeth day and night, 365 days a year, as many new cavities would have formed at the end of the year as were just restored during the previous year."

As children grow older and more independent, most of the messages they get from the adult world encourage them to eat food that is not best for their health. School cafeterias frequently serve meals rich in fat and low in whole grains. Television commericals employ the latest ad agency techniques to promote sugar-coated cereals and snack foods. The U.S. Department of Agriculture—over the objection of many nutritionists—allows schools to serve children nutrient-fortified cupcakes for breakfast in place of cereal and orange juice. Vending machines invite children (and adults) to buy soda pop, candy, and gum. Fast-food outlets specialize in meals that are almost devoid of vitamins A and C, two of the vitamins that many Americans consume too little of. Living in this kind of environment, children may be confused when their health teacher admonishes them to "eat good foods."

America's eating habits are epitomized by what is served at our standard celebrations: baseball games, carnivals, and picnics. What child would be caught at one of those affairs without a hot dog and soda pop? The child does not realize (and is not told), of course, that a diet with too high a fat content (including, for example, too many hot dogs) can contribute to the epidemic of heart disease and obesity with which this country is saddled.

Obesity is a serious medical problem. Dr. Ogden Johnson, former Director of Nutrition at FDA, has estimated that 40 million Americans are overweight or obese. In addition to being a severe social and psychological handicap, obesity is a major factor in cardiovascular diseases, mentioned earlier.

The fluffy white bun in which the hot dog is served is made from white flour, which lacks some of the nutrients that are present in whole wheat flour. Fiber is one substance that is almost entirely eliminated when the flour is refined. For several decades most researchers ignored this indigestible carbohydrate, disdaining it as mere "roughage." But evidence is mounting rapidly that fiber plays a crucial role in maintaining the health of the gastrointestinal tract (particularly the large intestine), in controlling caloric intake, and in excreting cholesterol.

British physicians, notably Drs. Denis Burkitt, Thomas Cleave, G.D. Campbell, and Hubert Trowell, have led the campaign to awaken the medical world to the importance of fiber. On the basis of field experience and laboratory studies they maintain that people who consume too little fiber—

and too much sugar—stand a high risk of developing obesity, diverticulosis, appendicitis, hemorrhoids, constipation, peptic ulcer, diabetes, heart disease, and cancer of the colon.

Although Americans do get a substantial amount of fiber from fruits and vegetables, Burkitt and Trowell believe that this fiber is not nearly as effective in maintaining health as that found in whole grains and legumes. Many physicians and nutritionists in the United States are now urging Americans to base a larger part of their diet on whole grains, nuts, bran, and other fiber-rich foods.

In their middle years, most Americans consume a diet that is reasonably complete as far as vitamins, minerals, and protein are concerned. The typical diet usually reflects eating habits formed in childhood, however, and is hazardously high in calories, sugar, fat, cholesterol, and salt, and hazardously low in fiber. Still, aside from dental problems and obesity, this diet usually causes no overt problems during the middle 20 or 30 years of most people's lives. Scurvy, pellagra, beri-beri, and other nutritional-deficiency diseases are almost unknown in the United States. After about age 40 or 50, however, the changes within the body that have been gradually and silently occurring over the decades begin to make themselves felt.

A heart attack or stroke is often the first sign that something is wrong. After the fact, physicians often urge dietary (and other) changes to prevent recurrences. The patient is ordered to lose weight and eat less cholesterol and less fat—especially the saturated fat found in meat and dairy products. The person who is around to make these changes in eating habits should consider himself lucky. The American Heart Association recommends reducing fat consumption and body weight *before* a heart attack drives home the message.

As old age approaches, signs frequently show up first—and painfully—in the large intestine. Every television watcher who suffers through the incessant commercials for laxatives surely knows that constipation or, euphemistically, "irregularity" affects millions of people. The commercials push brand-name panaceas, but vegetables, whole grain breads and cereals, and fiber-rich bran (which you can get in bulk from health food stores or as one of the all-bran cereals) can do the trick equally well. Of course, eating an adequate amount of fiber-containing foods all along would have helped prevent constipation from developing.

Many elderly Americans suffer from diverticulosis of the colon, and every year approximately 170,000 people are hospitalized for treatment. This often painful illness develops when pressure builds up within the large intestine, causing outpouchings, which frequently become infected. The prescription for prevention or treatment is the same: a diet high in fiber-rich foods.

To complete our description of a lifetime of eating, we return to baby food. This time around, though, the consumers are not infants, but the elderly who have lost their teeth as a result of decay and gum disease and can eat only semisolid strained foods. About 18 percent of all American adults have no teeth.

Ironically, some of the same companies that manufacture the foods that contribute to heart disease, constipation, and other illnesses of middle and old age have special lines catering to the sufferers of these illnesses. Individuals who have become constipated partly through eating sugar-coated flakes can switch to all-bran. Did high blood pressure result partly from heavily salted soups? The hypertensive patient can turn to dietetic low-salt soups (and pay a little extra for *not* having salt). Diabetics who once loved fruit canned in heavy sugar syrup must pay a premium price for fruit packed in water.

Despite the close relationship between diet and disease, no person, governmental agency, or private organization in the United States has had the mission or authority to develop a broad national food policy that would consider nutritional value as a top priority in the way our food is grown, processed, and distributed. As it is, our agricultural practices and eating habits have developed with little guidance from health professionals.

The importance of developing a coherent national food policy has gained much high-level support in the past year, largely because of rising food prices and an increasing awareness of nutrition. Famine overseas has also awakened many people to the moral obligations of the wealthy nations. The development of a food policy was given a boost last June [1974], when the Senate Select Committee on Nutrition and Human Needs held a hearing on a national nutrition policy.

Heard time and time again at the Senate hearing was the need for us to base a larger part of our diet on vegetables than we now do. As Frances Moore Lappé explained so eloquently in *Diet for a Small Planet,* growing soybeans and grain to feed livestock and then eating the livestock is a much less efficient way of producing food than eating the vegetable crops (see *Smithsonian,* January 1975). Huge amounts of fertilizer, energy, and food would be saved if Americans ate less grain-fed meat. More food could go to nations in short supply.

Serving as one cornerstone of a food policy should be the vast amount of knowledge that the world's researchers have produced in recent decades. We need to *apply* the findings of this research. One way of facilitating this would be to establish a Federal Nutrition Advocacy Agency, which could disseminate information to the public and professionals, and prod other governmental agencies to employ their resources to encourage better nutrition.

While awaiting the creation of such an agency, we can easily improve our own diets. For most of us, that means eating less fat, sugar, refined flour, and salt—and more fiber. In terms of foods, that translates into more whole grain foods, fruits, nuts, beans, and vegetables, and less meat and snack foods. A change to this kind of diet would mean better health for Americans and more food for the rest of the world and would give us less cause to worry about becoming what we eat.

|5| How Nutritious are Fast-Food Meals?

CONSUMERS UNION

Consumers Union, a nonprofit organization, provides the consumer with information and counsel on consumer goods and services. It both initiates and cooperates with individual and group efforts that seek to create and maintain decent living standards.

By 1980, if the present trend continues, Americans will eat half their meals outside the home. Doubtless we will eat many of those meals at McDonald's, Kentucky Fried Chicken, Hardee's, or at one or more of the many other fast-food chains that even now serve up some $10 billion worth of meals a year.

Reasons for the growing popularity of fast-food chains appear obvious enough. For one thing, the food is generally cheap as restaurant food goes.

The most frequently ordered meal at McDonald's—a "Big Mac" hamburger sandwich, french fries, and a chocolate shake—costs only $1.75. That's a bargain when you consider the saved time and effort of the persons who would otherwise cook and clean up at home. The food is filling. And, judging by the fact that customers return to the successful chains time and again, many Americans like the way it tastes.

But as fast food assumes an ever more significant role in the diet, it's appropriate to inquire about the nutritional value of such assembly-line eating. That's what CU [Consumers Union] concentrated on in this project.

We bought and tested meals typical of those served up at eight of the biggest chains in the country: Burger Chef, McDonald's, and Burger King, which specialize in variations on the hamburger theme; Pizza Hut; Kentucky Fried Chicken; Hardee's, which builds its meals around a pseudo-steak sandwich or hamburger; Arby's, which serves roast beef sandwiches; and Arthur Treacher's Fish & Chips, which specializes in breaded fried fish.

We will go into detail on our tests and results later. But first, some highlights:

• The meat in McDonald's "Big Mac" hamburger sandwich weighs about 25 per cent less than the meat in Burger Chef's "Super Shef" and Burger King's "Whopper." Yet the McDonald's meal provided ample protein (as much as Burger King's, for example).

• Pizza Hut is the protein champion by far (its "Supreme" 10-inch pizza contains plenty of cheese and other protein-rich foods). But none of the other seven meals tested was inadequate in protein.

• Nearly all the meals were too heavy on calories. Several of them provided almost one-half the daily ration of calories needed by the typical adult male. Thus, it's likely that a man who ate at one of these chains regularly, and also ate two other substantial meals a day, would put on weight, especially if he sat behind a desk most of the time between meals. (A deskbound woman would put on more weight because she needs fewer calories.)

• A lot of those excess calories come in a form almost useless from a nutritional point of view—sugar and other sweeteners that provide a quick shot of energy but no nutrients. Many of these "empty calories" are to be found in the beverage—either a "thick shake" (not to be confused with a *milk* shake, about which more later) or a cola drink.

• All the meals were deficient in at least a few nutrients usually considered essential in a well-rounded diet. A small nutrient deficiency is not a matter of great concern. But when a meal falls short in 10 essential nutrients, as Arthur Treacher's did, "Fish & Chips" lovers had best start thinking carefully about what they eat the rest of the day.

SOME NUTRITIONAL RULES OF THUMB

The accompanying table shows the total weight of each meal and the weight of the individual constituents. More significant are the columns showing the total calories and the amounts of protein, carbohydrate, and fat. Those columns summarize the nutritional pluses and minuses of each meal. Here's a simple guide to interpreting the nutritional information in the table:

Calories

As a guideline for the amount of calories one should consume each day, the National Academy of Sciences-National Research Council (NAS-NRC) has established a Recommended Daily Dietary Allowance (RDA) for both sexes and for various age groups and body weights. For the typical adult man between the ages of 23 and 50, the calorie RDA is 2,700; for children from 7 to 10, the calorie RDA is 2,400. (The "typical adult man," it should be noted, is 5 feet 9 inches tall and weighs 154 pounds. Bigger men need somewhat more calories; smaller men, somewhat less. Given equal size and weight, women need slightly fewer calories than men.) The calories, which are measurements of energy, come from three principal components of food—protein, carbohydrate, and fat.

Protein

Known as the body's builder and repairer, protein consists of a complex variety of amino acids. Meat, poultry, and fish are rich protein sources. So are milk and most milk products. (But not butter; that's largely fat.) Legumes—dried beans, peas, lentils, and the like—also have lots of protein, as do eggs and peanut butter. The NAS-NRC has established a guideline RDA for protein. For the typical adult man it would be 56 grams; for the typical 7-to-10-year-old child, male or female, 36 grams.

Carbohydrate

Carbohydrates are often associated with the empty calories of refined sugar. But carbohydrates also come from the starches in potatoes and cereal grains and the sugars natural to many other foods that contain a variety of essential nutrients—vitamins and minerals. A good daily diet should include some

THE EIGHT FAST-FOOD MEALS

The three hamburger meals are listed first, in order of amount of protein provided. The other meals follow in protein order. Descriptions of the meals with comments are on pages 58–59.

	Price	Total weight (oz.)	Meat weight (oz.)	Bread weight (oz.)	Potatoes weight (oz.)	Trimmings weight[a] (oz.)	Beverage weight (oz.)	Total calories	Protein (grams)	Carbo-hydrates (grams)	Fat (grams)
Burger Chef	$1.75	26.9	3.0	4.0	4.1	2.7	12.7	1300	47	181	41
McDonald's	1.75	18.7	2.3	2.9	3.5	1.5	8.6	1100	40	143	41
Burger King	1.70	20.6	3.2	4.0	2.6	2.2	8.5	1200	40	147	47
Pizza Hut	2.74	32.2	19.0[b]	—	—	—	13.2	1200	72	152	35
Kentucky Fried Chicken	2.08	22.7	7.9[c]	0.8	2.0	—	12.1	1300	65	141	57
Hardee's	1.89	21.1	3.2	2.2	4.9	0.3	10.4	1100	41	143	41
Arby's	1.95	22.9	2.7	2.8	2.9	2.3	12.2	1200	37	166	40
Arthur Treacher's	1.84	24.5	2.6	2.6[d]	4.7	—	14.7	900	22	101	42

[a]Trimmings include sauces, tomato slice, cheese, pickle, onion, lettuce, or cole slaw provided with the meal.

[b]Weight of total pizza.

[c]Including breading, but without bones.

[d]Weight of breading on fish.

bread and other grain products, as well as vegetables and fruit. If it does, it will include a certain amount of carbohydrate. But table sugar and other sweeteners are carbohydrate sources that contain only empty calories. There is no specific requirement for carbohydrates in the diet, nor has there been a guideline set for the amount of carbohydrate humans need daily, although the NAS-NRC Food and Nutrition Board has recommended 100 grams as a minimum. Nutritionists generally agree that the amount needed is low, but all our fast-food meals exceed 100 grams of carbohydrates—and thus, as only one of three daily meals, could contribute to a daily diet likely to be overly rich in carbohydrates. Your best guideline is to make sure your family's carbohydrates come mainly from fruit, vegetables, bread, and cereals, rather than from sugar or sweetened food.

Fat

This third source of energy is the one that's usually right before your eyes—on the meat, in the frying pan, in the bottle of oil, or as butter or margarine. It's the most concentrated source of energy, because one gram of fat is converted into nine calories, not the four calories that a gram of protein or carbohydrate produces. Thus, a little fat goes a long way, and a little more goes too far. You do need some fat; it's the only source of linoleic acid (an essential nutrient), and it's a carrier for vitamins A, D, E, and K. There are no guidelines for how much fat one should eat daily. Suffice it to say that most Americans get ample fat, usually far more than they need. Since fat converts into so many calories per gram, it's a good food component to cut down on if your daily diet includes more calories than it should.

Other nutrients

The body needs many vitamins and minerals as well as protein, and a well-balanced diet, one that contains a variety of foods, will include them all. Recommended Daily Dietary Allowances have not been established for every known essential nutrient. But our consultant did analyze the fast-food meals for a host of nutrients for which RDA's do exist. These include: folacin (folic acid), niacin, thiamine, riboflavin, pyridoxine, vitamins B_{12} and C, total vitamin A (both retinol and carotene), phosphorus, calcium, magnesium, iron, zinc, and iodine. Our consultant also analyzed the meals for biotin, pantothenic acid, and copper—nutrients for which the Food and Drug Administration has established labeling guidelines—and for total minerals, fiber, and moisture. We judged a meal deficient in a nutrient if it failed to provide one-third the daily allowance guideline.

~~~~~~

WHY WE DIDN'T FEED RATS THIS TIME

When CU reported on the nutritional value of breakfast cereals in the February [1975] issue, we noted that comparisons could best be made through studies of how rats fared on the cereals. Yet in this report on fast-food meals we compare the nutritional value of the ingredients without having fed the food to rats. How come?

Packaged cereal is a highly processed food. One can't assume that corn will behave like corn in the body once a manufacturer tortures it into *Quisp* or *Sugar Pops.* The food served by fast-food chains, on the other hand, is relatively "natural." We can measure the nutrients through recognized microbiological methods and predict their behavior in the body with accuracy.

Protein is a good example. We know the quality and biological availability of protein from ground beef, chicken, cheese, fish, and other foods. Therefore, a laboratory measurement of the amount of such natural foods present in a meal tells us enough of what we need to know about the adequacy of the protein content. But we don't know what the quality of protein in breakfast cereals is after the cereal-derived starches, flours, and grains have been processed. Some of these proteins may complement each other—and thus improve overall protein quality—and some may not. One good way to determine the quality of such artificial products is to feed them to growing animals and see how the animals make out.

~~~~~~

THE BEVERAGE PROBLEM

The nutritional booby trap common to all the fast-food meals we tested is the beverage. Both the shakes and the cola drinks contributed significantly to the general overabundance of calories and to the excessive amount of carbohydrate found in our analyses.

All the shakes are called "thick" shakes—perhaps because they are indeed thick, perhaps because the word "thick" and "milk" have a rough resemblance. They are rarely milk shakes. Milk shakes contain whole milk and ice cream; the sweet, heavy froths served at these fast-food chains usually do not. Judging by the fact that the shakes did contribute to the protein content of the meals, however, they no doubt do contain an appreciable amount of nutritious fat-free milk solids in addition to an appreciable amount of sweetener and chemical thickener. Our shakes averaged about

334 calories, most of them empty calories. (Note, by the way, that the table gives the weight of beverage in avoirdupois ounces, not the volume in fluid ounces. That's because the shakes are so thick and puffed with air that we couldn't measure their volume accurately.)

The cola drinks are, of course, familiar beverages that contain nothing of nutritional value. Our colas averaged 111 calories, all devoid of other nutrients. Cola drinks contain the drug caffeine (as they must by law to be labeled "cola"). The cola drinks we analyzed averaged about 30 milligrams (mg) of caffeine; a brewed cup of coffee contains about 100 mg of caffeine, on average.

~~~~~~

IODINE: A POTENTIAL PROBLEM

During our analyses of the meals served at fast-food chains, CU found one nutrient, iodine, present in surprisingly large quantity. On average, the fast-food meals tested for the accompanying report contained more than 30 times the Recommended Daily Allowance for iodine established by the National Academy of Sciences–National Research Council. Small amounts of iodine are necessary in the diet, mainly to prevent goiter. But no one has established how much is too much.

Can a continued high intake of iodine do harm? A recent review made by the Federation of American Societies for Experimental Biology for the Food and Drug Administration concluded that "adverse reactions to iodine in food are not a significant clinical or public health hazard." Yet little is known about a diet that contains as much iodine as we found in fast-food meals, nor did the review mentioned consider regular consumption of such high levels of iodine. It is known that too much iodine could affect the proper functioning of the thyroid gland. Thus, the review made for the FDA concluded that the amounts of iodine in the American diet should be evaluated periodically. We hope the FDA heeds the suggestion.

Where does all that iodine come from? Some of it may come from the iodized salt used in the preparation of the fast-food meals, but not all of it—or the meals would be inedible. There are two other likely sources: the rolls, bread, and breading made by bakeries that probably use high levels of iodates in their processes; or from residues of iodine compounds that may have been used to clean and sterilize food-processing equipment.

~~~~~~

Here, in summary, is the evaluation of the nutritional quality of each meal we measured.

BURGER CHEF

Our Burger Chef meal consisted of a "Super Shef" hamburger, french fries, and a chocolate shake. It would load children with half their total daily need for calories and come close to supplying half the calorie needs of an adult, too. The greatest nutritional drawback of the Burger Chef meal was its high carbohydrate content—higher in weight than that of any of the other meals. Most of those carbohydrates were empty calories of sweetness in the shake. (The same criticism can be made of the other shakes we tested; see pages 56–57). The meal was low in biotin, folacin, and pantothenic acid for adult and child; vitamin A for adult.

MCDONALD'S

We ordered a "Big Mac" hamburger, french fries, and a chocolate shake. The McDonald's meal provided less meat than the other burger meals and less total food. So perhaps the familiar advertising theme, "You deserve a break today at McDonald's," refers to the dietary break of slightly fewer calories than you get at the other hamburger chains. The protein content was more than adequate. The meal was low in biotin, pantothenic acid, and total vitamin A for both age groups.

BURGER KING

We bought the "Whopper" hamburger, french fries, and a chocolate shake. That meal contained more meat and less potatoes than the other two burger meals—and more fat, which probably came from the meat. As with the Burger Chef meal, calories came to half of a child's daily needs and nearly half of an adult's. The meal was low in biotin, folacin, pantothenic acid, and copper.

PIZZA HUT

Here we bought a 10-inch "Supreme" pizza—a pie appliquéd with tomato sauce, cheese, ground sausage, mushrooms, pepperoni, onions, and green pepper—and a cola drink. It provided the most protein of any of the meals, far exceeding a whole day's RDA for any age. Yet the total calories weren't unusually high, and the fat content was the lowest of all. This was clearly the best food buy, considering that pizza alone would provide a single meal's worth of protein for two persons. But it's by no means perfect. Surprisingly, considering its constituents, this meal was the only one that failed to have one-third the RDA for vitamin C for both adult and child. (The high baking heat probably destroyed the vitamin C.) The meal was also low in biotin and pantothenic acid for both age groups, and it contained more sodium than anyone on a sodium-restricted diet should have at one meal (see page 60).

KENTUCKY FRIED CHICKEN

Colonel Sanders' meal contained three pieces of fried chicken, french fries, a roll, and a chocolate shake. That added up to half the daily calorie need of the adult and to more than half of the child's needs. (But it's probably unlikely that many seven-year-olds could chew their way through all that food.) This meal contained considerably more meat than the hamburger meals and, as a direct consequence, a lot more protein—more than a whole day's RDA for adult and child. An excess of protein does no harm other than the harm done by the excess of calories likely to follow too much of any food component. (Note: we weighed the meat without the bone but with the breading—we just couldn't successfully separate the breading from the chicken. However, we believe the weight of the breading was not so high as to affect the general outlines of our findings.) With all that meat came more fat than in any of the other meals tested: The Colonel's frying process results in a greasy bird in hand; not only do your fingers need lickin', they need washin'. All in all, the Kentucky Fried Chicken meal represents a lot of food for the money, perhaps even a surfeit of food. The meal was low in biotin, folacin, and vitamin A for adult and child.

HARDEE'S

This meal consisted of a flaked and formed steak, a bun, french fries, and a chocolate shake. Calories, protein, carbohydrates, and fat were fairly comparable to that of the burger meals. And the steak was comparable to a hamburger (a "flaked and formed steak" is just shredded meat tenderized and formed into the shape of a steak). The meal was low in

biotin, pantothenic acid, and total vitamin A for both age groups.

ARBY'S

Arby's serves up sliced beef on a bun, two potato patties, and cole slaw (the roast beef plate). We also bought a chocolate shake. Arby's main contribution to fast-food technology appears to be its mastery of the art of paper-thin slicing. We counted an average of 28 slices of beef per sandwich, each slice *nine-thousandths* of an inch thick. But all those slices weighed only 2.7 ounces. That's an adequate portion of meat, but not a generous one. Thus the meal contained less protein than any of the other meals, although enough for one of three daily meals. Arby's meal also contained the second highest measure of carbohydrates, and, again, a lot of that was empty calories from the shake. It also fell short in biotin, folacin, pantothenic acid, total vitamin A, and copper for both age groups.

ARTHUR TREACHER'S

This meal contained two pieces of breaded fried fish, french fries, and a cola drink. That added up to the fewest total calories and the least amount of protein. We don't mourn the low calorie count, and there was still enough protein to provide one-third the daily needs of man and child. But this meal contained too little biotin, pantothenic acid, niacin, thiamine, total vitamin A, calcium, magnesium, iron, copper, and zinc for both adult and child.

Given the American appetite for shakes and cola drinks, and given the enormous advertising of cola drinks, one can hardly expect fast-food chains to refrain from offering them. Unfortunately, the ones we visited offered little other choice. Everyone would be better off, in our opinion, drinking water instead of the shakes and cola drinks served at all these establishments. If you can't wheedle a glass of water off the assembly line, unsugared tea or black coffee is the next best bet for an adult (neither offers any nutritional value, but neither do they add appreciably to the calorie count), and milk, juice, or a low-calorie soda, where available, would be better for children.

People on low-sodium diets face a problem at most fast-food chains. The specialty item is almost always presalted, and the potatoes are usually presalted. The Pizza Hut meal had the highest sodium content of all—four grams. That translates into about 1½ teaspoons of table salt—a full day's supply for a person on the mildest of sodium-restricted diets. The six meat meals each contained nearly one teaspoonful of salt, still a lot for someone on a diet. We found only negligible amounts of sodium in the Arthur Treacher's meal.

THOSE MISSING NUTRIENTS

The six nutrients most commonly in short supply in fast-food meals are: biotin, folacin, pantothenic acid, total vitamin A, iron, and copper. These nutrients, which perform a variety of functions in growth and life-support, are derived from many food sources, some of which would usually be part of almost any standard diet that includes a variety of foods. If you eat at a fast-food chain regularly, it would be wise to make sure that your other meals include such nutritious foods as beans, dark green leafy vegetables, yellow vegetables, and a variety of fresh fruits. That should overcome the nutritional deficiencies of fast-food meals.

| 6 | Protein Needs and Possible Modifications of the American Diet

D. MARK HEGSTED

D. Mark Hegsted is professor of nutrition at the School of Public Health, Harvard University. He is the editor of *Nutrition Reviews*, and since 1960 has been a member of various committees of the World Health Organization and of the Food and Agriculture Organization.

Copyright 1976 by The American Dietetic Association. Reprinted by permission from the *Journal of The American Dietetic Association*, Vol. 68, pages 317–320 and 325, April 1976.

The American diet is high in sources of animal protein. The total per capita cereal consumption in this country is also very high—most of it being consumed indirectly as animal products. Thus, a reduction in the consumption of animal products would reduce total cereal utilization and make more available for the rest of the world. Although this is true and although I feel that there are adequate reasons to modify the American diet, I believe that much of the recent discussion has oversimplified the argument and led many to unreasonable expectations about what can be accomplished.

There is a food-energy-population problem, and one cannot discuss these facets separately. We must recognize some hard facts. The major fact is that the world has approximately doubled its total food production during the past twenty-five years, but the nutritional problems of the developing countries have not been solved. Indeed, they are worse in many countries. We cannot indefinitely increase the food available—and increasing the food supply, even when it increases the per capita food supply, does not assure the food reaching the people who need it most.

The Green Revolution and other methods of increasing the food supply are supposed to—and indeed do—gain us time. However, much of that time has been squandered. We do not know how much time is left; we do know that it is finite.

It seems clear that the technology developed in the United States for food production is not directly exportable unless energy sources become cheaper. The cost of oil has more to do with the food supply and the cost of food than anything else.

Maximum food production in the United States is not only expensive in terms of energy but has many other attendant costs—increased pollution of all kinds, expenditure of irreplaceable resources, poor land usage, and so forth. It is not clear that we should "go all out" to produce food for the world.

In the long run, the food problems of the developing countries must, for the most part, be solved by the countries themselves. World trade and food donations can and should assist, but they can only provide a small part of the total food needs.*

It is difficult to state these facts without appearing callous and indifferent to the serious problems the world faces. I believe that we must do more to assist the world in the coming years. There are obvious limits, however, to which any country should mortgage its future if the only result is more hungry people. Making more food available does not place it in the mouths of those who are hungry. Conservation of energy by all available means, including modification of our food supply, is probably the most meaningful thing we could do rather than trying to feed the world with our expensive food supply. This should allow the rest of the world additional resources to solve its problems. However, even this is not likely to work at present, since both the supply and price of oil are artificially fixed by the producing countries.

THE PROTEIN MYSTIQUE

Protein needs are included in my title because of misconceptions and cultural patterns rather than nutritional reasons. Certain high-protein foods, particularly meat, have always occupied a special place in the diet. Protein, after all, is the stuff from which life is made. You will recall Liebig's theory that physical work "wore out" muscle, and protein was required to replace these losses. Fat and carbohydrate were utilized only to provide body heat. Inspection of the training tables of athletes demonstrates how little impact a century of investigation has had on this thesis.

More persuasive, perhaps, is the clear evidence that all populations—a few religious and philosophical groups excepted—want more meat when it is available. Meat, milk, and eggs are almost synonymous with the "good

---

*EDITOR'S NOTE: For a compelling elaboration of this point, see *Food First: Beyond the Myth of Scarcity*, by Frances Moore Lappé and Joseph Collins, with Cary Fowler (Boston: Houghton Mifflin Co., 1977).

American diet," and desires for this kind of diet are almost universal. This should make us cautious on two scores. First, regardless of scientific knowledge, it indicates the difficulty in modifying food practices. Unrealistic dietary recommendations which ignore these restraints are unlikely to be acceptable or very useful. Second, we should try to be sure that our knowledge is better than the "natural wisdom" of populations. It seems likely to me that man has not lived under affluent conditions with an abundant meat supply long enough to develop any natural wisdom, but at least we should be cautious, since nutritional knowledge is fragmentary.

The whole "protein mystique" was accentuated about a quarter century ago when it was recognized that kwashiorkor was a deficiency disease. It was first called "protein malnutrition" and later, when it was agreed that this was an oversimplification, "protein-calorie malnutrition." The emphasis of the nutritional establishment, however, remained the same, even though the etymologic niceties were observed, i.e., the major nutritional problem of the world was protein. Thus, the primary need is to increase the protein intake; thus our fortunate position in the world is related to protein; and so on. "Protein" and "nutritious" often seem almost synonymous. Continuous efforts are made to increase the protein content of foods in the American market even though no need can be demonstrated.

An increasing number of people are questioning these conclusions and the resultant prescriptions. The debate has been carried largely in the page of *Lancet* (1–6). As in most polemics, the proponents of either side tend to overemphasize the evidence which supports their views. The argument is not a new one, however. In 1959 (7), I concluded in a discussion of protein-calorie malnutrition that "investigators in this field have failed to identify the role of protein in the etiology of this condition."

MISCONCEPTIONS REGARDING MALNUTRITION

The debate over the role of protein in the etiology of malnutrition might be considered an academic exercise to provide an opportunity to compare the rhetorical abilities of various scientists or for the amusement of readers were it not that major policy decisions involving tremendous expenditures of money, energy, and time depend on the conclusions. Solutions to problems depend on a correct diagnosis. I believe there are a few major misconceptions which have led to incorrect diagnoses.

The occurrence of malnutrition primarily in young children rather than adults is attributed to their high protein needs. All estimates of needs show that very young infants require approximately 2 gm. protein per kilogram body weight—about the amount supplied by breast milk. The requirement per unit weight falls with age to approximately 0.5 gm. per kilogram body weight in the adult. All agree on this, although there is little factual data in between infancy and childhood. The published estimates of requirements in between these ages are largely extrapolation. The infant's requirement is thus approximately four times that of the adult; thus infants require high-protein diets; thus it is not strange that protein deficiency occurs at this age. This is not good logic.

Breast milk is a low-protein food. It contains only some 6 to 7 per cent calories as protein, less than in most cereals. The infant has high energy needs per unit weight. Consumption of enough food to meet these needs provides sufficient protein from relatively low-protein diets. Innumerable efforts over the past twenty years have been made to produce "high-protein foods" for infants and children, which are of dubious value since they are based on misconception—the misconception derived in part from our common nomenclature in expressing requirements which relate to body size and not to the food consumed.* They also derive from the ubiquitous use of the laboratory rat as a nutritional tool which, like most animals but not like man and other primates, does have a very high protein requirement for growth. In many ways, these are poor experimental models for this area of investigation.

Since the usual diet in many parts of the world where malnutrition is common is not very low in protein, one must conclude that if protein is a problem, it is the quality of the protein, not the quantity. However, current efforts to demonstrate that improvements in protein quality will be helpful are not promising. The exception to this generalization is probably those areas where cassava, bananas, and sugar are staple foods. A primary protein deficiency in such areas is likely.

NEED FOR KNOWLEDGE OF ENERGY METABOLISM

It is almost universally observed that total food (energy) intakes are low in countries where malnutrition exists. The causes, however, are not clear. In many places, it is not true that the children are starving and consuming every scrap of food available, although this, of course, occurs too commonly. The whole field of energy needs has made little advance since the

---

*EDITOR'S NOTE: See Comment at end of article.

studies of Atwater and others at the turn of this century. The tremendous advances that have occurred in our understanding of energy metabolism— the function of ATP [adenosine triphosphate, an energy-rich compound] and the delineation of many complex metabolic pathways, for example— have as yet had little practical impact on nutrition. This is a research area requiring development.

This is relevant to protein needs as well. The textbook tells us that "when calories are limiting, dietary protein is burned for calories." Various authors have arrived at diametrically opposite conclusions from the evidence. On the one hand, it can be argued that the addition of protein to diets when the energy intake is low is useless, since this will only provide calories—and expensive calories at that. On the other hand, one can just as legitimately argue that since protein is inefficiently utilized under such conditions, more protein will be required than when energy intakes are high or adequate. Again, I cannot discuss the evidence, but I must point out that estimates of protein needs are traditionally determined by feeding diets high in calories "to be sure that calories are not limiting" and tables of protein requirements assume an adequate energy intake. Are the standards applicable when caloric intakes are less than estimated energy needs? We really do not know. Small wonder that the etiology of malnutrition—the roles of calories and protein—is the subject of debate.

It would seem to be clear that suitable foods to replace breast milk are not generally available in the developing world and that the family diet is either inappropriate for young children or that they do not compete well for what is available. Special foods are needed if they can be appropriately distributed.

RELATIONSHIP BETWEEN PROTEIN AND CALORIE DEFICIENCIES

The other major misconception derives from our experience with vitamin deficiencies. In general, if a vitamin deficiency occurs, the usual diet can be assumed to be deficient. Thus, if protein deficiency occurs—and I do not debate this although some do—it is assumed that the usual diet is deficient in protein. This ignores many things that have been commonplace knowledge: that malnutrition is often associated with infections; that usual food patterns are not maintained during illness; that the indigenous therapeutic regimens are often such as to induce protein deficiency, and so forth. Protein deficiency can be induced rapidly, probably very rapidly, in marginally nourished children. The occurrence of protein deficiency may or may not be clearly associated with the protein content of the usual diet—nor is it clear that changing the protein content of the usual diet will modify the consequences which lead to kwashiorkor.

Traditionally, we have distinguished between marasmus as severe partial starvation and kwashiorkor as protein deficiency. It is doubtful that this is an entirely useful or a correct classification. In our studies with baby monkeys, which we believe are a reasonable model for research on this disease, animals restricted in either calories or protein become marasmic. The appearance is not very informative. Some—but only some—of the animals fed the low-protein diet develop the symptoms of kwashiorkor, i.e., edema, extensive dermatitis, and fatty liver. As in human infants, we do not yet understand why this is so. Some feel it is a breakdown in the adaptive responses of the organism (8, 9). However, the clinical diagnoses is not a sensitive way to distinguish between calorie and protein deficiency—biochemically, one may be able to do so. Of more interest, perhaps, will be the clinical and biochemical response observed when both protein and calories are limited. Although these studies are in progress, our current impression is that limiting the energy intake does not induce protein deficiency, even when protein intakes are marginal.

Without going through the detailed justification of the estimates of protein needs which have been presented many times (10, 11), one can say that there is no justification in such estimates for the high consumption of milk, meat, and eggs that is characteristic of Americans. The Ten-State Survey [a 1968–70 government survey of nutrition] revealed some groups with somewhat lower levels of plasma albumin than currently thought desirable. Just what this means is unknown but, disturbingly, they occur in poverty areas. The dietary data, on the other hand, indicate that the amount of protein per 1,000 kcal [kilocalories] is quite uniform for all groups. Thus, what appears to be low intake is associated with low food intake, not low-protein diets. The representativeness of the dietary data is unknown. Many of the low intakes of all of the nutrients that were obtained from 24-hr. intakes simply cannot be representative of the individual's intake. Whatever the significance, it brings us back to the relatively unexplored area of protein-calorie relationships.

NEED TO MODIFY THE AMERICAN DIET

I wish to turn briefly to the major reasons for a modification of the American diet. These relate to major causes of death and disability in our population—coronary artery disease, diabetes, intestinal disease, and so on. Every available study shows that hypercholesteremia is a major risk factor involved in heart attacks, and it is clear that it responds to dietary modification. The major evidence implicates excessive consumption of saturated fat and cholesterol. We are apparently involved in an endless debate over details.

It is now clear that cancer of the colon, diverticulitis, and perhaps other diseases of the intestine are much commoner in countries in which Western-type diets are consumed. Whether this is due to a deficiency of fiber or an overconsumption of meat, fat, sugar, and so on is probably not resolvable from epidemiologic data. One can anticipate that, in this field, as in heart disease, we are probably entering a protracted period of acrimonious debate.

The point that I would make is that there may never be clean definitions of cause and effect in these complex diseases. At some stage, decisions must be made on the basis of risk. We know what the risk is now. What are the probabilities that the situation will be made worse by modifying the diet according to best guesses now? What risk is associated with a decrease in consumption of meat and fat, particularly saturated fat and cholesterol, and greater consumption of vegetables, fruits, cereals? I submit that they are minimal. We could scarcely do worse than we are doing now.

The major reason for not modifying the American diet is that some industries would be adversely affected. Increased consumption of one food means lower consumption of another. Thus, the food industries adversely affected foster debate and confuse the public, and nothing is done. While the effect on the food industry is not a negligible problem, it is secondary and should not be permitted to delay progress forever. We must make recommendations based on the best knowledge available.

SUMMARY

The matter of protein needs is almost irrelevant in the discussion of appropriate modification of the American diet. Our total food supply system from the producer through the processor to the retail distributor is wasteful of energy and produces a food supply of less than optimal quality. The energy crisis may have a favorable effect on the food supply. We should and no doubt will contribute to the world food supply for a long time to come, but eventually the countries in need of food must solve their problems internally. In the long run, we can probably do more by attempting to conserve resources than by trying to feed the world.

References

1 Harper, A.E., Payne, P.R., and Waterlow, J.C.: Human protein needs. Lancet 1: 1518, 1973.

2 McLaren, D.S.: The great protein fiasco. Lancet 2: 93, 1974.

3 Altschul, A.M.: Protein requirements. Lancet 2: 532, 1974.

4 Brock, J.F.: Protein requirement. Lancet 2: 712, 1974.

5 Hansen, J.D.L.: Protein requirements. Lancet 2: 713, 1974.

6 Rivers, J., Seamen, J., and Holt, J.: Protein requirement. Lancet 1: 162, 1975.

7 Hegsted, D.M.: Protein requirement in man. Fed. Proc. 18: 1130, 1959.

8 Gopalan, C.: Kwashiorkor and marasmus: Evolution and distinguishing features. *In* McCance, R.A., and Widdowson, E.N., eds.: Calorie Deficiencies and Protein Deficiencies. Boston: Little, Brown & Co., 1968.

9 Rao, K.S.J.: Evolution of kwashiorkor and marasmus. Lancet 1: 709, 1974.

10 Energy and Protein Requirements. FAO Nutr. Meeting Rept. Series No. 52, WHO Tech. Rept. Series No. 522, 1973.

11 Food & Nutr. Bd.: Recommended Dietary Allowances. Eighth revised edition, 1974. Washington, D.C.: Natl. Acad. Sci., 1974.

Comment by Editor of the *Journal of The American Dietetic Association*

PROTEIN-ENERGY RATIOS

In his paper . . . Hegsted notes that, traditionally, protein requirements have been estimated in relation to body size. More recent data, however, indicate that they may also depend on caloric intake. Over the years, FAO/WHO Expert Committees have made recommendations for calories and for protein separately, and most recently (1973) for energy and protein in conjunction with each other.

Since the 1973 report, FAO and WHO have accumulated experience in the practical applications of these recommendations. Accordingly, in April 1975, these organizations and the Protein-Calorie Advisory Group of the UN sponsored a meeting of consultants in Rome. The report from this meeting, which appeared in the PAG Bulletin (Vol. V, No. 3), September 1975, summarizes present thinking.

For individuals or population groups having "moderate activity," a protein concentration of 5 to 5.5 per cent of energy would suffice to meet protein needs of almost all individuals who met their energy needs. For "light" activity levels, a somewhat higher ratio would be needed; correlatively, for "heavy" activity, a lower level might be sufficient. Exception may be the young infant, the pregnant woman, and the lactating woman, for whom the ratios are unlikely to be lower and may be higher (insufficient data are at present available to make generalizations for these groups).

It is emphasized that, where energy intakes are low and restrict desirable activity or performance, as in many developing countries, energy intakes should be increased to appropriate levels rather than protein-energy ratios adjusted to existing low levels of energy intake. It should also be recognized that whenever energy intakes are physiologically inadequate, protein utilization is impaired.

These safe protein-energy ratios are intended only for assessment of the individuals' diets and are not appropriate for comparison with national or average diet; the ratios are too low for that purpose.

The 1975 meeting reiterated the position set forth in the 1973 FAO/WHO report: The safe protein-energy ratios given above are based on predictions of the concentrations required to meet physiologic needs. They should be seen as a lower limit of acceptable dietary concentration, below which the risk of physiologic inadequacy increases. Preferred diets in many populations may provide higher concentrations.

| 7 | Food Additives—Food for Thought

JOAN Z. MAJTENYI

Joan Z. Majtenyi, a free-lance writer and editor, spent eight years doing research in peptide chemistry at Lederle Laboratories in Pearl River, N.Y. She was on the staff of *Chemistry* from 1968 to 1973.

From *Chemistry* 47 (May 1974), pp. 6–13 (chemical formulas have been omitted). Copyright © 1974 by the American Chemical Society. Reprinted by permission.

The average American consumes about $2\frac{1}{4}$ kilograms (5 pounds) of food additives each year. Many of these substances are both necessary and safe, but some people feel that a few additives have not been adequately tested and that many are used where not absolutely necessary.

What are food additives? Why are they added? How safe are they? These are questions consumers should be able to answer.

Distinguishing between a food ingredient and a food additive is sometimes difficult but, generally, a food ingredient is considered to be a natural nutritive component. Thus, sugar is an ingredient but saccharin, a synthetic sweetener, is considered an additive. Not considered additives are contaminants, such as pesticide residues that are unintentionally included in food, and adulterants—substances added to deceive the consumer. This article is concerned only with materials added intentionally by food manufacturers to prevent spoilage or to improve color, flavor, texture, or other characteristics. It is not concerned with nutrients which are sometimes added to food.

Before considering chemical additives, we should remember that foods themselves are chemicals. Milk, for example, is a mixture containing lactose, phosphatase, lactalbumin, folic acid, nicotinic acid, and at least 95 other chemicals. Also, food preparation involves chemical transformations and, during digestion, foods are broken down chemically into forms the body can use. Food spoilage, too, involves chemical reactions which can produce toxic substances or make food less nutritious or appealing. This is one reason for today's increased use of additives. Foods are often transported long distances from processing plant to market and stand for weeks on grocery shelves so that more preservatives are needed to keep them fresh. Another reason is the large demand for convenience foods.

SAFETY

To say that an additive is 100 percent safe probably will never be possible. Too many uncertainties are involved. Test results on laboratory animals often vary from species to species and may not be applicable to man. Small doses, though apparently harmless, may cause damage if they accumulate over a long period of time. Also, substances safe individually may present a hazard in combination. The only recourse is to see that additives are subjected to all available tests before use. In general, most scientists feel thorough studies should include both short- and long-term toxicity tests, including those to detect cumulative effects of cancer-causing substances, and experiments to determine effects on reproduction, such as birth defects (teratogenicity) and genetic mutation.

Many food additives have not been tested this extensively. One reason is that when these additives came into use, some techniques used today were not available. Another reason can be traced to the early history of food additive legislation. The first attempt to govern additives was the Pure Food and Drug Act of 1906 which stated only that additives should be safe for human consumption and serve a useful purpose. No provision was made for enforcement until a 1938 amendment. But even then the Food and Drug Administration (FDA) had to prove a substance harmful before it could act.

Finally, in 1960, another amendment stated that no chemical can be used unless the manufacturer proves to the FDA that it is safe. This was an improvement but did not cover additives already in use. Removing such additives from the market for periods of years until they could be tested was impractical. To solve this dilemma the FDA established a list of 687 chemicals which it felt were generally recognized as safe. This GRAS list, as it came to be known, included every thing from salt, vinegar, and spices to saccharin and sodium benzoate.

At present, the GRAS list is being reviewed as requested by President Nixon in 1969. As more of these compounds are tested thoroughly some may be found hazardous, as has already happened in the case of cyclamates, brominated vegetable oil, and several artificial colors. Until this review is completed it is difficult to assess fully the danger of these food additives.

Because experts disagree, a conservative approach seems justified. Accordingly, the following discussion indicates some additives that have not been tested as thoroughly as possible and describes briefly a few adverse testing results connected with them. Most of the discussion on safety is based on the views of microbiologist Michael Jacobson in *Eater's Digest* (6).

PRESERVATIVES

From earliest days food spoilage was a problem, and one of the first preservation methods was drying, effective because microbes, a major cause of food spoilage, need water to live. Foods low in moisture, such as grains and nuts, remain fresh for years because water content is insufficient to support microbe growth. Chemical preservatives were used early, too, including salt and wood smoke for meat and fish. Wood smoke inhibits microbe growth by coating meat with chemicals such as formaldehyde.

Today, refrigeration is a major factor in retarding bacterial growth but a wide variety of chemicals are used too. Calcium propionate and sorbic acid . . . prevent molding of baked goods. Sodium benzoate is used in many foods including salad dressing, margarine, and most soft drinks. All these preservatives except sodium benzoate have been tested and are considered safe. Sodium benzoate has not been examined for possible teratogenic effects.

Two preservatives that have been a source of controversy are sodium nitrite, $NaNO_3$, which, in the body, is converted to the nitrite. These substances are added to cured meats, especially pork products, for two reasons First, they prevent growth of *Clostridium botulinum,* an organism which causes the serious food poisoning botulism. Second, and some feel this is the major reason, is that nitrite reacts with myoglobin in meat to replace a grayish tinge with a healthy-looking red color. In the body, myoglobin both stores oxygen and enhances its rate of diffusion into the cells of skeletal muscle tissue. Also, sodium nitrite can react in the human digestive tract with secondary amines such as pyrrolidine to form nitroso compounds which have caused cancer in test animals (4).

Sodium nitrite can react with hemoglobin, impairing its oxygen-carrying ability. For adults, the low levels of nitrite used probably present no danger in this respect, but babies, who before the age of one year have less hemoglobin in their blood, could be endangered. A committee of the World Health Organization (WHO) stated that nitrites should not be added to baby food.

Some preservatives are designed to combat specific reactions; for example, rancidity of fats and oils which involves a chain reaction. First, fatty substances react with oxygen in air forming hydroperoxides. These hydroperoxides are unstable and can produce a few free radicals containing an unshared electron. These radicals act on some of the remaining fat molecules, breaking them into smaller oxygenated compounds called aldehydes and ketones which are responsible for the foul odor of rancid fat.

To retard oxidation of fat, manufacturers add small amounts of antioxidants which capture free radicals before they can do damage. Two antioxidants in widespread use are BHT and BHA (butylated hydroxytoluene and butylated hydroxyanisole). These substances are added to vegetable oils and shortening, cake mixes, snack foods, and cereals where they may be applied to the inside of packaging materials and migrate to the cereal itself.

Antioxidants can make a spectacular difference. In one test, potato chips were subjected to above normal temperature of 63°C. Chips without antioxidant became rancid in three days but those with antioxidant stayed fresh 26 days. Still, many question whether these chemicals really are needed under ordinary conditions. In fact, some plant oils contain the natural antioxidant vitamin E or α-tocopherol, and some brands of vegetable

USES AND SAFETY[1] OF SOME FOOD ADDITIVES

Additive	Function	Safety[2]	Examples of use
Adipic acid	Acidulant	Safe	Fruit drinks, gelatin desserts
Agar	Thickener	Safe	Frostings, ice cream
Algin, sodium alginate	Thickener	Unknown	Ice cream, cheese spreads
Ascorbic acid (vitamin C)	Preservative, anti-oxidant	Safe	Frozen fruits, yogurt
BHA (butylated hydroxyanisole)	Preservative, anti-oxidant	Question-able	Shortening, vege-table oil, cereal, convenience foods
BHT (butylated hydroxytoluene)	Preservative	Question-able	Same as BHA
Calcium propionate	Preservative in baked goods	Safe	Baked goods
Calcium stearoyl-2-lactylate	Emulsifier		Baked goods, dried egg whites
Carageen (carragheenan)	Thickener	Safe for adults, question-able for babies	Milk drinks, ice cream
Carboxymethyl-cellulose	Thickener	Safe	Ice cream, pie filling, diet foods
Citric acid	Acidulant	Safe	All fruit drinks, gelatin
Dextrin	Thickener	Safe	Candy, powdered mixes
Dextrose	Sweetener, browning agent	Safe	Bread, soft drinks
Dimethylpolysiloxane	Antifoaming, anti-splattering agent	Safe	Vegetable oil, wine, gelatin
Disodium guanylate	Flavor enhancer	Safe	Soup mixes, canned stews
Disodium inosinate	Flavor enhancer	Safe	Same as disodium guanylate
EDTA (ethylenediamine tetraacetic acid)	Preservative, sequestrant	Safe	Salad dressing, pickles, canned vegetables

[1]Information from (6).
[2]Safe, has been subjected to full range of tests with no ill effects noted; unknown, has not been fully tested; questionable, although not proved harmful, ill effects noted in some animal studies.

USES AND SAFETY[1] OF SOME FOOD ADDITIVES (continued)

Additive	Function	Safety[2]	Examples of use
Fumaric acid	Acidulant	Safe	Pudding, gelatin, soft drinks
Glycerol (glycerin)	Moisturizer, softener	Safe	Candy, baked goods
Glycerol lacto-palmitate	Emulsifier, surfactant	Safe	Cake mixes, convenience foods
Glyceryl monooleate	Emulsifier	Safe	Baked goods, pudding
Guar gum	Thickener	Unknown	Pudding, salad dressing
Gum arabic	Thickener, anti-crystallization agent	Unknown	Cake mixes, ice cream
Hydroxylated lecithin	Emulsifier	Unknown	Baked goods, margarine
Hydroxymethyl-cellulose	Thickener	Safe	Ice cream, pie filling
Lactic acid	Acidulant, preservative	Safe	Frozen desserts, soft drinks
Lactostearin	Emulsifier	Safe	Cake mixes
Lecithin	Emulsifier, antioxidant	Safe	Margarine, chocolate, ice cream
Mannitol	Sweetener, moisture inhibitor	Safe	Chewing gum, diet food
Mono- and diglycerides	Emulsifiers	Safe	Baked goods, candy, margarine
Monosodium glutamate (MSG)	Flavor enhancer	Causes discomfort in sensitive people; general safety questioned	Soup mixes, canned stews, soups
Polysorbate 60, 65, 80	Emulsifiers	Safe	Nondairy coffee creamers, frozen desserts
Potassium bromate	Ages flour	Safe	Flour

USES AND SAFETY[1] OF SOME FOOD ADDITIVES (continued)

Additive	Function	Safety[2]	Examples of use
Potassium citrate	Buffer	Safe	Imitation fruit juices
Potassium sorbate	Preservative	Safe	Cheese, jelly, mayonnaise
Propylene glycol	Moisturizer, solvent	Safe	Candy, soft drinks, marshmallows
Propylene glycol alginate	Thickener	Unknown	Frozen desserts, cheese spreads
Propyl gallate	Preservative, antioxidant	Questionable	Cereal, instant potatoes, vegetable oil
Sodium ascorbate	Preservative, antioxidant	Safe	Frozen fruits
Sodium citrate	Acidulant, antioxidant	Safe	Drink mixes
Sodium benzoate	Preservative	Safe, not tested for teratogenicity	Fruit juices, salad dressing, preserves
Sodium erythorbate	Preservative, antioxidant, gives red color to meat	Unknown	Bologna, frankfurters
Sodium nitrite and nitrate	Preservative, gives red color to meat	Questionable	Frankfurters and pork products
Sodium silicoaluminate	Anticaking agent	Safe	Salt, dessert topping mixes
Sodium sulfite	Prevents discoloration	Safe	Fruit juice, maraschino cherries
Sorbic acid	Preservative	Safe	Cheese, baked goods, mayonnaise
Sorbitol	Moisturizer, sweetener	Safe	Chewing gum, candy, soft drinks
Sorbitan monostearate	Emulsifier	Safe	Chocolate, frostings
Tragacanth	Thickener	Unknown	Salad dressing

oils, shortenings, and potato chips which are not treated with antioxidants stay fresh just as long as those that are. Also, the safety of BHT and BHA has been questioned. Although a high concentration of BHA proved nontoxic in short-term studies, the same concentration of BHT caused liver enlargement and raised enzyme levels in rats and dogs. Also, no long-term studies have been done to determine if these antioxidants could cause cancer.

Some Americans have as much as 3 ppm (parts per million) of BHT and BHA in their fatty tissues—six times as much as the average Englishman who eats less of these antioxidants. This might present no hazard and possibly do some good. The antioxidants may retard aging by capturing free radicals which are thought to play a role in this process. Nevertheless, any substance which accumulates in the body and has not been proved safe should be suspect. It is required that BHA and BHT be listed on product labels; thus, consumers can avoid them if they wish.

Another controversial antioxidant is propyl gallate, often used in conjunction with BHA and BHT. Some experiments have indicated that high doses of propyl gallate may affect kidneys and liver growth rate of rats and mice. Although no ill effects have been proved, evidence indicates that more detailed studies should be made. Propyl gallate is on the GRAS list; many products are available which do not contain the chemical and therefore it can be avoided.

Still another form of oxidation is catalyzed by enzymes present in fruits and vegetables. This is why cut surfaces of peaches and apples darken, a process which, as many cooks know, can be prevented by adding lemon juice, which contains ascorbic acid (vitamin C). Food manufacturers add ascorbic acid to items such as frozen peaches and fruit yogurts to prevent darkening.

Related to antioxidants are sequestrants, compounds used to bind metals, such as copper and iron, which act as catalysts to accelerate oxidation. Many of these sequestrants are chelating agents; that is, they are organic molecules having two or more active groups that can complex metal atoms. Thus sequestrants are used to prevent cloudiness in soft drinks by preventing iron or other metals in the water from reacting with other ingredients to form a precipitate.

One very effective sequestrant is ethylenediamine tetraacetic acid, or as it appears on food labels, EDTA. This compound has six unshared pairs of electrons and usually forms four stable chelate rings with the sixth electron pair bonded to a molecule of water. Like ascorbic acid, EDTA is used to prevent browning of fruits and vegetables, an enzymic reaction catalyzed by metals. EDTA is effective in very low concentrations from 0.0025 percent to 0.05 percent and, at such levels, has been shown safe in several thorough studies. Medically it is used to treat victims of lead poisoning because it bonds lead atoms in a form which can be excreted in the urine.

STABILIZERS

About 60 percent of today's food additives are designed to make food more appealing to the consumer. In this category are colors and flavors, as well as a broad range of chemicals that maintain stability of ingredients. The great increase in the use of this type of additive can be related to the growth of convenience foods—premixed and ready-to-eat concoctions ranging from chocolate pudding to sauce béarnaise and mixes which require addition of only one or two ingredients.

Emulsifiers

Many foods, especially prepared ones, consist of two systems—for example, an emulsion consists of one liquid dispersed in another; a suspension is a solid dispersed in a liquid; and a foam is a gas dispersed in a liquid. Eventually all these systems separate—less dense liquids float to the top, solids settle, and gas is lost. To delay such separation in food systems, manufacturers add an emulsifier, a special type of chemical called a surfactant that acts along the boundaries of liquids. For example, in a suspension of salad dressing, the emulsifier forms a thin protective coating around individual oil globules dispersed in the aqueous portion. This layer hinders globules from reuniting and delays separation.

One of the most popular emulsifiers is lecithin, which also has antioxidant properties. Lecithins are phospholipids . . . [and] are abundant in nature—those used in food technology come from soybeans. Also, lecithin is the substance in egg yolk which makes it possible to emulsify oil to make mayonnaise and butter to make hollandaise sauce. Actually lecithin, a source of choline, is a nutrient and appears to be completely safe.

However, less is known about hydroxylated lecithin, a derivative prepared by treatment with peroxide. A committee of the World Health Organization reported that the toxicology of hydroxylated lecithin has not been adequately studied.

Related to lecithins are the mono- and diglycerides. . . . These are extremely versatile emulsifiers, antistaling agents, and moisturizers. Like lecithin, they are natural materials which compose about 1 percent of natural food. Many derivatives such as acetylated, lactylated, citrated, and succinylated mono- and diglycerides are used, too, and, like the parent compounds, are safe. However, derivatives such as ethoxylated and sodium sulfoacetate mono- and diglycerides have not been studied thoroughly.

Some foods are both emulsions and foams. For example, whipped cream has butter fat dispersed in water and contains bubbles of air. Emulsifiers strengthen the walls of air bubbles and make foam last longer. Ordinary whipped cream lasts only a few hours but prewhipped toppings with emulsifiers can remain stable for weeks.

Emulsifiers are useful in bread and cake mixes where they produce a lighter, fluffier texture and inhibit staling by preventing crystallization of starch. In ice cream they keep butter fat from separating during freezing and they help nondairy cream substitutes dissolve in coffee. Among most commonly used emulsifiers for these purposes are the polysorbates composed of a polyoxyethylene sorbitan residue attached to a fatty acid. Polysorbate 80 is polyoxyethylene-20-sorbitan monooleate. . . . Polysorbate 60 and 65 contain monostearate and tristearate, respectively. The three polysorbates have been studied extensively and no hazard has been detected.

Related to polysorbates is sorbitan monostearate, frequently used in cakes, frostings, and toppings. It serves an interesting purpose in chocolate candy by coating the cocoa fibers, thus preventing the white haze or bloom which forms after chocolate has melted and resolidified. Although unappealing, this bloom, caused by cocoa butter rising to the surface, is harmless. Sorbitan monostearate has some nutritive value and no ill effects have been noted.

Emulsifiers do many other jobs and are difficult to classify. A great many are available and many perform more than one role. Some act as lubricants to make food less sticky. For instance, they prevent peanut butter from sticking to the roof of the mouth and reduce stickiness of caramel candy.

Moisturizers

Among the most useful moisturizers are polyhydric alcohols, most commonly glycerol, mannitol, sorbitol, and their derivatives. Depending on concentration, they can also soften, increase viscosity, and retard crystallization in candy. These additives are fully metabolized and converted by the body to some form it can use; therefore they are considered safe. Closely related is propylene glycol that serves as a solvent for oil-based colors in aqueous solutions.

Thickeners

The most common thickening agents used are polysaccharides from plant gums: algin, agar, and carageen (carragheenan) from seaweeds; acacia, tragacanth, locust, and guar from trees and seeds; and carboxymethylcellulose, carboxycellulose, and hydroxypropylmethylcellulose, prepared from wood and cotton. In addition to thickening foods, such as evaporated milk, frostings, and sauces, the gums perform such functions as giving body and mouth feel. For instance, soft drinks sweetened with saccharin feel thin compared to those sweetened with sugar. Adding gums restores body.

The physical properties of these gums vary slightly, making some especially suited to certain uses. Guar gum forms the thickest solutions and is used in ice cream, salad dressing, and doughs. Gum arabic is extremely water-soluble and is used to encapsulate flavors in dry mixes. Algin forms tough gels; it is used to prevent jellies from oozing out of pastries during baking. However, one disadvantage of algin gums is that it precipitates out of acidic foods. This was overcome by reacting algin with propylene oxide to produce propylene glycol alginate, a derivative which produces an acid-resistant gel.

Biological effects of these gums may vary too. Some, such as guar gum, are digested and others, such as agar, are not. Most of the natural gums and their derivatives have not been extensively tested, consequently their safety must be considered questionable.

Cellulose derivatives are becoming more popular. They are often used in diet foods because their bulk produces a full, satisifed feeling. They are not digested and, thus, are thought to be safe.

COLORS AND FLAVORS

Probably the most obvious type of food additives are the colors and flavors found in almost everything we eat. About 4 million pounds of synthetic dyes alone go into American food each year.

Colors

Color is an important factor in making foods appetizing. In fact, most people will reject food of a color different from what they are used to. Margarine is more acceptable when colored butter-yellow and soft drinks when they are colored bright fruit-like colors. Foods may be colored also to improve natural colors or to replace color lost in processing.

Once all colors came from natural sources and some still do. For instance,

much butter and cheese are colored yellow with annato, a dye from a tropical fruit. But today, 90 percent of food colors are synthetic, composed of
nine coal-tar derivatives, usually designated only by number, such as red 2*
and yellow 1. In 1970 over 3.5 million pounds of coal-tar dyes were certified
by the FDA for food use. Though many consumers feel reassured by the

*EDITOR'S NOTE: Red 2 was banned in 1976.

BEYOND RED DYE NO. 2

In hearings on food additives conducted
by the Senate Select Committee on
Small Business, January 13, 1977, Public Citizen Health Research Group
(HRG) advocated the immediate ban of
nine major food colors and called for
generally tighter regulation of the chemicals poured into our food.

Two days earlier, HRG had
petitioned FDA to ban the six permanently approved coal-tar dyes. HRG
submitted a detailed report on the
hazards of this group of chemicals and
the serious lack of safety evidence for
many other food dyes. Among the report's findings:

• Red No. 40, the popular replacement
of Red No. 2, causes cancer in mice.
• Citrus Red 2, used to dye oranges,
causes bladder cancer in laboratory
animals. The World Health Organization opposes its use in food.
• Yellow No. 5, most widely used of
food colors (almost 1½ million pounds

per year), might cause cancer. In addition, over 300,000 Americans could be
allergic to the dye.
• Blue No. 1, used in candy, beverages,
and baked goods in the U.S., is banned
in the United Kingdom and many
European countries. Animal studies
show it may be carcinogenic.
• Orange B, which colors the casings of
hot dogs and sausages, shows an
alarming similarity to Red Dye No. 2
(banned last year), and appears to
cause liver tumors in dogs.
• Red No. 3, more widely studied than
most food dyes, has been associated
with cancer, mutations, and thyroid
damage.

Three other coal-tar dyes (Blue 2,
Green 3, and Yellow 6), "provisionally"
approved by FDA, exhibit similar
hazards. Most of the 23 FDA-approved
non-coal-tar colors have never even
been tested for safety. And the large category of other food additives "generally

certified notice on labels, it is no indication of safety. Certified refers only to the purity of the dye.

Even though many coal-tar derivatives are known to be carcinogenic, these colors have not been tested thoroughly. In fact, 10 dyes once in widespread use have been banned because it was found they caused either cancer or other organ damage. The familiar violet dye once used to stamp inspected meat is now suspected of being carcinogenic also and has been replaced by a red dye.

~~~~~~

recognized as safe" (GRAS) have never been subjected to the rigorous scientific scrutiny both the law and the public health require.

Because of FDA's shoddy enforcement of scientific standards, Americans are exposed to over 5 million pounds of coal-tar dyes and hundreds of millions of pounds of other GRAS food additives each year. Many of these chemicals are simple "food cosmetics," with no nutritional or any other kind of benefit to the consumer. On this basis, HRG made the following recommendations before the Senate hearings:

• Immediately ban all coal-tar dyes.
• Abolish the "generally recognized as safe" concept. All food additives should be considered dangerous until proven safe by scientific studies.

• Disallow marketing of any new food additive unless it (a) has been thoroughly tested for all types of toxicity; (b) has more than just cosmetic benefit; (c) is better than an existing food additive of the same category.
• Take food additive testing out of the hands of industry. Industry should pay the bill; but reliable, closely monitored third parties should do the testing.
• Conduct a major "housecleaning" at the FDA Bureau of Foods. Critical, scientific, public health advocates must replace officials who are averse to confronting the food industry.

Hazards of Food Colors is available from Health Research Group, 2000 P Street, N.W., Washington, D.C. 20036.

~~~~~~

Three coal-tar dyes are in restricted use—each is permitted in only one food. Citrus red 2 is used only for coloring orange skins to make them more appealing to consumers. It is suspected of being carcinogenic and although the dye does not penetrate to the fruit itself, it could endanger anyone who sucked the peel or ate marmalade prepared from it. Happily, use of this dye is declining but as long as it remains on the market it is a potential hazard.

Another dye in restricted use, red 4, is permitted only in maraschino cherries. Tests in dogs indicate that high doses could damage adrenal glands and bladder. Orange B, the third restricted color, is used only in frankfurters.

Another problem associated with food coloring is the danger of allergic reactions. In some sensitive people, colorings cause symptoms of respiratory disorders, headaches, and intestinal disturbances. Those containing derivatives of salicylic acid have been linked to hyperkinetic behavior in children (5). Nevertheless, foods are not labeled to indicate exactly which dyes are present, and therefore they can be avoided by sensitive people only by avoiding colored foods completely. This is becoming more and more difficult as use of coloring increases.

Flavors

Once all flavors as well as colors were obtained from plants, such as vanilla and peppermint, but today flavor-producing components are made in the laboratory. Synthetics are both cheaper and more dependable, but some people think that some flavor is sacrificed. One reason is that flavor is a complex phenomenon—natural flavors contain impurities that may contribute subtle nuances to taste.

To reconstruct natural tasting flavors, food chemists also use many different chemicals, some of which are present in natural flavor and others which are not. One imitation cherry flavor, for example, contains 13 components. Because flavors are used in very small concentrations and because many of them are natural products, they are not as rigidly controlled by the FDA as other additives. But, considering that even natural flavors have been shown dangerous, such as sassafras used in root beer until it was found to be carcinogenic, some scientists feel that flavors have not been adequately tested and that more caution is advisable.

Sweeteners

Emphasis on weight control has led to a great increase in use of noncaloric sweeteners to replace sugar. Saccharin, a cyclic imide of benzene-sulfonic acid, has a sweetening power 300 times that of sugar but no food value.

Because of its great sweetness, drinks made with saccharin cost much less to produce—an added incentive to food manufacturers.

Saccharin might be safe but there have been some doubts. In 1951, one test indicated is caused kidney damage in rats and 1957 and 1970 tests, where a controversial technique was used, indicated it enhanced the tendency of cholesterol to cause cancer when implanted in bladders of mice. However, other more conventional tests did not confirm these findings and, in 1970, a committee of the National Academy of Sciences–National Research Council reviewed results and reports that saccharin is not a hazard. Nonetheless it was removed from the FDA GRAS list and is now used under an interim food additive regulation until results are known of several long-term toxicity studies now under way. Until then, many feel that only those who must should use saccharin.*

The synthetic sweeteners, calcium and sodium cyclamate, some 30 times sweeter than sugar, were popular for a few years because they have a less bitter aftertaste than saccharin. However, they were banned in 1970 after a test showed they caused abnormalities in chick embryos and bladder cancer in rats. These results have been questioned and cyclamates are being restudied. However, until they are proved safe they are not being used in foods.

Another sweetener, sorbitol, is a natural sugar alcohol prepared by hydrogenation of glucose. It is converted to sugar in the body and, thus, does supply calories but, because it is absorbed very slowly, blood sugar levels rise only slightly. For this reason it is useful for diabetics. Sorbitol is used in chewing gum to reduce tooth decay because bacteria which excrete caries-causing acid cannot metabolize it. Although very large amounts can have a laxative effect, sorbitol has been tested and shown to be safe.

Acidulants

A number of different acids are used to give tartness and tang to foods. The choice of which acid to use in a particular food is based on its physical

---

*EDITOR'S NOTE: A scientific panel, named by the Office of Technology Assessment to review the saccharin controversy for Congress, reported on June 7, 1977, that the artificial sweetener was a weak carcinogen that should not be regarded as safe for human consumption. The group, which cited studies showing saccharin had caused bladder cancer in rats, was unable to measure definitively the potential of the substance to cause cancer in humans. Although the FDA had been urging a ban on saccharin, the House of Representatives voted on June 21, 1977, to delay such a ban until September 30, 1978.

properties and cost. Citric acid is used about 60 percent of the time because it is extremely water-soluble and is quite inexpensive. Phosphoric acid . . . is preferred for soft drinks, and adipic acid is becoming popular for powdered drink mixes and gelatin desserts because it doesn't absorb moisture readily and the powders don't cake. Other acids in use are malic, tartaric, and fumaric acids.

Flavor enhancers

Most well-known of this type of additive is monosodium glutamate or MSG, which is known also under the brand name Aċcent. Although added primarily to enhance other flavors, it contributes a slight meaty flavor and consequently is used most often with meats, poultry, fish, and gravy.

As a derivative of an amino acid, MSG was thought for many years to be completely safe, but some question was raised in 1968 when it was found to cause such symptoms as headache, tingling in arms and neck, shortness of breath, and chest pain in some people (3). Because MSG is used liberally in Chinese cooking, these symptoms became known as Chinese restaurant syndrome.

Research has shown that MSG acts by stimulating nerve endings and that some people have low thresholds of sensitivity to it. In 1969, evidence was found that MSG damaged nervous systems of young mice and rats. Later, another study revealed high doses cause brain lesions in infant primates; however, this was not confirmed by later tests sponsored by the FDA. At present MSG it permitted as long as its presence is noted on the label. Manufacturers voluntarily stopped adding it to baby food because they agree it is unnecessary and had been included only to make the food appeal to mothers.

Other flavor enhancers becoming more popular today are the 5′-nucleotides, disodium inosinate and disodium guanylate. These are related chemically to nucleic acids, essential building blocks of life. These flavor enhancers are metabolized by the body to produce innocuous by-products and are considered safe.

The only other additives in this category are the maltols, which contain a pyran ring, a six-membered ring with one oxygen and two double bonds. Maltol was first isolated from birch bark, and small amounts are present in milk. To improve maltol's flavor-enhancing properties, chemists prepared the analog, ethyl maltol, which has six times the flavor-enhancing ability of maltol itself. Some testing has been done on both compounds with no ill effects observed, but additional studies are needed before they can be considered safe.

CONSUMER'S CHOICE

Surely it would be foolish not to take advantage of the many benefits food additives can bring. Preservatives have reduced danger of food-carried microbial disease, ensured great variety of foods all year round, and reduced waste due to spoilage. Other additives have made possible a variety of tasty, exotic dishes prepared quickly and conveniently. Still, any additional chemical taken into our bodies might present some degree of hazard. In weighing the benefits against the possible harm, any unnecessary risk, no matter how slight, seems too great. The most conservative approach, then, would be to use only those additives essential for health and at the lowest concentration needed to be effective.

In reality, such a turnabout by food manufacturers seems unlikely. However, concerned consumers can limit their intake of doubtful additives by reading labels and not buying products that contain them. With the wide range of products available today, this is feasible. For example, not all vegetable oils contain BHA, BHT, and propyl gallate, and not all frankfurters and sausage contain sodium nitrite.

Products which do not list ingredients must conform to a standard composition agreed on by government and manufacturers. This lists the ingredients that must be included in the product and also states which additives are permitted. These standards can be obtained from the government but they may not really help the consumer because manufacturers may not include all additives permitted in the product. Thus, consumers basing their choice on standard composition lists may avoid some products needlessly.

Consumers can reduce intake of additives also by limiting use of convenience foods because additives are more prevalent in them. Fresh vegetables with butter and a squeeze of lemon can be substituted for those frozen in a fancy sauce; recipes can be collected for desserts that can be quickly and easily prepared in place of ready-made and frozen ones. Consumers might also reevaluate how convenient some convenience foods really are. In the case of mixes, often only a few more minutes are needed to make a dish "from scratch." This way the consumer can be sure of avoiding unnecessary additives, will certainly save money, and may also get a tastier more nutritious product.

Suggested reading

1   Alexander, T., "Hysteria about Food Additives," *Fortune*, March 1972, p. 62.

2   Bernarde, M. A., *The Chemicals We Eat*, 1971, American Heritage Press, New York, N.Y.

3   *Chemistry*, 1969, 42(8), 5.

4   Ibid., 1972, 45(11), 23–24.

5   "Food Additives: Health Question Awaiting an Answer," *Medical World News*, September 7, 1973, p. 73.

6   Jacobson, M. F., *Eater's Digest*, 1972, Doubleday & Co., Garden City, N.Y.

PART II
Dietary Trends

Food is that which explains half the emotions of life.

—SIDNEY SMITH

Introduction to

Part II

By age 65, the average American will have consumed some 100,000 pounds of food, give or take a few tons. The quantity has, of course, little to do with the quality of nourishment. If an individual has managed to muddle through the decades in spite of nutritional neglect, that neglect will almost certainly be reflected in the state of his or her health by the age of 65, if not long before.

Knowledge is still murky concerning the extent to which body wisdom—that is, the regulating mechanisms in the endocrine system and the brain—sways food choices. Only in childhood are those choices made for us by someone else; after that, we are more or less on our own. Our possible course of action is to take this responsibility too seriously and become neurotic about it. Another, more commonly followed, is to be too lazy, self-indulgent, or misinformed to get on the right track and, once on it, to stay there.

The infant may be on the wrong track even before birth if the mother is undernourished during pregnancy. Each year in this country about 120,000 babies begin life malnourished, and some 35,000 die because of deficiencies in the prenatal diet. An infant deprived of adequate nourishment may never achieve full mental capacity.[1]

The choice of whether to breast-feed or bottle-feed is one that, according to the most recent studies, can be pivotal. Some 70 percent of American infants were breast-fed before World War I, but only about 5 percent were in the late 1960s. Yet by 1975, nearly 40 percent were again being breast-fed. Many pediatricians see the resurgence of breast-feeding as part of the "back-to-nature" movement; but whatever the cause, they are for it. For those who are not, Margaret Mead has a withering comment: if an American woman refuses to breast-feed it is "because her pediatrician, who would like to pretend he's feeding the baby himself, insists she shouldn't."[2]

Breast-feeding is the vital choice in poverty areas,

where there may be too little money to buy sufficient formula (if overdiluted, it can cause severe malnutrition), unclean water, little or no refrigeration, or inadequate home hygiene. But for the poor and affluent alike, breast-feeding may be preferable to formula-feeding if only because there are apparently some still unidentified components in human milk; no commercial formula has been able to duplicate it exactly. Then, too, milk varies so much from woman to woman that, scientists speculate, the milk of each mother may be designed especially for the needs of her infant.[3]

Marvelous as mother's milk may be, there is some question about its safety. Tests by the Environmental Protection Agency recently showed the milk of some nursing mothers to contain measurable, if small, amounts of industrial pollutants like PCBs and PBBs,* as well as residues of toxins that are breakdowns of chemicals widely used as pesticides in the past. (The levels of these residues are sometimes higher than those allowed by law for cow's milk.) Although the EPA stated that breast-fed infants were in no immediate danger and no adverse effects have been found thus far, absolute assurance is lacking. And the consolation? Infants have already picked up some chemicals while still in the womb, and, breast-fed or not, once on solid food they are apt to pick up quite a few more.[4]

In *Selection 8*, Jean Mayer describes the many advantages of breast-feeding, the cases in which it is not advisable, and the use of prepared formulas. In addition, he offers guidelines for introducing solid foods, both homemade and commercial.

The almost imperceptible overfeeding of an infant—which usually entails, among other things, too much salt, sugar, and fat—can predispose him or her to a lifetime of health problems. And during the formative years children may be subjected to so much "junk food" and convenience food (the difference is not always apparent) that pastel breakfast cereals soon seem as natural to them as a sunset. Knowledge about wholesome food is usually vague at best. Television commercials, vending machines, and supermarkets don't help. Unfortunately, even school lunch programs, however laudable their intent, have often been found nutritionally inferior. And when they do offer proper nourishment, students tend to make such poor choices within them that great quantities of the important nutrients go to waste.

---

*These are polychlorinated biphenyls and polybrominated biphenyls. The discharge of PCBs directly into waterways was barred in 1977, and Congress set a deadline of January 1, 1979, for an end to their manufacture.

Nutritionists have for some time been wringing their hands over the junk food young people eat. But now they have an additional worry: the dietary habits of those who refuse to eat junk food and resolutely adhere to exotic diets based on foods that have escaped technological tampering. Some of these diets have a good deal of merit; but when knowledge of how to use them is wobbly, severe nutritional deficiencies can crop up.

In *Selection 9,* Reva Frankle and F. K. Heussenstamm examine the reasons for the upsurge of nontraditional diet patterns and analyze the rationales, the programs, and the mistakes of advocates of vegetarianism, health foods, and "Zen" macrobiotics. They suggest new ways of providing conciliatory diet counseling for teenagers embarked on offbeat eating regimes.

In discussing the "Zen macrobiotic diet," the authors fall into a common error of both its critics and its adherents: they say that regimen number 7 is the ultimate goal of the diet, implying that one ends up eating nothing but brown rice forever. Michel Abehsera, who was trained in Zen cookery by George Ohsawa, the guiding light of Zen macrobiotics, states the rules this way:

> One begins with Number 7 . . . usually for ten days; one also goes back to Number 7 in case of illness. Numbers 6 to 3 should be where we spend most of our time. Those marked with minuses are slightly below the margin of safety, are resorted to occasionally in the search for variety, and are not recommended.[5]

In any case, Mr. Ohsawa did Zen a disservice by clapping its name on a diet that is strictly his interpretation—or misinterpretation—of ancient Zen dietary practices. (An old text emphasized the use of vegetables and seaweed, and recommended eating two-thirds of one's capacity during long meditation periods.) Though brown rice is nutritionally preferable to white, present-day Zen monasteries—George Ohsawa to the contrary—usually serve polished white rice. Zen Buddhists eat sparingly (and occasionally feast), use food with careful regard for its proper function, and do not waste or needlessly destroy it.[6] Daisetz T. Suzuki, the Zen Buddhist disciple who died in 1966 at the age of 95 as Japan's foremost authority on Zen, spent many of his later years in the United States, where he demonstrated no obsession about his diet and seemed perfectly content to go out for an occasional hamburger.[7]

The "new" vegetarians described in Selection 9 differ considerably not only from older vegetarian groups but also among themselves. Those, for instance, who are affiliated with groups are apt to be more extreme in dietary practices than the loners. To discount vegetarianism as a regime espoused only by fanatics and eccentrics would be very shortsighted. Vegetarianism has a long and mostly honorable history. It is true that Sylvester Graham, the noisy vegetarian zealot who in effect founded the modern American health movement in the early 1800s, is still the subject of mirth and ridicule (among his beliefs was that sexual indulgence, like condiments, could cause insanity). But many of Graham's extremist views on diet were based upon sound principles. The cornflakes and Grapenuts brigades that followed in his wake were, after all, harbingers of a positive future trend in American eating habits.[8] Dedicated vegetarians tend to be naturally careful eaters. Perhaps that is why they are rarely overweight, and appear to be healthier and may live longer than other Americans.

Janet Barkas, in an excellent history of the vegetarian state of mind, concludes:

> To become a vegetarian involves both a psychological predisposition and a distinct philosophical outlook. The recruiting efforts of religious and dietary fanatics are therefore contradictory to their desired end, for unless vegetarianism comes from the soul, it will be just another passing fad. Of course the idea must be exposed, but it cannot be indoctrinated. The basic issues involved are much too intricate and far-reaching to be overlooked or brushed aside. [The appearance of the fleshless diet] in contemporary societies is an indication of a positive questioning of traditional and age-old habits—a microcosm of the ideological conflicts facing thinking people of today.[9]

Vegetarians have as yet had little impact on the American way of eating, for our consumption of meat has soared in recent decades. During 1960–1970 the meat intake of the average American jumped from 190 to 236 pounds a year; between 1952 and 1972 per capita consumption of beef alone increased 80 percent. As noted in the Introduction to Part One, this state of affairs is both ecologically and physiologically unsound. There is no absolute evidence, however, that meat is nutritionally hazardous. Among the reasons it may be suspect is that sometimes high levels of the pesticides used on grain fed to livestock become concentrated in their flesh; there may also be residues of the six different hormones given legally to livestock in their feed or by injection.

Low degrees of meat-eating predominate in the three places in the world where people are renowned for longevity and remarkable health: the Andean village of Vilcabamba in Ecuador, the land of Hunza in the Karakoram Range in Pakistan, and the autonomous republic of Abkhazia in the Caucasus of the Soviet Union. Meat and dairy products play a minimal role in the total protein picture in Hunza (1.5 percent) and in Vilcabamba (12 grams daily). But in Abkhazia, where people allegedly live longer than anywhere else on earth, food from animal sources (with heavy emphasis on dairy products) accounts for 30 percent of the diet. The least meat is eaten by older people—who remain active members of their communities, as do their counterparts in Hunza and Vilcabamba, which may be one reason for their vigor and longevity.[10]

In *Selection 10*, Mervyn Hardinge and Hulda Crooks welcome the current trend toward vegetarianism. They distinguish the sensible vegetarian diet from the bizarre Zen macrobiotic diet, offer scientific evidence supporting vegetarianism, and succinctly survey some vegetarian regimes in other lands. The authors focus on the lacto-ovo-vegetarian diet, which is fairly simple to follow and has few nutritional snares. It is the vegans—those who shun all foods of animal origin—who are likely to be stumped when trying to figure out how to get the right kind and amount of protein plus sufficient vitamin B_{12}.* The main stickler is that the pure vegetarian must think of protein as coming from not just one or two sources but from the entire dietary. In *Selection 11*, Bronwen Godfrey neatly spells out how vegans can remain or become healthy on this more challenging, but basically simple diet.[11]

Many proponents of vegetarianism assert that their regime is crucial to ensuring an adequate world food supply in the future. Do you agree with them? Do you believe that a fleshless diet is nevertheless destined to remain the option of but a small minority of Americans? Is it or is it not realistic to expect over 200 million Americans to discard, or at least modify, their carnivorous bill of fare, if only because it makes ecological sense to do so? Taking both a world view and a personal view, Frances Moore Lappé in *Diet for a Small Planet* presents compelling reasons for adopting a lacto-ovo-vegetarian diet, perhaps supplemented occasionally with fish. She cautions, however, against trying to change lifelong habits overnight: "Never did [my family] swear off meat, vowing to make this a great sacrifice for the sake of mankind! Rather, meat began to play a smaller and smaller role in our diet as it was displaced by new and, frankly, more interesting ways of meeting our daily protein need."[12]

In contrast to the long-lived Hunzas, Vilcabambans, and Abkhazians mentioned above, the elderly in America—our fastest-growing minority—are all too often shunted aside as useless members of society. Easy victims of apathy and

---

*Curiously, strict Hindu vegetarians in India seem to be free of vitamin B_{12} deficiencies, but this is not true of those who have emigrated to Britain but remained on their customary diet. The apparent reason is that in India they inadvertently ate dried insects or insect parts harbored in their food.

depression, they may lose all motivation to eat properly. If they live alone, they may not bother to cook. If they have few teeth or ill-fitting dentures, they have trouble chewing. If they have no transportation, are arthritic, are partially deaf or can't see well, shopping becomes a major undertaking.

Because the elderly usually become less active and because they have a slower metabolic rate than when they were younger, they need fewer calories but require essentially the same amount of protein, vitamins, and minerals as when they were 25. (Some are apparently misdiagnosed as senile or schizophrenic when they are actually suffering pellagra induced by niacin deficiency.) Since every calorie must be worth its weight in nutrients, older people should eschew dietary frills and "empty" food.

Often afflicted with degenerative diseases that are not as yet curable, the aged are prime targets of health food charlatans who offer miracle cures and divest their victims of money better spent on wholesome food, medical and dental care, and recreation. "Above all," Jean Mayer counsels, "remember that, as the child is the father of the man, the middle-aged man is the father of the elderly. What happens to your nutrition and health in old age is very much the result of the practices and preparations of your preceding years."[13] And not only what you eat but how much you eat during the early years could have considerable bearing on how long you will live.

In *Selection 12*, Anthony Albanese summarizes the nutritional pitfalls of the elderly in America. He offers specific advice on how to erase at least some of the scars of past malnutrition and to sustain and perhaps even improve the health and vigor that still exist.

America's cornucopia of calories has led to the weightiest nutrition problem of all. Since 1900 the proportion of overweight people has tripled. The roughly 40 percent of Americans who are too heavy are inviting a host of ailments and a shortened lifespan. (According to insurance doctors, for every inch that your waist measurement exceeds that of your chest—not bust—your life expectancy decreases by two years.[14]) The majority of the middle-aged are too fat, as are more than 20 percent of children and adolescents.

Too many of us ignore or are unaware of the law of calorie reversal: with each passing decade after age 25, we burn 5 to 7 percent fewer calories. This means that by age 50 we require 12 to 17 percent less fuel, and by age 60 about 20 percent less, than at age 25. But food habits of earlier years die hard; although nature wants to gradually run the body on less fuel, many of us keep stoking up at the usual, or a higher, rate.

Lessened physical activity compounds the problem. In fact, inactivity may contribute even more to overweight than does overeating. As for mental exertion, someone has figured out that the energy needed for one hour of hard thinking could be supplied by half a peanut.

One of the tragedies of overfeeding children is that, since there are more fat cells in their bodies than in those of children of normal weight, they will be at a great disadvantage when trying to reduce later in life. Only the fat content, not the number of fat cells, is decreased during reducing; so these dieters must shrink each cell much more than is normal to hit the right weight level.

Torn between feasting and fasting, at any one time millions of Americans either are telling themselves to eat, drink, and be merry, for tomorrow we diet, or are more or less stoically reducing—usually suffering in silence and letting everyone know it. Each year some 50 million Americans try to extricate themselves from caloric chaos, spending some $10 billion in the process. A few even have their jaws wired shut, their ears stapled (on the assumption that ears have "obesity nerve endings"), their intestines shortened, or their fat surgically removed. Of those who lose weight on a fad diet, 85 to 95 percent gain it all back again.

In spite of the vast amount of published information on the caloric content of foods, misconceptions about "fattening" foods live on. Such foods as potatoes, bread, and bananas are, according to a persistent myth, fattening and have more calories than steak. The outstanding fallacy is that overweight is caused by fattening types of food rather than the amount consumed or what is consumed with them.

Reducing-diet guides keep rolling off the presses while the rolls of fat keep accumulating. A recent entry is Dr. Robert Linn's *The Last Chance Diet,* which has sold over two million copies. On this protein-sparing diet, the overeater is restricted to slurping up daily (for a total of 300 to 500 calories) a liquid formula of protein that is extracted from beef hides and heavily laced with cherry flavoring.* This diet and its imitators are based on a discovery by Harvard Medical School Professor George Cahill, Jr., and his colleague George Blackburn. They found that small amounts of pure protein could offset one on the major adverse effects of fasting: when the body is deprived of all nutrient intake, it begins to draw on its protein reserves as a source of energy. When pure protein is in-

---

*A few months after his book was published, Dr. Linn switched from beef hide to pigskin as the basis for his formula. He also dropped Prolinn, his original brand, and introduced E.M.F. (Enzymatic Modular Food). But the idea remains the same; and, as Dr. Linn has cautioned from the start, his diet should be undertaken only under medical supervision. Some nutrition authorities believe that no liquid-protein preparations should be used by dieters under any circumstances.

gested, the body's protein tissue is spared and the lean body mass need be only minimally destroyed for energy. But Cahill is not happy about Linn's clinical use and popularization of the discovery because of unknown risks and the question of long-term maintenance. Linn is an expert in behavioral modification as well as a nutritionist, and salesmanship rather than protein is said to be the key ingredient of his diet.[15] "When you deal with obesity," Cahill notes, "the more bull you throw in, the more people adhere to it. If you give them bracelets and let them join clubs, it works. If you charge money, the program's success doubles."[16]

The alacrity with which the diet-hungry latch on to "revolutionary," "sure-fire," and irrational schemes is amazing. To take just one instance: Dr. Abraham Friedman contends that by substituting sex for a 700-calorie snack, you can save 700 calories and work off an extra 200 calories while making love. Every three times you do this, he maintains, you'll lose over a pound. Deftly applying energy mathematics to this beautiful formula, Ronald Deutsch shatters it: "Actually, Friedman has miscalculated. Three of these combinations, at 900 calories per instance, would lead to only 2,700 calories lost, not the 3,500 which equal a pound. Unless, of course, Friedman is assuming some very energetic foreplay—say, on racing bikes." Friedman recently claimed he had lost 16 pounds during his marriage by practicing what he preaches. Says the relentless Mr. Deutsch: "According to Dr. Friedman's own data, this would suggest that 48 times [he and his wife] have substituted love for eating. For the sake of their marriage, one may well hope that either (a) they have not been married long or ... (b) neither is inclined to snack."[17]

How did those famous diets that don't work (in the long run) become so famous? Don Schanche provides some explanations, spiced with wit, in *Selection 13*. In the course of pointing out the major flaws in several popular diet books, he concisely covers the various causes of obesity, its extent among our population, and some sensible ways to combat it. He examines in particular the ketogenic diets, which are considered abominations by the medical profession in general. Among these, as Schanche notes, is the one touted in *Dr. Atkins' Diet Revolution*. Atkins insists that his diet has been used successfully by some three million people and that it is safe if followed under medical supervision. He suspects that attempts to discredit his work are carefully orchestrated: "The commercial interests of the majority of food advertisers of AMA [American Medical Association] publications (who are in the carbohydrate selling business) are best suited to perpetuation of the 'balanced' high carbohydrate myth."[18] Bearing in mind that Atkins's particular *bête noire* is refined sugar, and that health-minded vegetarians also tend to avoid sugar, do you think Dr. Atkins's views can be reconciled with those of vegetarians, almost all of whom are slim and eat relatively high-carbohydrate diets?

An increasing number of nutritionists, psychologists, and physicians believe that without behavior modification, without untying psychological knots, dieters will almost invariably backslide. Behavioral science, they say, must go hand in hand with nutritional science. The routes these new programs take include "mental dieting" (reprogramming the subconscious), relaxation and meditation techniques, and the monitoring of eating habits. Here the key to permanent weight loss is a change in one's style of life and a change in attitude toward food, toward other people, and toward oneself.[19]

On the assumption that fad diets fail because they focus on food rather than on eating habits, Michael J. Mahoney and Kathryn Mahoney in *Selection 14* present a seven-step method for using behavior modification to defy the calories.

Jack Osman takes a similar tack in his book *Thin from Within*. As he puts it,

Becoming thin from within is a rational process of getting your head together. Lifelong weight control involves more than just balancing your diet. It requires a lifelong balance of self-direction. Thin from within means you will no longer make excuses for what you are, what you feel, or how you look. Once you have gotten your head together, the substantial weight loss that will follow may strike you as the least of your gains.[20]

His advice ties in with psychiatrist Thomas Szasz's observation that "self-esteem and self-control vary directly: the more self-esteem a person has, the greater, as a rule, is his desire, and his ability, to control himself."[21]

References

1   "Mom's Diet: Key to Child's Growth," *Medical World News,* January 5, 1973, pp. 28–29; and Roger Lewin, "Starved Brains," *Psychology Today,* September 1975, pp. 29–33.

2   Margaret Mead, "Comments on the Division of Labor in Occupations Concerned with Food," *Journal of the American Dietetic Association* 68 (April 1976), p. 323.

3   "Is Breast-Feeding Best for Babies?" *Consumer Reports,* March 1977, pp. 152–153.

4   Carol Rasmusen, "The Debate on the Dangers in Mothers' Milk," *San Francisco Examiner,* August, 19, 1977, p. 27.

5   Michel Abehsera, *Zen Macrobiotic Cooking: Book of Oriental and Traditional Recipes* (New York: University Books, 1968), p. 4.

6   Philip Kapleau, comp. and ed., *The Three Pillars of Zen: Teaching, Practice, Enlightenment* (Boston: Beacon Press, 1967), pp. 37, 199. See also Edward Espe Brown, *Tassajara Cooking* (Berkeley: Shambhala Publications, 1973).

7 See, for example, Winthrop Sargeant, "Profiles: Great Simplicity," *The New Yorker,* August 31, 1957, p. 38.

8 Johanna T. Dwyer et al., "The 'New' Vegetarians," *Journal of the American Dietetic Association* 64 (April 1974), pp. 376–382; and Janet Barkas, *The Vegetable Passion* (New York: Charles Scribner's Sons, 1975). See also J. C. Furnas, *The Americans: A Social History of the United States, 1587–1914* (New York: G. P. Putnam's Sons, 1969), pp. 439–441; and Ronald M. Deutsch, *The New Nuts among the Berries* (Palo Alto, Calif.: Bull Publishing Co., 1977), pp. 25–35.

9 Barkas, *Vegetable Passion,* p. 193.

10 Ibid., pp. 177–178, 183; Alexander Leaf, "'Every Day Is a Gift When You Are over 100,'" *National Geographic,* January 1973, pp. 92–119; and Sabrina Michaud and Roland Michaud, "Trek to Lofty Hunza—and Beyond," *National Geographic,* November 1975, pp. 644–669.

11 *Laurel's Kitchen,* from which Ms. Godfrey's article is reprinted, is excellent not only as a cookbook for all types of vegetarians but also as a basic nutrition text. The classic primer on protein complementarity in vegetarian diets is Frances Moore Lappés *Diet for a Small Planet,* rev. ed. (New York: Ballantine Books, 1975).

12 Lappé, *Diet for a Small Planet,* p. 143.

13 Jean Mayer, *A Diet for Living,* Consumers Union ed. (New York: David McKay Co., 1975), p. 176.

14 James Trager,*The Bellybook* (New York: Grossman Publishers, 1972), pp. 472, 506.

15 Robert Linn, with Sandra Lee Stuart, *The Last Chance Diet* (Secaucus, N.J.: Lyle Stuart, 1976; New York: Bantam Books, 1977); and Susan Cheever Cowley, with Patricia J. Sethi, "The No-Food Diet," *Newsweek,* July 11, 1977, p. 74. See also Fredrick Stare and Elizabeth M. Whelan, "Dr. Fredrick Stare Rates the 10 Top Diets," *Harper's Bazaar,* July 1977, pp. 40–43; and Peter Bonventre with Susan Agrest, "The Protein Fad," *Newsweek,* December 19, 1977, p. 71.

16 George Cahill, quoted in Cowley, "No-Food Diet," p. 74.

17 Deutsch, *New Nuts among the Berries,* p. 214.

18 Robert C. Atkins, letter in *Today's Health,* January 1972, p. 70.

19 See, for example, Jack D. Osman, *Thin from Within* (New York: Hart Publishing Co., 1976); Elsye Birkinshaw, *Think Slim—Be Slim* (Santa Barbara: Woodbridge Press Publishing Co., 1976); Albert J. Stunkard, *The Pain of Obesity* (Palo Alto, Calif.: Bull Publishing Co., 1976); Frances Stern and Ruth Hoch, *Mind Trips to Help You Lose Weight* (Chicago: Playboy Press, 1976); James M. Ferguson, *Habits, Not Diets: The Real Way to Weight Control* (Palo Alto, Calif.: Bull Publishing Co., 1976); and Richard Tyson, with Jay R. Walker, *The Meditation Diet: The Relaxation System for Easy Weight Loss* (Chicago: Playboy Press, 1976).

20 Osman, *Thin from Within,* pp. 9–10.

21 Thomas Szasz, *Heresies* (Garden City, N.Y.: Anchor Press/Doubleday, 1976), p. 57.

THE YOUNG

| 8 |

A New Look at Old Formulas

JEAN MAYER

Jean Mayer, professor of nutrition at Harvard University from 1950 to 1976, is now president of Tufts University. An expert on the problem of human obesity, he has published some 650 papers and several books, the latest *A Diet for Living* (1975). Dr. Mayer has served as a consultant to several United Nations agencies. As chairman of the National Council on Hunger and Malnutrition in the U.S., he was instrumental in calling the nation's attention to the nutrition problems of its poor.

Reprinted from *Family Health/Today's Health,* October 1976, pp. 38, 40, and 78, by permission of Family Health Magazine. Copyright © 1976 Family Health Magazine.

During the last few years, conversations I've had with young mothers across the country, as well as the weekly stacks of mail that pour into my office, bear out the encouraging findings of some recent medical surveys: Growing numbers of American women, particularly among college-educated, upper-income groups, are returning to breast-feeding their infants. There also appears to be a growing preference for preparing solid foods for them from the family's own meals. With a few reservations, I think these trends augur well for the future health of our nation's children.

I was a hearty advocate of breast-feeding even during its darkest days when the indifference of obstetricians—combined with the blessings that hospital nursing staffs gave to widely advertised, "up-to-date," ready-prepared formulas—nearly doomed the practice to extinction except among the most "backward" of societies. Fortunately, new research fosters new attitudes, and people now realize that breast-feeding has many advantages—some of which we are only beginning to discover—for women who can nurse their babies (about 90 percent can) and for normal infants (who are the great majority).

There is, of course, the special emotional closeness between a nursing mother and her baby—which, like the new, gentler childbirth techniques, may well have a lasting psychological significance for the child. Breast-feeding is also convenient—and comparatively cheap (all you need is a little more food for the mother). The milk is ready-mixed, instantly available at the proper temperature, and in a sterile container. And the baby has the added advantage of being able to suck until he (or she) has had enough, without being urged to swallow the last drop.

Nutritionally speaking, breast milk is the ideal food for babies. It's been thoroughly consumer-tested—after all, human infants, by and large, have thrived on it for four million years. On the other hand, nature designed cows' milk for calves, which grow about three times as fast as babies, have a different pattern of development, and require different amounts of many nutrients.

Both breast and cows' milk (and most infant formulas, for that matter) have about the same number of calories—67 per 100 milliliters. Mothers' milk has less proteins; but the proteins it does contain are easier for infants to digest. And it has more carbohydrates in the form of lactose, a milk sugar. (Incidentally, most young babies have sufficient amounts of the enzyme lactase in their digestive tracts to be able to metabolize lactose.)

Human milk has about the same amount of fat as cows' milk, but it is higher in polyunsaturates (and thus also in the essential fatty acids) and is easier for babies to absorb. It is also slightly higher in cholesterol than cows' milk and, in fact, some investigators have suggested recently that although the baby's body can manufacture cholesterol, a moderate dietary supply may also be necessary—partly to aid the synthesis of bile acids and the steroid hormones (male or female sex hormones), and partly to spur the development of natural regulatory mechanisms for cholesterol metabolism.

But the situation with sodium is just the reverse. Cows' milk contains between 25 and 30 milligrams per liter, mothers' milk has only 7, and most formulas fall about midway between the two. This is a plus for mother's milk and worth considering when you begin flavoring your baby's diet with salt. Infants on milk and formula are already consuming generous amounts of salt. There is no question that a normal baby's kidneys can handle the extra sodium load—but is it necessary, or wise? A number of studies have shown that when baby rats from a strain that is predisposed to hypertension are fed a diet high in salt, even for a short time, they are more likely to develop high blood pressure in adulthood and at an earlier age. Although this doesn't prove that the same thing will happen to humans, we do know that some people are genetically predisposed to hypertension, and that salt intake certainly aggravates high blood pressure once it has developed. I definitely believe it is some cause for concern.

What about the other minerals? Except for copper, human milk is lower in most minerals and, in fact, has quite a bit less calcium and phosphorus than cows' milk does. But fortunately, the two to one ratio of calcium to phosphorus happens to be ideal for maximum absorption of calcium. However, both milks are very low in iron, which, like copper, is essential for the formation of red blood cells. Although babies are born with iron in their livers that should tide them over until they begin eating iron-rich foods, the amount the fetus is able to store is probably dependent upon its mother's own supply. Many young American women today are low in iron, and between 5 and 10 percent of women of childbearing age have iron-deficiency anemia. In any case, recent studies indicate that between 7 and 15 percent of children six months old have an iron deficiency. Most likely, pediatricians will prescribe an iron supplement for a breast-fed baby, and urge a mother who bottle-feeds to choose a formula that contains a readily absorbable form of iron, such as ferrous gluconate or ferrous sulfate.

Both human and cows' milk, unless they are fortified, also fall far short of the amount of vitamin D needed to prevent rickets in children who live in cold climates or smog-filled cities. So your pediatrician will probably recommend a daily supplement of 400 I.U. (International Units), too. Here, I must insert a word of caution, which I hope is not necessary. Both vitamin D and iron (and, indeed, all nutrients, including protein) can be dangerous if taken in excessive amounts. Do not try to prescribe your own supplements for your child: That job belongs to your doctor only.

In all other respects, the milk of a healthy, well-nourished woman (one cannot ignore the fact that a mother's nutritional state directly influences the amount and quality of milk she will produce) will provide her baby with all its nutrient needs for the first four, indeed the first six, months of life.

Of course, there are times when, for various reasons, it is either impossible or unwise to breast-feed. In such cases, if the baby is born full-term and healthy, with no food allergies or metabolic defects that make it unable to absorb one or more nutrients, you should look for a commercial formula based on cows' milk. Subject to your pediatrician's advice, it is usually better to choose one that reflects as closely as possible the composition of breast milk, with the addition of iron and vitamin D. Pay particular attention to calories. A number of studies, my own included, have found that young babies, unlike older children or adults, stop eating when they have a full stomach rather than when they have had the right number of calories in their food. (Calories yield energy, and we still don't know at exactly what point energy intake begins to regulate food consumption.) If, after a few weeks on a formula, your baby appears to be gaining too much weight in relation to length, your doctor may wish to prescribe a brand that is less rich in calories, or even less sweet.

When it comes to meeting special dietary needs, commercial formulas score high marks. For our young butterballs, there are low-calorie formulas; and for premature babies who are underweight, other preparations are high in calories. Some infants have difficulty absorbing fats, and for them there are formulas in which fat takes the form of medium-chain triglycerides (MCT); that is, it is already broken down for easy absorption. Still other commercial preparations contain only glucose, the form into which almost all carbohydrates are eventually broken down by the body. And for those few infants with lactose intolerance, formulas containing sucrose, another sugar, can be substituted. There is even one formula that leaves the choice of carbohydrate up to the physician.

What about those newborns who cannot digest milk proteins? Again, the prepared formulas offer healthy alternatives. There are formulas containing hydrolyzed casein, the main protein in cows' milk, in a readily absorbable form; and for newborns with an allergy to all milk proteins, soy-based or meat-based products are available.

In such special cases, formula feeding can make the difference between a healthy child and one who is chronically, even dangerously, ill. However, normal children have a better chance of staying healthy if they're breast-fed. The reason? Special protective factors in mother's milk. Babies are born with sterile intestinal tracts, which means they have no infection-fighting bacteria ready to battle for them. For the first few months of life, until they can build up their own defenses, newborns must rely on antibodies from their mothers for protection. We've known for some time that many of these antibodies are passed across the placenta before birth. But others—and we are just beginning to realize how important they are—are only present in breast milk and colostrum, the yellowish fluid that's excreted for the first few days before the milk itself starts to flow.

Why is colostrum so important? It is especially rich in immunoglobulins, antibodies that protect against the polio virus and various infectious bacteria. And it also contains leukocytes, the infection-fighting white cells, in as great a concentration as in blood. (Recent research indicates they are just as active and effective.) Studies within the last year suggest that leukocytes may provide key protection against necrotizing enterocolitis, a widespread, often deadly intestinal infection that strikes many newborns who have been given blood transfusions.

Human milk also contains a group of polysaccharides (complex starches known medically as the "bifidus factor") which, logically enough, promotes the growth of bifidobacteria. These friendly intestinal bacteria produce an acid environment that inhibits the growth of other dangerous microorganisms. Still other substances, including lactoferrin (an iron-binding protein that fights potent bacteria by depriving them of the iron they need for growth), and lysozymes, enzymes that combine with other factors to attack and destroy invading microorganisms, are a part of the storehouse of protection found in human milk. However well formulas can imitate or replace mothers' milk for other purposes, they cannot confer this kind of protection. It's especially important, then, to make sure that the ingredients you use in preparing a formula are kept refrigerated, that the utensils, bottles and nipples are scrupulously clean, and that any formula the baby does not drink is thrown away, rather than saved for another day.

Microbiological safety is equally essential when introducing solid foods. Enthusiastic as I am about the homemade variety, I must say that in this regard commercial baby foods have the advantage. It takes consistent and conscientious effort to maintain in a family kitchen the standards of cleanliness and sanitation observed by the big baby-food companies. But it can be done if you keep these rules in mind:

• Use only foods that are fresh and wholesome. Canned and frozen foods are usually salted (at an unknown level), and they may have additives, like monosodium glutamate (MSG) and nitrite, that are no longer allowed in commercial baby foods. Canned and frozen fruits, in particular, contain a good amount of sugar.
• Rinse all utensils—forks, knives, spoons, bowls, blender, cutting boards— in scalding, preferably boiling, water.

~~~~~~

BEECH-NUT, HEINZ MAKE CHANGES; GERBER DOESN'T

Things are changing for the better out there in baby-food land—but very slowly. When we last reported on baby foods (*Consumer Reports,* September 1975), we deplored the addition of salt, sugar, and modified starches to the commercial product. None of the additions are nutritionally necessary or good, we contended. The sugar and starches add nothing but empty calories. A high salt intake is suspected of predisposing infants to hypertension as adults, and a high sugar intake of stimulating a craving for sweets.

The homemade baby foods we made for that report generally proved nutritionally superior to similar commercial foods, primarily because the added salt, sugar, and starches in the commercial products took up a lot of room, displacing more nutritious ingredients.

Now for the changes: With great fanfare, Baker/Beech-Nut Corporation recently announced it was bringing out a line of "natural" baby foods. H. J.

Heinz Company quickly followed suit. The two firms, each of which have about 15 percent of the baby-food market, say they have taken *all* added salt out of their baby foods. And both companies say they have reduced the number of baby foods to which they add sugar. Meanwhile, Gerber Products Company, with about 65 to 70 percent of the market, continues to add salt and sugar to many of its baby foods.

Beech-Nut cites as a reason for its change to "natural" foods the severe criticism the baby-food industry has received from nutritionists over the possible long-range effects of excessive amounts of salt and sugar in the diets of infants. Certainly, that's one reason. Another is that Beech-Nut—and Heinz, too—obviously want to differentiate their products from those of Gerber, in order to gain more of the $450-million baby-food market. Whatever the reason behind their move, more power to them. No salt is better

~~~~~~

• Wash all food carefully, or peel it. Cook eggs, meat, fish, and poultry until well done. Eggs should have no hairline cracks and should be washed before they are broken.

• Use the same fresh foods you make for the rest of the family's meal, but separate the baby's portions and cook them without adding sugar, salt, MSG, or other seasonings.

• Don't taste your concoction and put the spoon back.

~~~~~~

than added salt, and less sugar is better than more.

But Beech-Nut and Heinz haven't gone far enough. A good many of their baby foods, like Gerber's, still contain added sugar or other sweetener. And many of their foods, like Gerber's, still contain modified starches. Here's the lineup, as calculated from figures provided by the companies:

Brand	Total number of baby-food products	Percent with added salt	Percent with added sweetener	Percent with added modified starches
Beech-Nut	131	0%	36%	46%
Heinz	108	0	33	49
Gerber	152	64	41	44

Then there's the matter of labeling. To their credit, both Beech-Nut and Heinz are labeling the *percentage* of added sugar or sweetener. In the Gerber products we bought, the ingredients—including any sugars—are simply listed in order of predominance. Less to Beech-Nut's credit is its claim: "No preservatives, no MSG or flavor enhancers, no artificial flavors or colors." That's all very nice, but Gerber and Heinz could say the same thing; none of the three companies use such ingredients in their baby foods.

~~~~~~

• Use vegetables such as beets, spinach, and carrots only occasionally, serve them just once when you prepare them, and don't store them—even in the freezer—for later feedings. These vegetables may contain a comparatively high concentrate of nitrates, which may, in rare cases, be converted to nitrites while the food is being stored or once it is inside the body.
• Store home-prepared baby foods in the freezer, even when you plan to use them the next day (incidentally, it is better to serve a variety, as you

would for other family members). Be as scrupulously clean in your freezing as you were in cooking. If you like, package portions separately on a sheet of scalded aluminum foil, or place food in individual pop-out ice-cube trays. Be careful not to defrost and refreeze a whole tray, or to partly defrost and then refreeze one serving while removing another. Freeze food no longer than one month.

Many women, for the sake of convenience, when they're too rushed to cook, or when they're traveling, like to combine homemade with commercial foods. That's fine—just keep in mind that the baby food section is much like the rest of the supermarket: Some of the foods are excellent, others are plain junk. So here are Mayer's Rules for Buying Baby Foods Wisely:

• Plain dry cereals are good foods that have one great advantage: They provide an iron supplement. Use them with milk (or if the pediatrician told you to count your baby's calories, water) instead of cereals with fruit, which are higher in calories and lower in nutritional value.
• Plain vegetables and plain meats are superior to creamed vegetables and meat combinations, both nutritionally and economically. The meats, particularly liver, are also good sources of iron.
• Fruits have added sugar and starch fillers, fruit juices have added sugar. Give your baby fresh fruits instead, and the real fruit juices, diluted with water.
• Don't add more salt to baby foods. Despite the fact that the level of sodium was voluntarily lowered by manufacturers in 1971, many vegetables, meats, high-meat dinners, dinners, and soups still have a concentration of that mineral that is considerably higher per calorie than the level found in cows' milk.
• Avoid baby desserts altogether.
• Read and compare the nutritional labels on the different brands for the best nutrient buys. If the manufacturer does not yet have such a label, write and ask him for nutritional information, including the amounts of salt, sugar, and food starch in his products. Baby-food manufacturers, incidentally, feel that food starch does no harm, that it keeps the food from separating in the jar, adds a pleasing texture, and dilutes the calories per serving. However, there is still some question as to whether babies even digest modified starches.

And finally, no matter which type of food you choose for your baby, there are several things a young mother should remember. Above all, don't abandon iron supplements even though you begin your baby on solid foods, unless your pediatrician advises it. And by the sixth month, if not before (again, ask your pediatrician's advice), if your local water supply is not naturally or artificially fortified with one part per million of fluoride, you should start giving your infant fluoride supplements as well.

Many mothers ask about the virtues of skim milk for infants. Although it does provide more than four times the estimated requirement for protein, it will put some strain on a baby's kidneys, and it does yield less than the estimated requirement for essential fatty acids. You'll be wiser to cut calories by other means, and reserve skim milk for children past two years of age. On the other hand, although 2 percent milk is higher in protein and lower in fat and the essential fatty acids than whole milk, it is probably not harmful for infants.

There, in brief, are my feelings about the best ways of feeding our young babies. They are practices I myself would follow if my children were still infants. And I would also try to start one more trend: I would not introduce solids until at least the fourth month. No doubt they are well tolerated, even in the first few days of life, but they are expensive, unnecessary, and can promote the habit of overeating and an early liking for sweet or salty foods. If there is ever a case for being well behind the Joneses—this is it.

9

Food Zealotry and Youth: New Dilemmas for Professionals

REVA T. FRANKLE and F. K. HEUSSENSTAMM

Reva T. Frankle is coordinator of the Nutrition Division, Department of Community Medicine, Mount Sinai School of Medicine, New York City; and instructor, Programs in Nutrition, Teachers College, Columbia University. F. K. Heussenstamm is associate professor of education, Teachers College, Columbia University.

Reprinted from *American Journal of Public Health* 64 (January 1974), pp. 11–18, by permission of the American Public Health Association. © 1974 by the American Public Health Association, Inc.

". . . You can eat anything your heart desires
From organic rice to bagels and lox
We've got one more bowl, for one more soul
And you can sleep here in this cardboard box. . . ."

"Soul Pad"
The Coasters
Copyright: Date Records

INTRODUCTION

"Can't you hear me talking to you?" is an alternatively plaintive, sometimes angry recurrent theme in adolescent communications that are directed to adults, and the dramatic upsurge of youthful interest in "alternative life styles" is reverberating through the popular culture. One can hear it in their music, read it in their newspapers, and see it in their behavior in every community.

Compounding the data on grievous malnutrition often found among members of low income families,[1-7] other researchers have found evidence of nutritional deficiencies among the children of the privileged and more affluent sectors of the society.[8-11] Nutritionists have studied these issues,[12-14] but today they are confronted with compelling new dilemmas. Our data indicate that a growing group of teenagers and youth, with diverse motivation, are adopting new eating patterns, some of which are extreme, faddish, eccentric, or grossly constricted, and because these patterns are different from those of the majority of our society, they may aggravate and exacerbate the relationships between adolescents and their parents, and between adolescents and adults in general. The conflicts stimulated in their adoption of atypical dietary patterns are symbolic of a variety of youthful postures interpreted as outright affrontery by many adults. For those whose responsibility involves the planning of preventive health care and education of adolescents, these challenges to accepted practice are being accelerated at such a rapid rate that many physicians, nutritionists, and public health workers, to name only a few of those whose vocations demand sensitivity and awareness, are losing touch with the very clients that they are motivated to serve.

ALTERNATIVE THEORIES AND DIRECTIONS

Conflicts with some adolescent and youthful clients is seen as inevitable as a consequence of new thinking about the nature of man, of society, and their relationships, according to Keniston.[15] In his examination of the two major camps of theorists dealing with "the youthful opposition," he criticizes first one group and then the other and suggests a series of more viable alternative directions for exploration. Youthful critics of contemporary society—and nutritional deviance is only a small part of the behavior which many adults find so disturbing—are classified as either "counterrevolutionary" or "revolutionary" by Keniston. His careful apologia for grouping such diverse men as Brzezinski, Bell, Kahn, Feuer, Shils, Bettleheim, and Lipset into one group is understandable; nevertheless, the careful analysis he makes of their writing is valuable. These men comprise the group who feel that dissident youth are "counter" to the important forces emerging in postindustrial, technetronic society. The other group of contemporary theorists—those concerned more with consciousness and culture—view youth as the revolutionary vanguard of the new society. Reich, Slater, Hoffman, Roszak, and Hayden are cohorts among the proponents of this second position.

The counterculture is seen by the latter as a consequence of the exhaustion of cultural, historical, and institutional forces at work in the West. This posture further assumes that "new values, new aspirations, and new life styles" not only are possible, but are mandated. The counterculture further is lauded as "an expression of . . . latent possibilities, a rational effort to remedy . . . failings . . . in some sense . . . logical fulfillment." Today's youthful "nutrition seekers" largely fall into this new "expansion of consciousness" movement according to our observations. In sharp contrast to the apathetic soda-and-candy-bar self-destructive and self-neglecting teenagers about which health care specialists and nutritionists have been appropriately concerned in the past, responsible adults are now confronted with what can only be described as food zealots, eager to act on new (to them) philosophical and moral premises in regard to care of the physical vehicle. The basic premises on which countercultural cuisine is based are extreme self-consciousness about food intake, and self-control and self-denial in dietary decisions, grounded in either purported scientific knowledge or religious faith. Regardless of which direction the apostles are moving, it is difficult to classify or categorize them neatly. On one hand are those youngsters who suggest that the most important reasons for their concern about their diet are improvement of their health and physical appearance, vitality, and longevity, and on the other hand are those for whom the "purpose of food is to become one with nature" because "from food are born all creatures, which live upon food and after death return to food," according to the placemat of one "health" restaurant in Manhattan.

NONTRADITIONAL DIET PATTERNS

Three major types of diets have been adopted by the atypicals within the purview of this article, although there are not always clear-cut distinctions among them. The first group are vegetarians; the second, advocates of organically grown and health food; and the third group are followers of the Zen macrobiotic regimen. Vegetarianism is a diet dependent entirely, or in large part, on the plant kingdom. Usually, the dietary pattern falls into one of three groups: (1) vegans, whose diet contains no animal foods whatsoever, (2) lactovegetarians, who eat no meat or fish but who include milk and cheese products, and (3) ovolactovegetarians, who eat an all-vegetable diet supplemented with dairy products and eggs. In addition, there is still another group known as "fruitarians" whose mainstay is raw or dried fruits and nuts. In a recent *New York Times* article, 29-year-old Dr. Andrew Weil described himself as a former 230-pound meat-eating doctor who is now a 175-pound vegetarian already leaning toward a fruitarian diet.[16] Historically, the roots of the proponents of such diets can be found in the Scriptures. Oriental religions, including Hinduism, Brahmanism, Buddhism, and Jainism, have as a basic tenet the belief in the transmigration of souls, thus, the reverence for animal life.

Hardinge and Crooks, of the Department of Pharmacology of Loma Linda School of Medicine, in their historical study of nonflesh dietaries, trace the origin of the vegetarian movement in America to Reverend William Metcalfe and 41 members of his church who landed in Philadelphia in 1817.[17] After 1850, sanitariums were established from which a health food industry eventually grew and this history provided Ronald Deutsch with material for his popular book *The Nuts among the Berries.*[18] Severe interpretations of Catholicism led to the founding of ascetic Trappist monasteries within the ranks of the Catholic Church. In the United States today these priests limit their dietary to only whole wheat bread, cereals, fruits, vegetables, and milk.[17] Another group, adherents of the religion of the Seventh-Day Adventist Church, follow a largely ovolactovegetarian diet. They have been the most cooperative in scientific investigations and it is mainly through them that any clinical and biochemical assessment of the nutritional status of non-flesh-eating populations has been made known. Studies conducted at the Loma Linda School of Medicine were reported in a series of articles which dealt with: (1) nutritional, physical, and laboratory studies;[19] (2) dietary and serum levels of cholesterol;[20] (3) dietary levels of fiber;[21] (4) dietary fatty acids and serum cholesterol levels;[22] (5) proteins and essential amino acids.[23] The subjects of these studies were lactovegetarians, vegans, and nonvegetarians.[23a, 23b]

> Widely differing dietary practices appear among vegetarians and near-vegetarians. A reasonably chosen plant diet, supplemented with a fair amount of dairy products, with or without eggs, is apparently adequate for every nutritional requirement of all age groups.[24,24a]

Researchers found no significant difference between these three groups in terms of height, weight, and blood pressure, although the pure vegetarians more closely approximated their ideal weight. The differences between the groups were not statistically significant for total protein, albumin, and globulin measurements. Slight differences were observed for hemoglobin, hematocrit, and erythrocyte counts. As would be expected, the serum cholesterol was higher in the nonvegetarian group, while the fiber intake was higher in the vegans and the lacto-ovovegetarians.

In the final study, "the amounts of essential amino acids, as well as of cystine and tyrosine in the diets of vegetarians and non-vegetarians, [indicate] all groups met and generously exceeded twice their minimum requirements."[23] However, Ellis et al. report that the mean serum vitamin B_{12} level was lower in 26 vegans than the controls in their study. This is the nutrient most likely to be deficient in the vegan diet.[25]

RATIONALE FOR ALTERNATE DIET PATTERNS

A third group of vegetarians in this country are those who have a strong belief in nonviolence and benevolence toward animals. Among them are found an aging population of fanatical opponents to orthodox medicine and the antivivisectionists. At the other extreme are the newest adherents of vegetarianism, dissident youth, who list among their various reasons for the adopting of nonflesh dietary: the desire to avoid animal products contaminated by fallout, growth hormones, and antibiotics; fear of poisoning by glandular secretions generated in animals who die in terror; the desire to preserve animal life, to become nonviolent, to practice religious convictions; the desire to improve their nutrition, to cook more creatively, to promote the ecology movement by reducing the waste products of animal slaughter; the desire to purify the body, to live a more organic natural life, and/or to save money by growing their own vegetables. All of these reasons are reported in some combination in a study of 60 teenage clients of the Los Angeles Free Clinics.[26]

Organic food proponents

Not all youthful food revisionists are vegetarians, by any means. Some can be described as proponents of organically grown, natural, or health foods. In December, 1971, at a two-day public hearing on health and organic foods in the New York City Office of Consumer Affairs chaired in the New York City Office of Consumer Affairs chaired by Commissioner Bess Myerson, panelists James Turner, Fred Stare, Jean Mayer, and Glen King agreed that the term "organic" food is erroneous in that all foods are carbon compounds and therefore organic in nature. They suggested that the preferred terminology is "organically grown food." Robert Rodale, who also testified at the hearing, defined organically grown food as food fertilized with manure rather than chemical fertilizers, grown without application of pesticides, and processed without the use of food additives.

The public outcry of the natural food movement has been amplified by the aggressiveness of some of the new youth who find in their study of food-growing and processing practices further evidence of disenchantment with the Establishment. These militants reject the findings of both the United States Department of Agriculture and the Food and Drug Administration and turn instead for positive sanctions to exposé types of books and articles like *Ramparts'* "Food Pollution"[27] and Turner's *The Chemical Feast,*[28] for which Ralph Nader wrote an introduction. They consult with health food

~~~~~~

TYPES OF "FOOD FADDISTS" AND THE PATTERNING OF SELF-NEEDS THEIR FEEDING PRACTICES SERVE, AS DESCRIBED BY BEAL*

Type of food faddist	*Need served by the fad*
1. Miracle seeker	Patterning need to establish stability regarding health, energy, and so on. Accomplished by diets intended to forestall aging or restore organism to health. Ego defense need to re-establish positive self-concept and feeling of self-worth.
2. Antiestablishmentarian	Self-realization need to express self in a manner consistent with self-concept and value system.
3. Super health-seeker	Ego defense need to forestall aging process. Accomplished by diet intended to give super health. Self-realization need to present front of strength and health.
4. Distruster of medical profession	Ego defense need to establish control over own destiny and not be dependent on unknown others.
5. Fashion-follower	Ego defense and patterning need to establish an identity to gain approval and acceptance from others.
6. Authority-seeker	Self-realization need for recognition of self-competency, provided by apparent knowledge in area of food information.
7. Truth-seeker	Patterning need to process existing claims concerning nutrition.
8. One concerned about uncertainties of living	Patterning need for anchors and stability concerning the world.

*Based on V. A. Beal, "Food Faddism and Organic and Natural Foods," paper presented at National Dairy Council Food Writers' Conference, Newport, R.I., May, 1972.

Reprinted from Robert Schafer and Elizabeth A. Yetley, "Social Psychology of Food Faddism," *Journal of The American Dietetic Association* 66 (February 1975), p. 131, by permission of The American Dietetic Association. Copyright © 1975 by The American Dietetic Association.

~~~~~~

store proprietors for medical and dietary advice which is often exotic when compared with the traditional advice of nutritionists and physicians.

Health food stores

Curious about health food store operations, one of the authors found during her two weeks of employment in a health food store, located in a suburban high socioeconomic status community, that the retailer and his employees acted as "medicine men," prescribing various foods, herbs, and teas plus vitamin and mineral supplements to meet the health needs of the customer. One 40-year-old male customer said:

> "I have been diagnosed as having cancer of the lymph glands. I take a lot of medication as prescribed by my physician at a New York City hospital. It isn't helping me. I would like to change my eating habits. I tried the macrobiotic diet but I like orange juice too much. Being restricted to 8 ounces of fluid is murder! I have tried the barley water you suggested last time. What do I do?"
>
> "Chico-san Rice, organically grown . . . no chemicals or poisons," was recommended by the store employer.

"Do you have anything for constipation?" The observer could not hear the answer, as it was an intimate conversation. The employee's comment afterward was, "She is so overweight and consumes so much of a high carbohydrate diet that I just gave her a colloidal suspension. It will do the trick." On other occasion, beet juice was recommended for a colostomy patient. Ten other stores in New York City and two in Westchester County were visited, with growing conviction that when the retailer assumes the role of physician, professional medical care is often delayed.* Peter New and Rhea Priest also studied patrons of health food stores. They identify one group as "general users" (those who purchase a variety of products, such as wheat germ and molasses, marketed in health food stores) and a second group as "unitary users" (those who subscribe to a philosophy linked to particular health food diets, e.g., vegetarianism). Twenty-four members of each group were interviewed. The interviewers conclude that:

> The use of health foods is but one manifestation of a feeling of unrest and dissatisfaction among the users. The nutritional value of health food, as such, is not really the key issue. Health food is symbolic of a continuing search by the users for peace of mind.[29]

---

*R. T. Frankle, personal observation, 1970.

Further, they suggest:

> The challenge in studying health food users rests in recognizing that, although use or misuse of health foods, with all of their attendant claims and counter-claims, is an important issue with regulatory agencies and nutritional groups, that is not the single issue. A more crucial problem is understanding the social psychology involved in the use of these products especially in the meaning of health foods for the users.[29]

Ecological issues

Natural food adherents have some powerful allies within the field of ecology, e.g., biochemist Barry Commoner, Director of the Center for the Biology of Natural Systems at Washington University in St. Louis. He feels that soil husbandry in the United States is suffering under the emphasis on chemical fertilizing, the use of synthetic pesticides, fungicides, and other powerful long-lived compounds which are a threat to intricate natural balances.[30]

Personal relations within this movement are stressful. Organic, natural, or ecological types of youngsters are running head-on into the health food traditionalists who have been

> highly integrated into [their] own circle of membership but largely isolated from the rest of society. . . . The natural healthers were ofter rejected by outsiders as "nuts" and the ordinary adherent of the movement often concealed his health beliefs from others, even close acquaintances and relatives, to avoid their rejection. In the last few years, events in our society have severely disrupted the isolation of natural organizations. The hippie phenomenon, the consumers' rights drive, and the ecology movement have transformed the natural healther's relationship with the rest of his society.[31]

Assaults on polluting practices of the larger society for financial gain by the Ehrlichs,[32] Commoner,[30] and other ecologists have partially legitimized the philosophical foci of older members of the health food movement and have given them greater visibility, and a plethora of new health food stores and restaurants have sprung into existence throughout the country. Many have been started by youngsters, e.g., the short-lived "Love and Serve," a railroad diner at the Greenwich, Connecticut, station.

Communes intent on growing their own "untainted" food, and in which "the communion of food" is central to their new life style, are appearing in both remote rural and suburban areas. According to a December, 1971, *New York Times* article, group cooking has assumed a pivotal position in almost all of the 40 communes visited by Lucy Horton, who reported that "many people moved into the country because they wanted to eat organically and found that impossible to do in the city."[33] The writers note with interest the other influences of these younger converts to natural foods, e.g., supermarkets in the metropolitan areas of the country are beginning to move whole wheat flour and wheat germ into new sections marked "Health Foods." They are also raising the prices, which makes these highly nutritious items less available to the low-income shopper, an irony to say the least.

Campus cafeterias respond

Universities as widely separated as Yale, University of California at Los Angeles, Friends World College, Stonybrook, Goddard, and Marlboro have been forced to go into the health food business, making available cafeteria lines where health foods and packaged dried fruits and nuts, for example, are also available. Yale's health food restaurant opened in October, 1970, and by November, 1971, it was serving dinner to roughly 10 percent of Yale's 4,800 undergraduates. "Brown rice," says Mr. Dobie, Director of Food Services, is favored as "the perfect food. It is four parts Yin and one part Yang."[34]

Ingesting a balance of Yin and Yang foods is one of the basic tenets of the Zen macrobiotic diet, the most rigorous of the three styles being adopted by some teenagers and youth. For a detailed description of the Yin-Yang theory and dietary rules, refer to writings by Ohsawa, Chen, and Nyoiti.[35-40*]

THE MACROBIOTIC DIET

The term "macrobiotic" means "the way of long life" and is believed to be a technique of rejuvenation. The macrobiotic diet, outlined by George Ohsawa (1893–1966), was originally a series of 10 stages, each progressively more constricted than the preceding one.

Table 1 prescribes a percentage of combinations of the amounts of cereals, vegetables, soup, animal foods, salads and fruits, desserts, and drinking liquid which must circulate in a balance of spiritual energies represented by the Yin and Yang symbols.[40] Contemporary followers have compressed the diet into seven stages. Ohsawa insisted that following his principles would enable an individual to overcome all forms of illness, which he attributed to excesses in the diet.

---

*EDITOR'S NOTE: Ohsawa and Nyoiti are one and the same. George Ohsawa, a Parisian, was born in Japan as Sakurazawa Nyoiti.

There are 11 preparatory dietetic instructions:

1 Do not eat chemical white sugar and avoid everything that is sugared.
2 Look for the minimum quantity of water that is necessary to your existence and that will require you to urinate no more than three times per day.
3 Use the least possible amount of animal products, especially if you reside in a warm climate or if you are going to visit one.
4 Avoid industrial foods, particularly those with colored dye stuff, imported from afar. A free trade economy violates the laws of the universe in our diet and consequently undermines our health.
5 Avoid fruit.
6 Your diet must include 60 to 70 per cent of cereals and 20 to 25 per cent of well cooked or baked vegetables.
7 Avoid potatoes, tomatoes, and eggplants.
8 You must season dishes with salt and use vegetable oil in a tropical climate.
9 The culinary preparation may be by French, Chinese, or Indian methods.
10 No vinegar.
11 Masticate food as thoroughly as possible, on average of about 30 times each mouthful.[40]

Ohsawa explained that his philosophy was based on the "Unique Principle of the Far East," according to which everything in life is faith.

Internally this faith is a clairvoyance . . . which clearly sees and comprehends everything through infinite time and space. Externally, it is a manifestation of universal love or supreme judgment, enhancing all antagonisms and transferring them into oneness, distributing the eternal joy of life to all, forever.[37]

Ohsawa proclaims that this universal logic, the "very key to the Kingdom of Heaven," can be further realized if the macrobiotic diet is followed because "adherence to a macrobiotic regimen would not only ward off all human ailments, but could arrest, and even cure, these ailments, no matter how seriously advanced the condition."[40]

The diet is, then, a part of an entire life style which seeks total awareness and harmony with the world and embodies a religious philosophy. The disciplined convert is expected to move from the minus diets to diet number 7

TABLE 1   MACROBIOTIC DIET*

No.	Cereals	Vegetables	Soup	Animal	Fruits, Salads	Dessert	Drinking Liquid
				Per Cent			
7	100	—	—	—	—	—	Sparingly
6	90	10†	—	—	—	—	Sparingly
5	80	20	—	—	—	—	Sparingly
4	70	20	10	—	—	—	Sparingly
3	60	30	10	—	—	—	Sparingly
2	50	30	10	10	—	—	Sparingly
1	40	30	10	20	—	—	Sparingly
−1	30	30	10	20	10	—	Sparingly
−2	20	30	10	25	10	5	Sparingly
−3	10	30	10	30	15	5	Sparingly

*From Reference 40.

†Refined vegetables. In other regimens vegetables are not refined.

with the promise of reaching enlightenment or Nirvana. Fred Stare, Chairman of the Department of Nutrition, Harvard University, recalls that

> Dr. Timothy Leary, a guru of a different type, once said that macrobiotic food is the only kind that enables one to hallucinate. It could be that increasing numbers of young people, from Cambridge to Berkeley, are "turning on" by turning to brown rice instead of pot and other drugs. Better than drugs, for sure—but still dangerous to health.[11]

Nutrition assessment problems

It is well known to nutrition and medical professionals that some forms of euphoria experienced and interpreted as religious experience may be, in reality, one of the clinical signs of malnutrition.

Evaluation of the adequate nature of this diet in terms of essential nutrients is difficult as intake depends upon the level of the diet (the stage), the length of adherence, and the individual interpretation of the dictates of the master by a disciple. The ultimate goal is to reach regimen number 7, which is 100 per cent cereals—"the easiest, simplest, wisest and swiftest way back to health . . . if you are suffering from some chronic ailment."[40] This stage is low in protein, lacks some of the essential amino acids, vitamin A, ascorbic acid, vitamin D, and many minerals. One confounding variable is that the percentage composition of the nutrients of the various rices sold in the health food stores is not known. As seen in Table 1, the diet starts where the individual is most apt to comply because he ingests a more varied intake of food groups; however, even in this stage there are omissions of basic required nutrients.

In an effort to become more knowledgeable in macrobiotic methods of cookery, the senior writer enrolled in a 10-week class taught by an approved graduate of the Michio Mushi Center, formerly located in Brookline, Massachusetts, which teaches "Zen" cookery. She found that: (1) there is reverence in the handling of the food, which is considered a gift from God; (2) vegetables are chopped into extremely small particles, so that an increased surface exposure tends to increase nutrient losses, as a long cooking time is suggested; (3) fluids are restricted to eight ounces per day; (4) due to the restricted fluid intake any fluid remaining after vegetable cookery may not be utilized; (5) the recommended intake of salt is very high and, in addition, high sodium extracts such as tamari and soy sauces are used excessively; (6) deficiency in ascorbic acid occurs as a result of the avoidance of high vitamin C fruits; (7) use of milk is discouraged; thus, an excellent source of protein, calcium, phosphorus, vitamin D, and riboflavin is denied the follower. Conversations with reported followers of the Zen macrobiotic diet and Taoist macrobiotic proponents, who differ in marked respects, indicate individual variation and many do eat citrus fruits even though the diet prohibits it.

Extravagant claims

Although there is cause for concern about inadequacy in terms of the total nutritive quality of the diet, a more serious problem stems from extravagant claims made on behalf of the diet as a cure-all for a variety of diseases. In one instance, it was claimed as a cure for arthritis. The patient, on brown rice and various low-calorie levels of the macrobiotic diet, lost 74 pounds. She was able to walk again, but she was a poor nutritional risk. "I couldn't believe it. It did work. There has been a change in my entire physical, mental, and spiritual health which made the cure possible. I do smoke still but if you don't eat red meat, the badness in the cigarette isn't absorbed. My gray hairs are gone. The Bancha tea [roasted green tea] is a real cure."*

The dangers of the diet are dramatically highlighted in a review of six cases of death or near death in testimony presented to the Passaic County Grand Jury.

> The concepts of the Zen Macrobiotic diet present a public health nutrition problem and they are dangerous. Individuals consuming this diet for a considerable period of time could develop anemia and eventually would develop vitamin deficiencies and, if continued, irreversible tissue damage. This diet can result in death. . . . An individual consuming this diet would in a few weeks develop scurvy because of the lack of vitamin C. It takes only from three to five weeks to develop scurvy. He would develop osteoporosis and this would come about because of the lack of calcium in the bone structure and such an individual would be in definite negative nitrogen balance. All individuals need a good amount of nitrogen. . . . This results in tissue damage and death.[41]

Further condemnation of this diet comes from Sherlock and Rothschild:

> A woman who embraced the Zen Macrobiotic philosophy with its rigid nutritional system was completely bedridden and near death with the classical manifestations of scurvy and severe folic acid and protein deficiency. This rigid diet is a threat to life and should be condemned.[42]

---

*R. T. Frankle, personal observation, 1970.

Some former adherents have already abandoned the diet; according to Horton, "Zen Macrobiotic food was dead and had disappeared from virtually all commune tables."[33]

SUMMARY

In summary, three major kinds of nonstandard eating patterns are being adopted by many adolescents and youth: some degree of vegetarianism; emphasis on health, natural, or organically grown foods; and the Zen macrobiotic diet. We do not have an accurate count of the numbers. One of the cardinal rules in diet counseling is to ascertain where your patient is at the moment. How and what is he eating? On what basis are food choices made? For this reason, it is essential that professionals who work with adolescents become knowledgeable about the atypical diets that have been described. An awareness of the basic tenets of the counterculture will make it possible to provide nutritional education that is both meaningful and relevant. Based on the literature cited, a dietary intake consisting of a variety of fruits and vegetables, whole grain cereals, nuts, legumes, and seeds appears to be nutritionally adequate, although it is preferred that at least eggs and milk products be included. Sensitivity to and recognition of the emotional significance of food on the part of professionals will help to establish rapport because to some of these youngsters the spiritual value of food is important and meaningful. It is crucial to understand the social psychology involved in the uses of these foods. A better understanding of the motivations promoting youth to adopt new or different diet patterns is critically central to today's nutrition education.

> Nutrition is one of those rare comprehensive arts and sciences whose many disciplines, ranging from food technology and cultural anthropology to biochemistry and medical epidemiology, fit together into a beautiful mosaic. Food, because it is one of the major determinants of human ecology, can act as a potent and effective vehicle for health . . . the reason is simple; everyone eats.[43]

It is possible that conciliatory discussion of diets and nutrition can help bridge the generation gap, but we have found "they listen least to those who preach the most," especially when the lessons are void of emotional content.

> Good health is linked in the unconscious with basic needs for survival, security and master. Ill health is connected with fears of bodily disintegration, dissolution and death. In the course of growing up in almost all cultures, what children put

into their mouths or any part of their bodies is strongly connected with good and evil. "Eat this, it's good for you." "Don't put that in your mouth, it will make you sick" . . . are among the early aspects of child-rearing. " 'Good' food is 'pure,' 'clean,' 'wholesome'; 'bad' food is 'impure,' 'dirty,' 'poisonous.' " To eat well is to be secure, healthy and happy; the converse means insecurity, starvation and death. Little wonder that when psychotics experience a weakening of their ego boundaries, one of their commonest delusions is of being poisoned.[44]

New directions

Some adolescents are eager to talk about food. They appear anxious to learn the meaning of good nutrition. Erhard reports an innovative approach used while working with the hippie culture in the San Francisco Bay Area, where traditional approaches of presenting nutrition education proved inadequate. "The technique of appealing to their faddish orientation worked better than the lecture approach using the 'basic four' or talking about nutrients in the usual way. . . . 'Rap' sessions provided the best medium for educating these groups."[45,45a]

Perhaps even the new nutrition labeling program proposed by the Food and Drug Administration will help the youthful consumer select a more nutritious diet. Instead of "turning the kids off" out of sheer boredom and repetitiveness, a more comprehensive and acceptable approach may add interest and vitality to our efforts. The concern of professionals to reach adolescents was emphasized in the November, 1971, National Nutrition Education Conference in Washington, D.C., which had as its theme: "Youth-Nutrition-Community." The objectives of the Conference were to:

- Look at youth today—his values, life styles, eating habits, health;
- Look at youth in his environment—physical, biological, social;
- Identify effective ways of working with youth in providing support in the development of his food habits.

Youth involvement

We feel that teenagers may be even more effective teachers of their peers than adults. Programs in San Diego and San Francisco begun by youth themselves have proved highly effective in drug education and have reduced drug abuse among youthful clients beyond all expectations. Models developed for youth-tutoring-youth programs are highly effective.[46]

It is strongly recommended by the writers that all agencies which serve this age group empanel a board of teenage advisors with whom adults can pilot-test new program plans, instructional materials, and promotional ideas and from whom they can elicit more information about youthful eating patterns. Panels should cut across racial and ethnic lines as well as socioeconomic levels. Before beginning any new programs and to revitalize the existing ones, we are obligated to ask the potential consumer for his opinions. We must end unilateral (meaning adult-determined) decision making about nutrition education and "teach them what they want to know."[47]

References

1   Schaefer, A. E., and Johnson, O. C. Are We Well Fed? . . . The Search for the Answer. Nutr. Today 4:2–11, 1969.

2   Frost, J. L., and Payne, B. L. Hunger in America: Scope and Consequence. In Nutrition and Intellectual Growth in Children. Bulletin 25A, Association for Childhood Education International, pp. 5–18, 1968.

3   Citizens Board of Inquiry into Hunger and Malnutrition. Hunger USA. In Nutrition and Intellectual Growth in Children, Bulletin 25A, Association for Childhood Education International, pp. 19–24, 1968.

4   Briggs, G. M. Hunger and Malnutrition. J. Nutr. Ed. 1:4, 1970.

5   Ten State Nutrition Survey in the United States, 1968–1970. Preliminary Report to the Congress. U.S. Department of Health, Education and Welfare, April, 1971.

6   Loyd, F. G. Finally, Facts on Malnutrition in the United States. Today's Health 47:32–33, 80, 1969.

7   Ullrich, H. D. Hunger in America and Nutrition Education. J. Nutr. Ed. 1:5, 1969.

8   Everson, R. Bases for Concern about Teenagers' Diets. J. Am. Diet. Assoc. 36:17–21, 1960.

9   Heald, F. (ed.). Adolescent Nutrition and Growth. Appleton-Century-Crofts, New York, 1969.

10 Hodges, R. E. and Krehl, W. A. Nutritional Status of Teenagers in Iowa. Am. J. Clin. Nutr. 17:200–210, 1965.

11 Stare, F. J. The Diet That's Killing Our Kids, Ladies Home J. 87:70, 1971.

12 Huenemann, R. L., et al. Food and Eating Practices of Teen-Agers. J. Am. Diet. Assoc. 53:17–24, 1968.

13 Leverton, M. The Paradox of Teen-Age Nutrition. J. Am. Diet. Assoc. 53:13–16, 1968.

14 Wharton, M. A. Nutritive Intake of Adolescents. J. Am. Diet. Assoc. 42:306–310, 1963.

15 Keniston, K. Youth and Dissent: The Rise of a New Opposition. Harcourt Brace Jovanovich, New York, 1971.

16 Sokolov, R. A. Meat-Eating, 230-Pound Doctor Is Now 175-Pound Vegetarian. New York Times, Aug. 12, 1971.

17 Hardinge, M. G., and Crooks, H. Non-Flesh Dietaries. I. Historical Background. J. Am. Diet. Assoc. 43:545–558, 1963.

18 Deutsch, R. M. The Nuts among the Berries. Ballantine, New York, 1961.

19 Hardinge, M. G., and Stare, F. J. Nutritional Studies of Vegetarians. I. Nutritional, Physical and Laboratory Studies. Am. J. Clin. Nutr. 2:73–82, 1954.

20 Hardinge, M. G., and Stare, F. J. Nutritional Studies of Vegetarians. II. Dietary and Serum Levels of Cholesterol. Am. J. Clin. Nutr. 2:83–88, 1954.

21 Hardinge, M. G., Chamber, A. C., Crooks, H., and Stare, F. Nutritional Studies of Vegetarians. III. Dietary Levels of Fiber. Am. J. Clin. Nutr. 6:523–525, 1958.

22 Hardinge, M. G., Crooks, H., and Stare, F. J. Nutritional Studies of Vegetarians. IV. Dietary Fatty Acids and Serum Cholesterol Levels. Am. J. Clin. Nutr. 10:516–524, 1962.

23 Hardinge, M. G., Crooks, H., and Stare, F. J. Nutritional Studies of Vegetarians. V. Proteins and Essential Amino Acids. J. Am. Diet. Assoc. 48:26–28, 1966.

23a Dwyer, J. T., Mayer, L. V. D. H., Kandel, R. F., and Mayer, J. The New Vegetarians. J. Am. Diet. Assoc. 62:506, 1973.

23b Register, V. D., and Sonnenberg, L. M. The Vegetarian Diet. J. Am. Diet. Assoc. 62:257, 1973.

24 Hardinge, M. G., and Crooks, H. Non-Flesh Dietaries. III. Adequate or Inadequate. J. Am. Diet. Assoc. 45:537–542, 1954.

24a Raper, N. R., and Hill, M. M. Vegetarian Diets. Nutr. Prog. News, U.S.D.A., July/August, 1973.

25 Ellis, F. R., Path, M. R. C., and Montegriffo, V. M. E. Veganism, Clinical Findings, and Investigations. Am. J. Clin. Nutr. 23:249–255, 1970.

26 Heussenstamm. F. K., and Forman, M. Teenage Vegetarians: A Study of Motivation and Practice. Paper, 1971.

27 Zwerdling, D. Food Pollution. Ramparts 9:31–37, 1971.

28 Turner, J. The Chemical Feast. Grossman, New York, 1970.

29 New, P. K-M., and Priest, R. P. Food and Thought: A Sociologic Study of Food Cultists. J. Am. Diet. Assoc. 51:13–18, 1967.

30 Commoner, B. The Closing Circle. Knopf, New York, 1971.

31 Hanson, R. R., and Roth, J. A. Health Nuts and Hippies: Old and New Movements Meet. Paper read at annual meeting of the American Sociological Association, 1971.

32 Ehrlich, P. R., and Ehrlich, A. H. Population, Resources and Environment. Freeman, San Francisco, 1970.

33 Sokolov, R. A. The Food Is at the Heart of Commune Life. New York Times, Dec. 2, 1971.

34 Treaster, J. B. Yale versus Those Mushy Vegetables. New York Times, Nov. 15, 1971.

35 Ohsawa, G. Macrobiotics: The Art of Longevity and Rejuvenation. Ohsawa Foundation (n.d.).

36 Ohsawa. G. Zen Macrobiotics: The Philosophy of Oriental Medicine. Ignoramus Press, Los Angeles, 1965.

37 Ohsawa, G. The Book of Judgment: The Philosophy of Oriental Medicine, Vol. 2. Ignoramus Press, Los Angeles, 1966.

38 Ohsawa, G. Zen Cookery: The Philosophy of Oriental Culture, Vol. 1. Ignoramus Press, Los Angeles, 1966.

39 Chan, W. T. (ed.). Source Book in Chinese Philosophy. Princeton University Press, Princeton, N.J., 1963.

40 Nyoiti, S. You Are All Sanpaku (trans. W. Dufty). University Books, New York, 1965.

41 Zen Macrobiotic Diet Hazardous: Presentment of the Passaic Grand Jury. Public Health News, 46:132–136, 1966.

42 Sherlock, P., and Rothschild, E. O. Scurvy Produced by a Zen Macrobiotic Diet. J.A.M.A. 199:130–134, 1967.

43 Christakis, G. The Tailored Product—Need for Changing Foods—Food as a Vehicle for Health. Paper presented at 15th Annual Joint Education Conference, Food and Drug Law Institute, Food and Drug Administration, 1971.

44 Marmor, J., Bernard, V., and Ottenberg, P. Psychodynamics of Group Opposition to Health Programs. Am. J. Orthopsychiatr. 30, 1960, as quoted by V. W. Bernard in Am. J. Public Health 55:1145, 1965.

45 Erhard, D. Nutrition Education for the "Now" Generation. J. Nutr. Ed. 2:135–139, 1971.

45a Frankle, R. T., McGregor, B., Wylie, J., and McCann, M. B. The Door, a Center of Alternatives: The Nutritionist in a Free Clinic for Adolescents. J. Am. Diet. Assoc. 63:269, 1973.

46 Gartner, A., Kohler, M., and Riessman, F. Children Teach Children: Learning by Teaching. Harper and Row, New York, 1971.

47 Byler, R., Lewis, G., and Totman, R. Teach Us What We Want to Know. Connecticut State Department of Education, 1969.

THE VEGETARIANS

| 10 | ## Is a Nonflesh Diet Adequate?

MERVYN G. HARDINGE and HULDA CROOKS

Mervyn G. Hardinge is dean of the School of Health, Loma Linda University. A lecturer and writer, he is also editor of *Life and Health*. Hulda Crooks is a dietitian affiliated with Loma Linda University.

Reprinted from *Vegetarianism*, Supplement to *Life and Health*, 1973, pp. 20–23, by permission of *Life and Health*. Copyright © Review & Herald Publishing Association 1973.

CURRENT TRENDS

Today's awakening in vegetarianism is unique. In the past, advocates of a meatless diet have tended to be mature men with a background of experience in philosophy, religion, or science. But our current phenomenal upsurge of interest in vegetarianism and healthful living is not spearheaded by gray-bearded philosophers or diploma-heavy men of science. Rather, young Americans of high school and college age are in the vanguard. All over the country students are joining the search for a simpler, more natural way of life.

ZEN MACROBIOTIC DIET

But unfortunately, some of these young people lack sufficient knowledge of nutrition to select a well-balanced meatless diet. A few are even experimenting with extremes, such as the rigid Zen macrobiotic diet, which is a threat not only to health but to life itself.[1] The highest level of perfection of this bizarre diet consists in restricting one's food to cereals only, and this mainly rice, and the water intake to as little as possible. This unphysiological and dangerous program must not be confused with any reasonable vegetarian diet compounded of a variety of wholesome foods.

YOUNG PEOPLE ARE LEADING OUT

The diet revolution is making an impact in many areas. Food service directors and dietitians are besieging vegetarian food factories for help in the know-how to provide the students with tasty, adequate, meatless meals.[2]

Even ivory-towered Yale University is reported as responding to the quest of youth for a more wholesome diet than that which conventional society offers.[3] Both Yale and the University of California at Santa Barbara are providing vegetarian cooking for those students who desire it. Longtime favorites like roast beef and mashed potatoes must now make room for lentil and soybean patties, pinto bean goulash, and whole-grain products. Fresh, quick-cooked vegetables have taken the place of overcooked, mushy ones poured out of a can. Fried foods are losing favor, and whole-grain bread is made of unbleached whole-grain flours without chemical additives.

But what about this diet revolution? Is a nonflesh diet adequate?

EVIDENCE FROM SCIENCE

Many studies of vegetarians, their food intakes and health, have been reported in recent years. Wherever an adequate food supply is available, the average vegetarian dietary presents no problem. In areas where the diet depends almost entirely on one kind of food, however, a better balance is needed. Thus, young children suffer from marasmus and kwashiorkor when taken off the breast and fed on thin cornmeal gruel or on mashed roots such as cassava, taro, or similar bulky, refined foods. These are low in protein and, though relatively high in calories, they lack some essential nutrients. In parts of Asia where white rice is the mainstay of the diet, beriberi is a problem among adults as well as among children. The cause is a lack of thiamin (vitamin B_1) lost in the milling of the grain. But these grossly deficient diets are not to be compared with any reasonable practice of vegetarianism.

Evidence as to the adequacy of well-selected vegetarian diets is beyond dispute. Scientists found that foods eaten by lacto-ovo-vegetarians were very similar to those used by nonvegetarians, except that they did not use meat.[4] The nonvegetarians had a much higher protein intake. No benefit could be shown from the larger intake of the nonvegetarians, even in the growth rate of adolescent boys and girls. The amount of protein in the blood was the same in all groups whether they used meat or not, but the vegetarians had the advantage of a lower blood cholesterol. Their diet also provided more unrefined foods such as whole-grain bread and cereals and more fresh fruits and vegetables, which added a desirable amount of bulk to their diet. This was especially true of the pure vegetarians.

HUNZAS

The longevity and remarkable health of the Hunzas is common knowledge. In 1964 Dr. Paul Dudley White, famous heart specialist, visited this small "roof of the world" principality and studied its people.[5] The diet, he noted, is spartan; the mainstays are fruits, nuts, vegetables, and grains (barley, wheat, millet), with a little milk from goats. Meat, primarily mutton, is eaten only once or twice a year.

Dr. White and an associate, Dr. Edward G. Toomey, studied twenty-five Hunza men believed to be 90 to 110 years old. Even at this advanced age they found "normal blood pressure, normal blood cholesterol levels, and normal electrocardiographic patterns."

OKINAWANS

During World War II an autopsy study of Okinawans showed similar results.[6] The native diet consisted mainly of plant foods. The low incidence of deficiency diseases and the natural longevity and fertility of these people led the investigators to conclude that the native diet, mainly nonflesh, was excellent.

OTOMI INDIANS

The food pattern of the Otomi Indians of the high plateaus of Central Mexico has also been proven to be sound.[7] It consists mainly of tortillas (a thin, flat, unleavened cornbread), beans, peppers, and various local foods in each locality. Clinical study showed these people to be uncommonly healthy; none were overweight, and high blood pressure was a rarity.

NORWEGIANS

In 1966 a comparative study of 116 healthy vegetarians and a comparable number of healthy nonvegetarians was reported from Oslo, Norway. Yale University participated in this study.[8]

The protein intake of the lacto-ovo-vegetarians was only a little less than that of the ordinary Norwegian diet, but a much larger proportion of it came from plant foods. The blood protein values of the two groups showed no significant differences.

The bread of the vegetarians contained more whole grain than did ordinary bread, and the diet was rich in complex carbohydrates (starch, pectin, fiber, and cellulose) and low in refined sugar. Thus it was higher in substances that tend to lower blood cholesterol (the complex carbohydrates and unsaturated fats) and lower in factors that have been found to raise the cholesterol level (saturated fats, dietary cholesterol, sucrose, and total calories). The intake of minerals and vitamins was high among the vegetarians due to the generous use of unrefined foods and of fresh fruits and vegetables. Fewer vegetarians than nonvegetarians were overweight.

BRITISH

Studies of British lactovegetarians (those who use milk, but not flesh foods) showed that their calcium intake is greater than that of the average nonvegetarian, perhaps due to the fact that muscle meat contains very little calcium.[9] Also, the bones of the vegetarians contained significantly more calcium than those of nonvegetarians of the same age.[10] At the approach of seventy, no further loss of bone minerals occurred in the vegetarians, while bones continued to weaken in the nonvegetarians.

UNDERDEVELOPED AREAS

A very convincing evidence that a flesh-free diet can supply basic needs is the tremendous population increase in countries where meat is scarce. It is in the underdeveloped regions, where the diet consists almost wholly of plant foods, that the human crop is so heavy. The high fertility rates of the world are not in countries richly supplied with animal foods, but in Latin America, Africa, India, and the Middle East where the diet depends mainly on cereal grains and vegetables.[11]

SHERPAS

Then there are the Sherpas, dwellers of the harsh, stony uplands of the eastern Himalayas, whose fabulous strength and endurance as carriers for Everest expeditions have been so highly extolled. In his autobiography, *Tigers of the Snows*,[12] Tenzing Norgay, the famous Sherpa who accompanied Sir Edmund Hillary, first to set foot on top of the world's highest peak, says of his native diet: "Potatoes are our biggest crop and form the basis of much of our food, just as rice does for the Indians and Chinese."

Potatoes and barley, Tenzing Norgay says, grow up to 14,000 feet elevation and wheat to 10,000. From their flocks of sheep and goats and their herds of yak these people obtain milk and cheese with which to supplement their potato and cereal diet. Meat is seldom eaten, and the stricter Buddhists among them eat none.

APPALACHIA

An experiment just reported from the Department of Human Nutrition at the Virginia Polytechnic Institute, Blackburn, Virginia, found no protein lack in 7- to 9-year-old girls fed diets in which cereal grains and legumes provided nearly all the protein. The diets simulated those of low-income Southern families. Supplementation with several essential amino acids failed to improve the protein adequacy of the diet. The authors conclude that widespread fortification with amino acids is not justified.[13]

NUTRITIONISTS SAY

Many years ago Dr. E. V. McCollum, research scientist at Johns Hopkins University, concluded: "The lactovegetarian diet, or combination of vegetable foods and milk, is . . . easy to plan so as to be highly nutritious and to promote optimal health."[14] Noted scientists around the world today support Dr. McCollum's conclusion.

As Dr. Robert Harris said at the time he was professor of biochemistry at the Massachusetts Institute of Technology:

> Both the vegetarian type and the carnivorous type of diet can adequately feed mankind. The realization of this fact by those who struggle with the food problem of the world is of terrible importance. There is not sufficient land in the world to feed all mankind the animal protein diet now consumed in the United States. . . . People may prefer to eat diets rich in animal protein, but those diets are not necessary, and most people cannot afford them.[15]

SO . . .

What then is today's answer to those who ask if a nonflesh diet can meet human nutritional needs? It is a clear "Yes." Such a diet is wholly suitable for human nutrition on the highest level, not only for ordinary living but also during periods of stress as in pregnancy, breast-feeding, and growth of the young. It is also adequate, as the Sherpas have demonstrated, to prepare young men to endure the most severe stress that can be laid on the human body—extreme altitude, almost unbearable cold, supreme endurance, and elephantine strength.

A well-formulated lacto-ovo-vegetarian diet is adequate for every nutritional requirement. No longer need anyone fear the day when beefsteaks and pork chops may have to give way to plant proteins.

References

1   Council on Foods and Nutrition. Zen macrobiotic diets. *J.A.M.A.* 218:397, 1971.

2   Vegetarianism is "in" on campus. *Univ. Observer,* November 18, 1971, p. 6.

3   Meatless meats invade Yale. *The Southwestern,* December, 1971 (Southwestern Union College).

4   M. G. Hardinge and F. J. Stare. Nutritional studies of vegetarians: 1. Nutritional, physical, and laboratory studies; and 2. Dietary and serum levels of cholesterol. *J. Clin. Nutr.* 2:78–82; 83–88, 1954.

5   E. G. Toomey and P. W. White. A brief survey of the health of aged Hunzas. *Amer. Heart J.* 68:842, 1964.

6   P E. Steiner. Necropsies on Okinawans: Anatomic and pathologic observations. *Arch. Path.* 42:359, 1946.

7   R. K. Anderson, J. Calvo, W. D. Robinson, G. Serrano, and G. C. Payne. Nutritional appraisal in Mexico. *Amer. J. Pub. Health* 38:1126, 1948.

8   K. Kirkeby. Blood lipids, lipoproteins, and proteins in vegetarians. *Acta. Med. Scandinav.* 179, Supp. 443: 56–60, 1966.

9   F. R. Ellis and P. Mumford. The nutritional status of vegans and vegetarians. *Proc. Nutr. Soc.* 26:205, 1967.

10 F. R. Ellis, S. Holesh, and J. W. Ellis. Incidence of osteoporosis in vegetarians and omnivores. *Amer. J. Clin. Nutr.* 25:555, 1972.

11 72.6 million more people in 1970. *War on Hunger* 4:4, 1970.

12 T. Norgay and J. R. Ullman. *Tiger of the Snows.* New York: G. P. Putnam's Sons, 1955, p. 14.

13 R. P. Abernathy, S. J. Ritchey, and J. C. Gorman. Lack of response to amino acid supplements by preadolescent girls. *Amer. J. Clin Nutr.* 25:980, 1972.

14 E. V. McCollum, Orent-Keiles, E., and H. G. Day. *The Newer Knowledge of Nutrition.* New York: Macmillan Co., 1939, p. 563.

15 R. S. Harris. Presented at the International Congress on Vitamins in Havana, Cuba, Jan. 25, 1952.

| 11 | Four Food Groups for the Vegan

BRONWEN GODFREY

Bronwen Godfrey is a registered nurse with experience in coronary care and family-practice nursing. A vegetarian since her teens, she has had a longstanding interest in nutrition; she wrote this section in consultation with experts at the University of California.

From *Laurel's Kitchen: A Handbook for Vegetarian Cookery and Nutrition,* by Laurel Robertson, Carol Flinders, and Bronwen Godfrey. Copyright © 1976 by Nilgiri Press, P.O. Box 477, Petaluma, Calif. 94952. Reprinted by permission.

The diet of the vegan (pronounced *vej-an* as in *veg-*etable) is the vegetarian diet in its purest form, made up exclusively of plant foods without any foods of animal origin at all. It represents a direction in diet which many people find more and more appealing with the passage of time, as they become less dependent on animal foods and more aware that it is possible to be completely well nourished without dairy products and eggs. It is, however, a diet with limitations which can be serious. These limitations must be completely understood and carefully compensated for.

. . . Plant foods can be balanced so that their protein pattern is more than adequate in meeting human needs. A diet which gets 60 percent of its protein from grains, 35 percent from legumes, and 5 percent from leafy green vegetables will be adequately balanced with respect to protein.* If you get the total *amount* of protein you need in these proportions, there will be essential amino acids to spare.

Because legume protein is necessary for balancing grain protein in the absence of animal foods, legumes must be a staple in the vegan's diet. The Four Food Groups for the vegan, then, are Grains, Legumes, Vegetables, and Fruit. From these groups the vegan must be careful to select foods rich in the nutrients which are usually best supplied by milk—specifically, calcium and riboflavin. The diet *must* be supplemented with vitamin B-12.

Grains should be the predominating food in the vegan's diet, as in the diet of any vegetarian. Yeast-raised or naturally leavened whole-grain bread

---

*Conversation with Doris H. Calloway, Professor of Nutrition, University of California, Berkeley, 6 November 1974.

should be eaten generously, as it is a dependable source of many scarce minerals like iron and zinc. Of course, the total amount of grain foods needed to provide the necessary 60 percent of the diet's protein will depend on the protein concentration in the foods chosen. Grains vary greatly in their protein concentration, from about 8 percent protein for uncooked rice and corn to about 14 percent for uncooked hard spring wheat. More calories must be eaten of the foods low in protein to get the same 60 percent of your protein requirement. This presents no problem as long as the whole diet has enough calories to meet your energy needs. In the example on the following page, about two and a half cups of various grains and four slices of bread supply the average male vegan's grain protein needs. When calories are restricted, however, as they are in a low-calorie weight-reducing diet, getting enough grain protein is more of a problem, and the person should concentrate on the higher-protein grains. Nut and seed protein may be counted as grain protein because it has similar strengths and weaknesses.

One cup of cooked beans has enough protein to supply the legume protein requirement (35 percent of the total requirement) for most people. Beans have a higher concentration of protein than grains (uncooked, about 20 percent) and they only double their size when cooked, whereas grains triple. So the one-to-three ratio of bean to grain *protein* becomes more like a one-to-six ratio of *servings* of cooked beans to grains. Soy milk, which is high in protein, is often a staple food for vegans. Two cups of it can nearly meet the need for beans. If it is fortified with vitamin B-12 and calcium, it can make a great contribution to the nutritional safety of the vegan diet as well as make it more interesting.

The vegan will want to eat plenty of fresh dark green vegetables. One serving is enough to round out the protein balance of the diet, but leafy greens are also good sources of riboflavin, a nutrient usually supplied most efficiently by milk. In addition, the dark green leafy vegetables without oxalic acid—mustard, turnip, and dandelion greens, collards and kale, and both romaine and loose-leaf lettuce—supply another milk-concentrated nutrient, calcium. They also supply iron.

Fruits, of course, are important to the vegan for vitamin C, just as to anyone else.

Vitamin B-12 is the really critical nutrient in the vegan diet, since it cannot be found in any plant food in sufficient quantities to meet human needs— and B-12 deficiency is a serious matter. A simple way to get your B-12 is in fortified soy milk. However, commercial soy milk products are often de-

FOUR FOOD GROUPS FOR THE VEGAN

BALANCING PROTEIN		Men	Women
For the vegan, the four food groups and their proportions are determined by the formula for vegan protein balance:	60% from grains	33g	28g
	35% from legumes	20	16
	5% from leafy greens	3	2
	Total protein RDA	56g	46g

GRAINS

33 grams grain protein for men; 28 grams for women. Include 4 slices of bread, 3 to 5 servings of grain, and 1 serving of nuts or seeds every day.

EXAMPLE:

	Protein(g)	Calories
1 cup oatmeal	5	132
1 cup brown rice	5	232
1/2 cup cracked wheat	3	108
1/4 cup sesame meal	4	130
2 slices commercial whole wheat bread	5	122
2 slices rye bread (made with whole-wheat, rye, and gluten flour)	11	244
	33	968

LEGUMES

20 grams legume protein for men; 16 for women. Include 1/3 cup beans and 2 cups fortified soybean milk OR 1 1/4 cups beans plus other sources of vitamin B-12 and calcium every day.

EXAMPLE:

	Protein(g)	Calories
2 cups soy milk	15	312
1/3 cup navy beans	5	75
	20	387

VEGETABLES

4 or more servings of good-quality vegetables every day (3 grams protein). Include 2 substantial servings of dark leafy greens for calcium and riboflavin.

FRUIT

1 to 4 servings a day. Include a raw source of vitamin C.

LIMITED NUTRIENTS AND GOOD SOURCES

Vitamin B-12   Two cups fortified soy milk, fortified nutritional yeast, or a vitamin pill.

Calcium   Fortified soy milk, leafy greens without oxalates, sunflower seeds, unhulled sesame seeds,* blackstrap molasses

Riboflavin   Beans, green leaves, certain nuts, nutritional yeast, wheat germ

---

*EDITOR'S NOTE: Unhulled (brown) sesame seeds contain oxalates of calcium, which may be toxic. So although hulled (white) sesame seeds offer less calcium, they are generally preferable.

signed primarily for the meat-eating child who is allergic to milk rather than for the vegan, so check the label to see what percent of the recommended dietary allowance (RDA) for B-12 is met by a glass of that particular product. If it is 10 percent, you'll need ten glasses to meet the RDA, and you can suspect that the manufacturer had the allergic child in mind. Because commerical products are expensive and heavily sugared, you may wish to make your own soy milk, which you can flavor and fortify yourself. If you prefer, alternative ways of getting vitamin B-12 are to use nutritional yeast which has been grown on B-12 enriched media or to take a vitamin pill. Pills generally come in high dosages, so you may need only one a week. The RDA level may also be supplied by daily multiple vitamin pills: again, check the label to see that it lists at least 2 micrograms of B-12.

Because the pure vegetarian diet contains a lot of vegetable fiber, many people have trouble eating enough food to meet their caloric needs. While a carefully chosen whole-food diet can be adequate for adults, children probably need supplemental sources of calories from easily digested, non-bulky foods. One of the most effective ways to supply this is to add sweetener to your soy milk. Another is to use oil in cooking, and margarine on your bread. Adequate calories keep the body from burning its protein supply for energy.

To those who are just entering the widely varied world of meatless cookery, the vegan's diet may seem a little odd. Cooking with soy milk for soup bases and making grain dishes without eggs is a real challenge to your cooking skill. But more and more of our friends have been experimenting with this challenge—and finding that with loving care, the vegan diet can be not only nourishing but delicious as well.

THE ELDERLY

| 12 | ## Nutrition and Health of the Elderly

ANTHONY A. ALBANESE

Anthony A. Albanese is director of the Nutrition and Metabolic Research Division of the Burke Rehabilitation Center (White Plains, N.Y.) and of the Geriatric Nutrition Laboratory of the Miriam Osborn Memorial Home (Rye, N.Y.). He is also associate editor of the *New York State Journal of Medicine* and editor in chief of *Nutritional Reports International,* and has published over 240 articles in the field of human nutrition.

Reprinted from *Nutrition News* 39 (April 1976), pp. 5 and 8. © 1976, National Dairy Council. Courtesy of National Dairy Council.

Today the care of the fastest growing minority, the aged, presents the greatest challenge—to create health to correspond with the duration of life. The acceptance of geriatrics as a specialized segment of medicine has focused particular attention on nutrition of the aged.

A common nutritional pitfall of the elderly is the gradual but progressive development of apathy toward other individuals, toward their environment, and particularly toward food. The aged individual living alone all too often limits nutritional selection to easily prepared foods with a high carbohydrate content such as bread, jam, jelly, and easily prepared cereal foods. Such narrow diet selection does present nutritional difficulties if it persists.

Dietary studies of the Ten-State Nutrition Survey and numerous biochemical studies have disclosed that many outwardly normal persons

past the age of 50 are definitely deficient in proteins, one or more B vitamins, vitamins A and C, iron, and calcium.[1] The adverse effects of environmental malnutrition are frequently aggravated by 1) a decrease in rate of
protein synthesis, 2) reduced carbohydrate metabolism resulting in decreased glucose tolerance, and 3) inferior utilization of lipid substances, frequently reflected in hyperlipidemia.

In this connection it may be pointed out that faulty nutrition manifests
itself in a stepwise order in the following conditions: tissue depletion,
biochemical changes, functional changes, and anatomical changes.

We can only review here selected clinical and biochemical observations
related to variation in intake of specific nutrients.

Water

Maintenance of fluid balance is essential to distribution of nutriments to the
ultimate cellular units, elimination of wastes, and innumerable physiochemi-
cal processes. Calculations of average water requirements from our data on
persons 65–90 years of age disclosed that normal fluid balance can be
maintained with a daily water intake of 1.3 quarts for the average 132-
pound individual.

Calories, carbohydrates, and fats

One of the important considerations in the nutrition of the aging and aged is
the food energy content of the diet. An excess of caloric intake over needs
induces overweight—a burden to the cardiovascular system—which accelerates development of degenerative disease and shortens the life span.

Unfortunately, the decreased energy expenditure of age is not always
followed by decreased calorie intake because food habits tend to remain
unchanged. This results in varying degrees of obesity, which is the most
prevalent form of malnutrition in this country today.

Much has been written of the causal relationship of increased intake of
sugar and fats to the incidence of cardiovascular disease; nonetheless, the
subject remains controversial for lack of *hard* experimental data. Our 10-
year study with 135 "healthy, normal" elderly women showed that when
corn or peanut oil margarines were substituted over a five-year period for
conventional animal and hydrogenated vegetable shortenings in preparation
and serving of all meals, blood cholesterol levels decreased significantly in
most women during the first 18 to 24 months but rose to the prior five-year
baseline level within 36 to 48 months.

Proteins

In the elderly, liberal amounts of good-quality proteins are especially important to counterbalance the prevailing catabolic processes of age. Dietary animal proteins provide the nitrogen and all the essential and nonessential amino acids needed for the formation of both hard and soft tissues. Vegetable proteins are frequently deficient in one or more essential amino acids. In the presence of adequate amounts of animal-derived proteins, cereal proteins can profitably and economically provide a fair percentage of the total protein of the diet. In our two-year clinical study, 87 underweight (20 percent) elderly male and female convalescent patients received a daily dietary supplement containing 560 calories and 40 grams of milk protein for periods of three weeks and showed an average increase in body weight of 4.4 pounds. The control group of 122 equally underweight elderly convalescents gained 2.1 pounds. The hospital diet offered approximately 2,000 calories, with 65 grams of protein per day.[2]

Iron

The complexities of iron absorption and its metabolic control are not yet fully understood. Because of the high incidence of anemia and difficulties of attaining adequate intakes of iron from ordinary mixed diets, recommendations have been made to fortify staple foods with iron. The elderly living on low-cost diets with little animal protein seem to be particularly vulnerable to development of nutritional anemias. A combination of nutritional anemias may coexist in elderly persons, most often iron-deficiency anemia and deficiencies of either folic acid or vitamin B_{12} or both. Folic acid deficiency may also be found in conjunction with ascorbic acid deficiency, since both of these vitamins are found in fresh fruits and vegetables. Thus, it is important to ascertain the presence of each factor in anemic patients prior to therapy.

Vitamin C

The many functions of vitamin C have not been completely elucidated. Further study is needed, especially in the elderly who bear a lifetime of nutritional shortcomings. Available evidence indicates that vitamin C may be intimately involved in the aging process. While there may be confidence in the amount of vitamin C to prevent overt deficiency symptoms, we are less sure about the nutritionally optimal amounts needed for other purposes, including slowing down the process of cell aging. Biochemical data suggest that

~~~~~~

DIET AND LONGEVITY: THE LINK CONFIRMED

There is ample evidence that overeating early in life leads to irreversible obesity. . . . There is also evidence, from M. H. Ross of the Fox Chase Cancer Center in Philadelphia and from G. Bras of the Rijks University in Utrecht, Netherlands, that overeating early in life predisposes one to cancer.

Now Ross and Bras report in *Science* [Oct. 10, 1975] that overeating also shortens life-span.

Such a finding is hardly surprising, but scientific confirmation is valuable. As Ross explains it: "Obviously there are all sorts of ways to shorten life-span. But diet is apparently the only way we know of to date that will increase the length of life of a warm-blooded animal. I think that what we have done here is confirm the fact that under natural conditions there is a relationship between dietary habits and life-span, whereas in previous work the study was always on animals under some kind of stress."

What Ross and Bras did, essentially, was allow 121 rats to select their own diets after the first 21 days of life and to follow these diets until they died. The rats, like people, selected widely varying amounts and choices of foods. There was a dramatic correlation between how much the rats ate and how long they lived. The average life of a rat is 630 days. The rats in the study lived anywhere from 317 days to 1,026 days.

Length of life was inversely related to the amount of food consumed. However, the magnitude of the food intake effect changed with age. It was maximum during age period 100 to 199 days and by midlife it was negligible. If the amount of food was not considered, a low-protein diet early in life was more likely to be associated with a short life-

~~~~~~

vitamin C may exert a protective role because of its ability to synergize the antiperoxidative activity of vitamin E.

Calcium

Because of the many metabolic and nutritional functions of calcium and their relation to the high incidence of osteoporosis in the elderly, further investigation of the needs of this nutrient is indicated. Osteoporosis constitutes a major orthopedic disorder in about 25 percent of post-menopausal women.

There is strong evidence that long-continued inadequate intake of calcium may lead to osteoporosis. Some osteoporotics show increased bone regeneration and a high retention of calcium when placed on high-calcium

~~~~~~

span than a high-protein diet was. The importance of sufficient protein early in life for longevity was underscored by the fact that many of the short-lived rats who ate little protein early in life often ended up eating more protein later in life than did the long-lived rats. What seems to be an attempt to make up for early protein deprivation is, however, apparently unsuccessful.

Ross believes the study has implications for human diet and life-span. "It's what you eat during the early phase of life that counts," he says. "An ample diet and a nonexcessive rate of increased body weight is apparently conducive to a long life." He is reluctant to extrapolate further because of the complexities of mammalian nutrition. For example, the rats in his and Bras's study were from different genetic backgrounds and obviously had different caloric needs as well as different food preferences. So saying that so much protein early in life would be good for all rats (or people) would be risky, to say the least.

Nonetheless Ross and Bras will probably continue to shed light on the influence of diet on life-span. Since they submitted the *Science* paper for publication, they have found that they can predict, on the basis of what rats eat and how fast they grow, how long they will live. "We are now trying to see whether imposing a change on such animals truly increases their life-span," Ross says.

~~~~~~

diets. Intestinal malabsorption syndromes, which frequently occur in the aged, reduce calcium bioavailability in the face of an adequate intake. This problem may be overcome in most instances by raising calcium intake, so that the amount absorbed is increased proportionately. It is the change of balance of various hormone systems associated with the onset of menopause which causes a major and progressive loss of bone in women of 45+ years. Calcium retention is adversely affected by emotions, inactivity, or immobility which increase with age.

Vitamin D increases calcium absorption, particularly under conditions of low intestinal tract concentrations. Adequate intake of vitamin C appears to be essential for biosynthesis of collagen—bone protein.

A U.S. Department of Agriculture survey of 5,500 "normal" females showed that the estimated calcium consumption averaged approximately 450 milligrams per day in the age group of 45+ years. In our studies we observed a high incidence of subnormal coefficients of bone density and spontaneous fractures for 313 females over 55 years of age.[3] In another study with "healthy normal" elderly females, average age 80.2 years, whose calcium intake from self-selected regimens was 450 ± 50 milligrams per day, we found x rays showed that bone loss reversal was evident following calcium supplementation of 700–800 milligrams per day for periods of 12–36 months. Coincidentally, a decrease in serum cholesterol levels occurred with improved bone density.

Over the 25 years of our studies in geriatric nutrition, we have found that elderly individuals frequently raise the especially pertinent question: "At my age, what benefits are yet available from adequate nutrition?" In answering, it must be frankly recognized that either the benefits or the blights of past nutrition are already recorded. Although in the advanced years many of the scars of past malnutrition cannot be eradicated, others may be improved in greater or lesser degree. Effort, therefore, should be directed toward detection of nutritional failure in the elderly patient and toward the application of proper nutritional therapy. Even in the last period of life, good nutrition offers its rewards. Further advance of the aging processes and of chronic degenerative disease may thus be retarded. Existing degrees of health and vigor thereby are sustained and, in many instances, may be improved. Also, good nutrition appears to work on the favorable side of longevity, even though but a few years remain.

References

1   *Dietary levels of households in the U.S. Spring 1965.* 1968. Agric Res Ser, USDA, Cons and Food Econ Div.

2   Higgons, R.H., and Albanese, A.A. 1957. Management of malnutrition of convalescence. *NY State J Med* 57: 2951.

3   Albanese, A.A., Edelson, A.H., Lorenze, E.J., III, Woodhull, M.L., and Wein, E.H. 1975. Problems of bone health in elderly: ten-year study. *NY State J Med* 75:326.

THE OVERWEIGHT

| 13 | Diet Books That Poison Your Mind ... and Harm Your Body

DON A. SCHANCHE

Don A. Schanche, formerly a newsman, has held editorships with *Life, The Saturday Evening Post,* and *Holiday.* As a free-lance author, he contributes articles to many national magazines.

From *Today's Health,* April 1974, pp. 56–61. Reprinted by permission.

A few months ago two fit-looking men appeared on a television panel show in Houston. The subject was dieting and nutrition.

One of the panelists was a physician who was deeply concerned about the millions of gullible, overweight Americans who swallow spurious diet books almost as readily as they gulp down food.

The other was a self-proclaimed "successful" dieter who boasted that he owed his strikingly lean shape to the best-selling book *Dr. Atkins' Diet Revolution: The High Calorie Way to Stay Thin Forever,* by Robert C. Atkins, M.D.

Visually the show was a standoff, but verbally it turned into a real contest. If one could judge from the reactions of the panel's moderator and the small studio audience, the glib dieter won, hands down. The physician's sober warnings against the potential hazards of Atkin's discredited high-protein, low-carbohydrate diet were no match for the sparkling wit and evident success of the high-calorie advocate.

But viewers missed the show's ironic sequel. The very next day the seemingly healthy dieter called his fellow panelist and urgently asked for a professional appointment. Sheepishly, he explained that while rising from his morning bath he had blacked out, struck his head on the tub, and very nearly drowned.

As it turned out, he had suffered a spell of what doctors call "postural hypotension"—a dramatic drop in blood pressure when one shifts from a supine to a standing position—when he stood up in the bathtub.

Most low-carbohydrate dieters—and there are many millions in the United States—know the feeling: a slight dizziness when rising from a chair or getting out of bed. In this man's case it was more severe. His brain momentarily lacked sufficient blood flow to sustain consciousness. He was lucky to survive with only a bad headache.

The cause, according to the physician, was *Dr. Atkins' Diet Revolution*, a book that has been condemned by the Council on Foods and Nutrition, of the American Medical Association, as being not only "without scientific merit," but fraught with hazards.

Reduced blood pressure is but one of a number of ill effects directly traced to Atkins's and other immensely popular diets which promise that you can lose weight and inches while consuming all the calories you want. All you must do, the diet books say, is stick to copious servings of protein and fats—such as eggs, meat, and cheese—and stay away from carbohydrates, such as bread, potatoes, and sweets.

One of the worst problems (and, paradoxically, the greatest lure) of such diets, according to Philip L. White, Sc.D., Secretary of the AMA Council, is that they "create a situation that is not dissimilar to the metabolic pattern of diabetes." The high-fat, low-carbohydrate diets trigger an abnormal body response called ketosis, the increased production of compounds called ketones—usually associated with conditions of impaired metabolism, such as diabetes. In normal quantities, ketones play a routine part in the body's metabolic process. But when they flood the system in excessive quantity, they suppress appetite.

Presto! Diet magic. Since the dieter no longer is stuffing down all the calories he *thought* he wanted to eat, he loses weight.

But, like the rueful TV panelist who toppled in the tub, he or she may end up paying a very high price in general health for this seemingly magical ketogenic effect. Even if he succeeds in maintaining the weight loss (less than 10 percent of dieters achieve that goal), he still may be in trouble.

Physicians have reported hundreds of cases of men and women hospitalized from the side effects of such dieting programs. One example, that of an old-fashioned case of scurvy in a young women dieter, was recently mentioned to me by Theodore B. Van Itallie, M.D., the internationally known nutrition expert and professor of medicine at New York's Columbia University.

Among other health problems directly linked to low-carbohydrate diets are fatigue, apathy, dehydration, calcium depletion, kidney trouble, and threatening elevations of blood lipids (cholesterol and triglycerides) which are associated with heart disease. Therefore, according to C.E. Butterworth, Jr., M.D., the AMA Council's chairman, "the full impact . . . may not become apparent to an individual's health until many years later."

As a druggist once said to an unsteady but pleasure-bent young sailor who anxiously ordered a bottle of Dramamine and a box of contraceptives, "If it makes you sick, why do you do it?"

Because, says Dr. Van Itallie, this is the "Age of Caloric Anxiety." The anxiety stems from the inherent conflict between our thin standards of beauty and desirability, to which Americans are conditioned from childhood, and our fat standard of living. Not just plump. Fat!

Between 25 and 45 percent of us are officially obese (that is, more than 20 percent overweight) according to Richard F. Spark, M.D., of Harvard Medical School. Our diets, even among the nonobese, are tilted out of balance—too many of the wrong kinds of calories.

Fat, for example, constitutes 43 percent of the average American's daily calories (50 percent among college students and businessmen surveyed by the U.S. Department of Agriculture). Nutrition experts say it should be 30–35 percent, at most.

One out of five of us skips breakfast; and many of us snack around the clock, mainly on foods which are high in calories and low in nutritional value. Per capita consumption of such "empty" foods as potato chips and sugared soft drinks has doubled during the last two decades.

At the same time, the energy crisis notwithstanding, we're more sedentary than ever. For every jogger, hiker, and tennis player you see working off his excess calories, there are 20 soft bodies parked behind a table or a TV set.

"We have inherited a body made to hunt—to run after deer and club them—not to sit at a desk," says [nutritionist] Jean Mayer. . . .

It is no wonder that we are anxious about our weight and that in our anxiety we have spawned a $10 billion industry that caters, often irresponsibly, to our wishful hope of getting off that fat.

The industry that has sprung up promotes everything from "hot pants" (worthless rubber sweat-suits whose overuse can drain vital body minerals such as sodium and potassium and cause congestive heart failure) to luxurious fat farms (where pampered dieters often lose more money than weight). The most conspicuous and widely used products, for which Americans apparently have an insatiable appetite, are diet books and pamphlets.

No one knows just how many diets there are, because so many circulate in mimeographed and handwritten private editions. But there are literally hundreds of diet books on the open market, and they sell by the millions, annually. Except for Bibles and dictionaries, nothing in the history of world literature has surpassed them in volume.

A few of the more recent offerings, such as *How Sex Can Keep You Slim,* by Abraham Friedman, M.D. ("reach for your mate instead of your plate"), probably won't hurt you, which is more than can be said for the vast majority of weight-loss regimens. The idea behind the book is that sex, not overeating, is the better substitute for the unsatisifed emotional needs of many overweight people. Psychiatrists say that emotional food-stuffing is a lot more complicated than that, but at least sex is less fattening than a bedtime snack.

"It sounds like a real fun way to reduce," says Dr. White, who can manage simultaneously to place his tongue in cheek and lift his eyebrows over Dr. Friedman's assertion that the average sex act consumes more than 200 calories of energy (roughly equivalent to jogging a mile). More seriously, Dr. White adds that "there's no real harm in a book like this, except the economic loss to the person who buys it and fully believes what he reads— and the unwanted pregnancies that may result."

Two others of the emotional genre, minus the joys of sex, are *Think and Grow Thin,* by Morton Walker, M.D., and Joan Walker, and *The Psychologist's Eat Anything Diet,* by Leonard Pearson, M.D., and Lillian R. Pearson. These books joined *The Thin Book by a Formerly Fat Psychiatrist,* by Theodore Isaac Rubin, M.D., on the self-help shelf. Any one, or all three of them, may actually benefit dieters who have the strength and emotional maturity to recondition themselves psychologically as well as physically. All, in different ways, try to help the reader establish his own internal signals to tell him when enough is enough. But the fact that 90 percent of American dieters fail to maintain their weight loss after *any* diet, even a medically prescribed one, indicates that few can manage such a psychological flip-flop without professional help.

But those are tough, demanding books, as is *The Truth About Weight Control: How To Lose Excess Pounds Permanently,* by Neil Solomon, M.D., with Sally Sheppard. Dr. Solomon, of Johns Hopkins University Medical School, . . . offers no magic and no gimmicks—just sound, nutritional advice for people who are willing to work at sensible, healthy weight control.

Unhappily for our national state of health, the public, by its overwhelming dollar-vote in the diet-book marketplace, still opts for fads and gimmicks that do little good and can do much harm. Last year, for example, Senator George McGovern's Select Committee on Nutrition and Human Needs turned up 51 new "egg and grapefruit" diets, all of which were at least figuratively fruitless and distressingly alike.

The diets were variations of an old perennial that usually surfaces under the name "Mayo Diet," even though no identifiable Mayo, including the prestigious medical center of that name, has ever had anything to do with it.

The bogus "magic" of the diet is the false implication that grapefruit, because of its tart, acid quality, has the extraordinary property of "dissolving" body fat. No food can do that. A grapefruit merely adds 110–120 calories, plus some healthy nutrients such as vitamin C, to the dieter's plate. Eggs, as every dieter knows, have high protein content and are one of nature's richest producers of cholesterol—one of the chief villains of cardiovascular disease.

Fortunately, most people who try such high-protein fad diets (or their opposite numbers: low-protein/high-carbohydrate) do not stick with them very long, so they probably do little immediate harm. But persistent dieters who go off-again on-again in a never-ending cycle of fat chasing can suffer from what Dr. White and Dr. Solomon call a "yo-yo" or "roller-coaster" effect. Its process was demonstrated in a recent experiment at the Harvard University School of Public Health. The results of blood tests on student volunteers revealed a surprising organic response to dieting. The cholesterol levels would rise a little higher with each dieting experience—almost as if the body were taking two steps down the weight ladder for each three steps up the blood-fat ladder. The experiment was curtailed to avoid doing permanent harm to the subjects, because such incremental increases in blood lipids can be dangerous.

That danger is one of many reasons why medical experts and nutritionists are virtually unanimous in singling out diets that are high in fat and protein and low in carbohydrates for special condemnation. These are the ketogenic diets, such as *Dr. Atkins' Diet Revolution.*

Careful scientific analyses of the diets and their hazards have received such widespread publicity that almost everyone, by now, must know of their dubious qualities. Yet ketogenic diets remain at the top of the list of best-sellers and promise to stay there until all of us drop in our bathtubs.

Actually, none of these popular diets is "revolutionary," nor do they differ much from one another. All stem, in fact, from the same source, a slender pamphlet published in 1863.

That was the year that William Banting, a portly Londoner, slimmed down on an experimental diet prescribed for him by a surgeon named William Harvey (not to be confused with the revered physician William Harvey, who first described the mechanism of blood circulation two centuries earlier). Harvey drastically restricted Banting's carbohydrates but let him eat all the meat and dairy products that he craved. In tribute to his doctor, Banting wrote "A Letter on Corpulence Addressed to the Public."

Almost a century later, Banting's diet became the foundation of an immensely profitable, quasi-literary trade in ketogenic weight-loss plans, most of them written by men who, like Banting, knew little or nothing about the hazards of their course of eating.

The best-known among the early entrées were the so-called Air Force Diet (variously and falsely attributed to both the Canadian and U.S. Air Forces); *Calories Don't Count* (which earned its author, Herman Taller, M.D., a mail-fraud conviction); and *The Drinking Man's Diet* (which merely added the numerous "empty" calories of booze to its adherents' low-carbohydrate meals).

Sales of these books, while brisk, were relatively small potatoes by today's standards. In a way, they were to diet-book publishing what an advance man is to politics: merely paving the way for the two biggest and most profitable ketogenic diet acts of all time.

The first came in 1967, when Irving Stillman, M.D., a Coney Island physician, and his highly visible ghost-writer, Samm Sinclair Baker, brought out *The Doctor's Quick Weight Loss Diet.* It was soon followed on the doctor's profitable quick-publishing schedule by four warmed-over spin-offs: *The Doctor's Inches-Off Diet; The Doctor's Teen-Age Diet; The Doctor's Quick Weight Loss Diet Cookbook;* and a 25¢ abbreviated version in pamphlet form.

The books and pamphlet have so far sold 20 million copies and are still going strong, according to Baker. And he adds that the indomitable ketogenic collaborators are readying another number, *Dr. Stillman's 14-Day Shape-Up Program,* which promises to puff its way onto the best-seller lists by midyear.* The book's "new" quality is that it adds exercise to the old diet, along with the astute observation that if you do your 15-minute daily workout in front of a television set, it won't turn out to be so boring.

Stillman and Baker may stand alone in terms of sheer productivity and sales, but they will never top Atkins in record-setting impact. Within a year after his revolutionary version of the same old diet was published, he had sold more than a million hardcover copies, at $6.95 apiece. Industry sources say that's an all-time record for *any* hardcover book of *any* kind.

Curiously, when the AMA's Council on Foods and Nutrition took the unprecedented step of issuing a warning against the book (as well as some of the others mentioned above), *Diet Revolution* experienced only a "brief and spotty lag in sales," according to the publisher, David McKay Company. Then it took off again.

When the paperback version hit the stands last fall, it moved even faster. Bantam Books reports that Dr. Atkins is now in his fourth paperback edition, with 2.45 million copies in print—all of which suggests that there are vast numbers of us who will swallow anything in our quest for fashion-model figures.† For reasons which no one has satisfactorily explained, there seems to be a mystique to the psychology of overweight and dieting that even trips up usually skeptical scientists.

A few years ago, for example, many professional readers of the normally somber *Journal of the New York Academy of Sciences* pondered a weighty

---

*EDITOR'S NOTE: This was Dr. Stillman's last book. He died in 1975.

†EDITOR'S NOTE: Mary Ann Crenshaw is equivocal about the Atkins diet in her book *The Natural Way to Super Beauty* (New York: David McKay Co., 1974). By following the diet, she writes, she at first became slim and healthy but then ran into trouble. So she delved further into weight-reducing formulas and concluded that kelp, vitamin B_6, and cider vinegar help the pounds roll off and that lecithin shifts the desired weight around to where it's supposed to be. And thus was another popular diet born. According to nutritional scientists, Crenshaw's formula (which is available in one capsule in health food stores and some drug stores) has no scientific basis. If one loses weight on Crenshaw's "super diet," it may well be because her singular quartet is being used in conjunction—as she recommends—with a low-calorie diet.

psychological monograph that purported to shed new light on "the relationship between eating habits and personality traits." The article disclosed several startling psychonutritional findings, one of which was attributed to an exhaustive psychoanalytic study of a group of asparagus-eaters.

Its author reported that people "who spontaneously attack and eat the *tip* of the asparagus first are likely to be immature, fearful, dependent, and unable to defer gratification—even briefly.

"Those individuals who proceeded from stem to tip," on the other hand, "rated high in such personality parameters as frustration-tolerance, self-security, and confidence. . . . In the American psychosocial tradition, [they] showed faith in the future, confidence in the Judeo-Christian ethic, and a conviction that delayed gratification is morally correct."

The title of the paper was "Freud Eggs." It was an obvious spoof. Yet the journal's chagrined editor reported that many of his scientist readers took its findings seriously.

While that may say something about the humorlessness of some scientists, it probably says more about the general public's apparent eagerness to believe anything in print that links food with emotional hang-ups. There is plenty of evidence to support the link in at least some obese people, although most overweight Americans can blame their life-styles, not the hang-ups, for excess pounds and inches.

Unless we have deep-seated problems or extreme obesity, most of us ought to be able to shape up on our own, without expensive psychiatric attention or diet books that play Russian roulette with our metabolism. All one really requires, say experts such as Dr. White, Dr. Van Itallie, and Professor Mayer, is a balanced, nutritious, low-calorie diet. Eat normal foods but less of them. On such a meal regimen of 1,000 to 1,200 calories a day, the average chubby American will lose between two and two-and-a-half pounds a week and learn something about healthful eating in the process.

You've heard that before, right?

Well, if it's not for you, try eating your asparagus from stem to tip, then reach for your mate. It can't hurt.

| 14 | Fight Fat with Behavior Control

MICHAEL J. MAHONEY and **KATHRYN MAHONEY**

Michael J. Mahoney is associate professor of psychology at Pennsylvania State University at University Park. Kathryn Mahoney, his wife, was a social worker before turning to the Clinical Psychology Program at Penn State, where she is a doctoral candidate. For the past few years she has worked with her husband in the study and treatment of obesity.

Americans hunger for diets. The average person goes on—and off—1.4 diets per year. In the search for slimness, dieters drink gallons of water, diet colas, and grapefruit juice; munch on rice, carrots, and celery; and satiate themselves with yogurt and cottage cheese. The rush to slimness .often has physical costs. Diets can cause headaches, dizziness, diarrhea, fatigue, indigestion, skin disorders, and constipation. And there are psychological costs: dieters often suffer from irritability and depression. They sacrifice, agonize, and lose sleep, but they seldom stay thin. The problem is that permanent weight control requires focusing more on behavior and less on food.

For everyone, including those who say, "I was meant to be fat," "Obesity runs in my family," or "I have a hormone problem," being overweight means consuming more calories than the body uses. Adults require a minimum of about 1,200 calories a day for good health; those who get less risk serious health problems. How many calories a person needs above the 1,200-calorie level depends upon his metabolic rate, how active he is, and his present weight.

Vicious spiral

Calories that are not needed to maintain body processes or to move us about are converted into fat. The fat-conversion formula varies from person to person, but the average is one pound of fat stored for every 3,500 excess calories. A little over 100 extra calories a day—a handful of peanuts or a glass of beer—and in one month the eater is one pound heavier. Eating both peanuts and beer means two extra pounds. In a year, it's possible to go from thin to plump without ever being gluttonous.

Occasional binges add up the same way. A person may eat sensibly all week, but if he helps himself to extra servings of cake on the weekends, extra pounds will slowly appear. Most people become less active as they grow older, and this has the same result as eating more. With additional pounds to carry around, people become still less active, add more fat, and so on in a vicious spiral interrupted only by periodic stints of dieting. Maintaining a sensible weight does not mean a lifetime of carrots and celery, nor does it require hours of painful calisthenics, but it does mean keeping calorie consumption and activity in harmony. It's like balancing a checkbook, and the human body is a fierce accountant.

Most diets are lists of do's and don'ts, but they usually tell us nothing about *how* to do the do's and avoid the don'ts. The implication is that the answer is will power; it's the dieter against the chocolate-cream pie. Trouble is, as many dieters have discovered, the pie seems to get stronger as they get weaker. All too often, dieters resist temptation long enough to shed the unwanted pounds, and then go back to the old habits that put on those flabby ripples in the first place.

Permanent weight control requires an entirely different focus: you must concentrate on behavior, not will power or a magic list of permissible foods. It is your daily eating and exercise habits, the input and output of energy, that must be changed.

Changing your behavior does not require that you endure hunger pangs or the nausea, headaches, and other side effects of many diets. But it does require effort and a long-term commitment. Realistic changes in behavior will result in slower weight loss, and if you do establish new behavior patterns, you will keep the pounds from coming back.

We have worked with hundreds of overweight people over the past five years. Out of that work we have developed the SCIENCE program for permanent weight control. Since we know that behavior is the villain that keeps people fat, many of our techniques are those of the behavior therapist. In fact, we ask our overweight clients to study their own eating and exercising habits the same way a behavior therapist might study the tics of a neurotic patient. The SCIENCE approach consists of seven simple steps:

1 specify the problem,
2 collect data,

3 identify patterns,
4 examine possible solutions,
5 narrow options and experiment,
6 compare current and past data, and
7 extend, revise, or replace solutions.

Specify the problem

If you are overweight, you are doing something wrong. The goal if to find out what. You may be eating too much, eating the wrong kinds of foods, or exercising too little. The more overweight you are, the more likely it is that you are doing all three.

Collect data

You need to have an objective measure of what you actually do. Many overweight people complain about the unjustness of their condition and back it up with "facts": "I had only *one* egg for breakfast," or "I starve myself and still gain weight." Such statements may get you sympathy, but they won't get you thin. While it may be true that you had only one egg for breakfast, it is also true that you had two chocolate eclairs as a midnight snack. The point is, you will have to keep an honest record of your eating habits in order to know the changes that are necessary.

Dieters are used to counting calories, and that information is helpful. But other facts are equally important. Keep a record for one week of when and where you eat, as well as what and how much. Also keep track of your exercise habits—the amount of time spent walking, jogging, doing calisthenics, playing tennis, etc. Remember that the purpose of data collecting is to get an objective measure of what you ordinarily do, so make no special effort to exercise more or eat less during this period.

Identify patterns

After a week of data collecting, you are ready to search for the source of your energy imbalance. You might begin by computing the average number of calories you eat in a day, and checking that number against the number you need for your desired weight (see box, page 156). If the numbers agree, your problem may be more a matter of inactivity than of overeating.

Most overweight people will find they consume too many calories. The problem is to find out where those calories come from. For example, the hypothetical sample dieter's diary shown is like many of the diaries we get

Sample dieter's diary

Monday, October 1

8:30 2 pieces buttered toast, 1 bowl corn flakes with milk (light sugar), 2 cups black coffee

10:30 4 peanut-butter cookies, cup black coffee

12:45 tuna-fish sandwich on whole-wheat toast, dill pickle, glass of milk (10 oz.)

2:15 cup of coffee, half piece of toast with peanut butter

4:30 2 peanut-butter cookies

6:00 1 serving corn, 2 servings fish, 1 small boiled potato, 2 cups coffee

9:20 1 Coke (16 oz.) and about 25 potato chips

10:30 1 cup chocolate ice-cream

Tuesday, October 2

8:30 1 bowl corn flakes with milk (light sugar), 2 cups black coffee

10:00 Coke and doughnut

12:15 (restaurant) BLT sandwich, small serving cole-slaw, cup of coffee

3:00 4 peanut-butter cookies, 1 Coke (16 oz.)

6:00 2 servings rice casserole, small salad with dressing, 1 slice buttered bread, 1 cup coffee

9:00 1 Coke (16 oz.) and 6 vanilla wafers

10:00 1 glass milk, 2 pretzel sticks

from our obese clients. While it shows sensible eating at meals, it also reveals a tendency toward recreational eating. Many people take a morning break and have coffee and doughnuts with their friends. In the afternoon they have candy or pie during breaks from studying or other monotonous work. In the evening they munch on potato chips and cookies while watching TV or reading. These are the people who often complain at meals, "See,

I eat no more than Mary, but she stays thin and I get fat; all I have to do is look at a piece of cheesecake and I gain weight." The hard data of a diary will often convince the weight watcher that he is doing more than just looking.

In our society, food is often connected with recreation. We go out for coffee, invite friends over for drinks, celebrate special occasions with cakes or big meals. We can't think of baseball without thinking of hot dogs and beer, and eating is so often an accompaniment to watching TV that we talk of TV snacks and TV dinners. Just as Pavlov's dogs learned to salivate at the sound of a bell, the activities we associate with food can become signals to eat. Watching TV becomes a signal for potato chips; talking with friends becomes a signal for coffee and doughnuts; nodding over a book tells us it's time for pie and milk.

Examine possible solutions

The next step is to decide which inappropriate behaviors are easiest to change. For the hypothetical case shown above, the following solutions seem reasonable:

1 reduce the number of snacks,
2 when at home, snack only in the kitchen,
3 exercise at times when snacking might occur,
4 snack on low-calorie desserts, and
5 join an exercise class.

After listing possible solutions, the next step is to select those that seem most likely to succeed. It is tempting to make a list of perfectionistic rules, especially if you aren't hungry at the moment. This should be avoided. Remember that if you were perfect, you wouldn't be fat. Rigid rules, such as no snacks, no high-calorie desserts, are bound to be broken eventually, and that leads to a sense of failure. Stick with rules you think you can follow.

For example, some people cannot stand diet desserts; it makes little sense for them to try substituting diet colas and diet cookies for tastier snacks. Similarly, a thin roommate is apt to show little enthusiasm for the idea of having only diet desserts in the house. On the other hand, a roommate might be induced to buy snacks that are the weight watcher's least favorite foods. And while a person who hates exercise is not likely to suddenly become a jogging enthusiast, he might succeed in substituting short walks for pies and candy as afternoon breaks. Since moderate exercise tends to lessen appetite, the walks might also mean eating less at meals.

Compare current and past data

It is not enough to come up with possible solutions; you must see if the solutions work. Continue to keep track of your habits for at least three weeks; by then you should be able to tell whether your plan is working. Do not search for immediate results in the mirror or on the bathroom scale. Most bathroom scales are too inaccurate to measure subtle weight changes, and your daily weight fluctuates slightly anyway. We recommend that you check the scale no more than twice a month. The goal is to change your behavior, and if you do that, the pounds will take care of themselves. It is often helpful to convert your data from the diary to charts. . . .

After three or four weeks you should have enough data to see trends. If

~~~~~~

HOW MUCH SHOULD YOU WEIGH?

Many people try to determine how much they should weigh by reading height-weight tables, but since these tables often indicate average weights rather than optimum weights, the figures tend to be too high. There is, however, a formula for estimating your healthiest weight.

Adult women of average build can compute their ideal weight by multiplying their height in inches by 3.5 and then subtracting 110 from the product. Thus, a woman who is five feet tall should weigh about 100 pounds ($60 \times 3.5 - 110 = 100$). For men of average build the formula is height in inches times four, minus 130. A six-foot man should weigh about 158.

It is reasonable to make allowances for bone structure and muscularity: even if Woody Allen and Rosie Grier were the same height, they should not weigh the

same amount. But be careful that in making these allowances, you don't mistake fat for muscle. And remember that if you are 30 pounds overweight, it is unlikely that the difference is all in your bones.

The amount of food you need to maintain your ideal weight depends upon how active you are. Begin by rating yourself on the scale below:

13	very inactive
14	slightly inactive
15	moderately active
16	relatively active
17	frequently, strenuously active

If you are a sedentary office worker a housewife you should probably rate yourself a 13. If your physical exercise consists of occasional games of golf or an afternoon walk, you're a 14. A score your plan shows signs of working, then you should continue the program or extend it to include other solutions. If your plan is not working out, you will have to reexamine your data and look for other solutions. You should also check your record to see if you have developed any bad habits while working on adopting good ones: e.g., you may find that while you were able to cut down on snacks, you began eating more at meals.

When you apply the SCIENCE method to your own eating and exercise habits, you may find that your problems are much different from those discussed above. You may find that you are a social eater and eat whenever you are with friends. Or you may find that you can't resist the sight or fragrance of food, so that you eat whenever food is available.

~~~~~~

of 15 means that you frequently engage in moderate exertion—jogging, calisthenics, tennis. A 16 requires that you are almost always on the go, seldom sitting down or standing still for long. Don't give yourself a 17 unless you are a construction worker or engage in other strenuous activity frequently. Most adult Americans should rate themselves 13 or 14.

To calculate the number of calories you need to maintain your ideal weight, multiply your activity rating by your ideal weight. A 200-pound office worker, for example, needs 2,600 calories a day; a 200-pound athlete needs 3,400 calories.

To estimate how many calories you are getting now, multiply your current weight times your activity level. If your weight is constant at 140 pounds and you are inactive, you are consuming about 1,820 calories a day (13 times 140). Subtract the number of calories you need for your ideal weight from the number of calories you are consuming, and you will know the size of your energy imbalance.

To reach your ideal weight, we recommend that you correct your calorie imbalance slowly. It's a good idea to lose no more than one percent of your current weight a week. Cut your daily calorie consumption by two times your current weight and you should achieve that goal. Regardless of your weight, you should not get less than 1,200 calories a day. Reducing by much more than one percent of your body weight a week could mean destruction of muscles and organs as well as fat. The same is true of diets that prohibit all fats and carbohydrates.

—Michael and Kathryn Mahoney

~~~~~~

Many obese people find themselves obsessed by thoughts of food. Thinking about food makes them hungry, which, in turn, makes it difficult to stop thinking of food. The SCIENCE method can be applied to changing thinking habits as well as overt behavior. Keeping a record of your thoughts about food will tell you when, where, and under what circumstances your thoughts turn to food.

Housewives, for example, often find that they think about food primarily when working in the kitchen. One obvious strategy for them might be to avoid the kitchen whenever possible. Maybe someone else in the family can wash dishes or fix meals once in awhile. Or they might prepare simple meals that can be put together in minutes. Other people find that they think of food primarily when talking to weight-conscious friends. They talk about their latest diets, how much weight they have lost or gained, or the new diet dish they've discovered. A solution might be to ask their friends to help by not discussing food; if that doesn't work, they might try changing the subject whenever the conversation shifts to food.

Eating by the clock

Another common problem of obese people is the inability to listen to their bodies. They eat because food is available or because it is time to eat. For example, Richard Nisbett, at the University of Michigan, found that when he offered food to thin people, they ate as much as they wanted and then stopped, but obese people were influenced by how much food was put in front of them: if they were given one sandwich, they were satisfied with that, but if they were given three sandwiches, they ate them. Many of us learn as children that we must clean our plate; children are starving in India, and somehow we are made to feel that any wasted food will contribute to their misery.

Clocks can also push people to eat. At Columbia [University], Stanley Schachter and Larry Gross rigged two clocks so that one ran fast and the other ran slow. They began the experiment at 5 p.m. By 5:30, the slow clock registered 5:20 and the fast clock showed 6:05. When overweight people were given a chance to snack, they ate an average of twice as much when the clock told them it was after six than when they thought it was 5:20.

If your own data tell you that you are easily influenced by such external cues, you can set up a plan to avoid them. For example, try taking smaller portions of food at meals. If you are still hungry, you can make the effort of going back for seconds, but you will be eating because you want the food, not just because it is on your plate. You can also make it a practice to put foods out of sight; don't leave candies, nuts, or crackers around the house. If you find that you listen to the clock rather than your stomach, you might try going without a watch or rearranging your schedule so that when it is time to eat you are busy with something.

How you eat can also influence how much you eat. If, after studying your own eating habits, you find that you are one of the faster forks around, you might take steps to slow down. Put your fork down between bites, chew each mouthful thoroughly. One reason that eating fast is bad is that it doesn't give your body a chance to react to the food you've eaten. By the time the body is able to say, "that's enough," you've already had too much. A simple solution that works for many is to eat what seems a reasonable amount and then leave the table for 30 minutes. If you are still hungry after half an hour, go back to the table and resume your meal. You may find that you no longer feel hungry.

No magic involved

Exercise is often a neglected factor in weight control. In a study of obese adolescent girls, Jean Mayer found that the girls actually ate less than their thin classmates, but they were also far less active. The fact is that exercise is almost 50 percent of the weight-control formula: taking off excess weight means eating less or exercising more. In most cases it is advisable to do both. Staying active does not necessarily mean spending hours on the tennis court. If your personal data convince you that you are not active enough, try working more exercise into your day: walk instead of ride, take the stairs instead of the elevator, go to the bowling alley instead of a movie, play golf on Saturday afternoon instead of watching others play it on TV.

There is no magic to the SCIENCE method. It is a program that is based on well-grounded behavior-modification principles and it can mean the end of dieting, but it demands concentration and serious effort over a long period.

It means making permanent changes in your lifestyle, and some of those changes may be hard to take. But the reward, in many cases, is better than a sequence of slothful plumpness and desperate diets. You have a strong chance of joining the world of the permanently thin.

For more information, read:

Mahoney, Michael J. and Kathryn Mahoney. *Permanent Weight Control: A Total Solution to the Dieter's Dilemma*, Norton, 1976.

Mahoney, Michael J. and Carl E. Thoresen. *Self-Control: Power to the Person*, Brooks/Cole, 1974, paper.

Thoresen, C. E. and Michael J. Mahoney. *Behavioral Self-Control*, Holt, 1974, paper.

Part III
Prevention
and Therapy
through Nutrition

*. . . I have watched a good
many triumphs of nutritional
therapy. I have regarded
every one of them as a mon-
ument to a failure —for what
nutrition cures, it ordinarily
prevents.*

—CARLTON FREDERICKS

Introduction to

Part III

A few food fanatics, oblivious of the possible multiple origins of disease, go so far as to claim that *all* diseases are caused by improper nutrition. Many illnesses, however, are unquestionably diet-*related,* and poor diet can lower the resistance to any disease. And yet, nutritional therapy is ordinarily applied only as a last resort, if at all. The relation between diet and illness is seldom seriously considered, especially since penalties exacted by faulty nutrition may not show up for a decade, or two or three—when the deterioration of one's health is usually broadly attributed to "getting old."

Malnutrition has become commonplace among both the poor and the affluent. The Senate Select Committee on Nutrition and Human Needs (whose pronouncements are not universally endorsed by nutritionists) recently warned that current eating habits "may be as profoundly damaging to the nation's health as the widespread contagious diseases of the early part of the century."[1]

This country leads the world in both fabricated foods and degenerative diseases. Since 1950, life expectancies for adult males have been greater in almost 30 nations than they have been in the United States. Americans spend more on health care—an estimated $160 billion in 1977—than the people of any other country. Some nutritionists say that possibly a third or more of that bill is the result of poor nutrition.[2]

Many adults who claim to be healthy simply because they have no specific disease consider it no mean feat to haul themselves out of bed, make it to the office, and remain fully conscious until the coffee break. Accustomed to instant foods and instant pain-relievers, they expect disease will be instant too: if there are no immediate bad effects from the food they so carelessly ingest, the stuff must be okay. Still they dole out over $1 billion a year for laxatives (there are about 700 brands to choose from) and hundreds of millions of dollars on Alka-Seltzer, Rolaids, and other digestive consolations.

"The most basic weapons in the fight against disease," observes biochemist Roger J. Williams, "are those most ignored by modern medicine: *the numerous nutrients that the cells of our bodies need.* If our body cells are ailing—as they must be in disease—the chances are excellent that it is because they are being inadequately provisioned."[3] In treating a disease, according to Williams, top priority would best be given to those medications that most resemble the biological weapons of nature. The basic fault of alien chemicals is that

> they have no known connection with the disease process itself. They tend to mask the difficulty, not eliminate it. They contaminate the internal environment, create dependence on the part of the patient, and often complicate the physician's job by erasing valuable clues as to the real source of trouble.
>
> If this sounds extreme, let me put the case as simply and bluntly as I can: Do you really believe you have headaches as a result of your system's lack of aspirin?[4]

All this is not meant to imply that, if you're sick, you might as well forget the doctor and try to cure yourself with decent food and a lot of nutritional supplements. What it does mean is that good nutrition should not only help lower the incidence of sickness but also, when you do need medical attention, effectively complement any treatment the doctor prescribes.

No one can in fairness say that the medical profession fails to adopt new diagnostic and treatment methods. But, historically, it has tended to accept new ideas that don't conform to its biases with the alacrity of a felled ox. Advances in therapy and cure that have come from outside the field of medicine (for example, with Pasteur) as well as those that have originated within it (for example, with Semmelweis) have often been denounced and ridiculed by the medical opinion-makers of the day. (This is not to suggest that all new ideas are good. What is involved here is healthy skepticism versus outright condemnation.)

Fortunately, the seemingly implacable defense of the status quo is slowly crumbling with regard to nutrition. Some prominent leaders in the medical community now admit that nutrition has been almost completely neglected in the profession, and the number of nutrition-oriented doctors is slowly growing.

Still, as Carl Pfeiffer and his colleagues point out in *Selection 15,* "most American physicians have not yet recognized that nutrition is an essential part of good medicine."* The authors survey the extent and causes of malnutrition and plead for an emphasis on nutrition in preventive medicine. They champion the concept of orthomolecular therapy, which, as Selections 16 through 18 reveal, has already stirred up a controversy that could rage for years.

---

*See also Selections 31 and 37 and page 399.

Whether taken in megadoses, as in orthomolecular therapy, or in lesser amounts, vitamin and mineral supplements have become a central issue in American nutrition. Most proponents of supplements contend that personal experiences are their guide; they scorn some of the professional nutritionists and Food and Drug Administration spokespersons who claim that supplementation is a waste of money and possibly hazardous. "Vitamins," Atkins and Linde contend, "do not compete with drugs within your body. But they do compete in the marketplace—and for this reason an economic war is being waged, and your bodies are the battlefield."[5] Drug companies are covering all the bases: Squibb, for instance, has advertised that as a trustworthy, old-line firm it "has marketed vitamin products since 1875"—no mean feat, since vitamins were not discovered until almost four decades later.[6]

Opponents of supplementation, including many physicians, stress the dangers of vitamin toxicity, although any such dangers pale by comparison with the innumerable and hazardous side effects of the thousands of drugs doctors prescribe. In their book *Panic in the Pantry,* Whelan and Stare present a detailed list of the incredible number of supplements one woman took, to her detriment.[7] Isolated cases such as this frequently appear in the literature. One could just as easily cite the case of British author Barbara Cartland, a vigorous septuagenarian whose works number over 220 and who in her seventy-fourth year dashed off 19 novels and a cookbook while serving as president of England's National Health Association. She takes 90 vitamin pills a day *plus* ginseng and a personal formula of vitamins and dried sheep brains.[8]

Naturally, there are inherent dangers in taking too much of anything (one woman recently died from drinking too much water).[9] What is the margin of safety? According to one source, the margin is tremendous: "The few studies to date which seem to support a vitamin A and vitamin D toxicity potential used fantastically large quantities to demonstrate an ill effect. You'd have to sit down and plan your own demise to take a damaging dosage of these nutrients."[10] Toxicity, nevertheless, is a matter of individual variation; it is most apt to occur when vitamins are taken singly rather than in combination as nature intended. It is probably a toss-up as to which is more exaggerated, the need for vitamins or their toxicity.

Jean Mayer maintains that, if your physician recommends it, one vitamin pill a day—containing no more than the RDAs—is sufficient. As to megavitamins, he cautions that

> in normal amounts, vitamins are food; at five, ten, a hundred, or a thousand times the normal level, vitamins are drugs and should be treated accordingly. . . .

. . . If the history of the development of our science is a dependable guide, there may be nutrients performing significant duties for us that we have not yet identified. In particular, there may be minerals functioning heroically to our benefit and all unknown to us. If they exist, we are getting them from the varied diet we enjoyably consume. Attempting to depend on "appropriate capsules" might deprive us of substances that we now have and will continue to need.[11]

If you read Selections 16, 17, and 18 in sequence, you might do well to keep in mind an observation made by F. Scott Fitzgerald in his novel *The Crack-Up*: "The test of a first-rate intelligence is the ability to hold two opposing ideas in the mind at the same time, and still retain the ability to function."

In *Selection 16*, Dr. Robert Atkins and Shirley Linde explain why they believe supplements are necessary, discuss the roles of specific vitamins and minerals, and show how to tailor an individual vitamin and mineral program. Disagreeing with their views, Ronald Deutsch in *Selection 17* sums up an array of arguments against vitamin supplements, delivers some blows to orthomolecular therapy, and along the way deals unequivocally with the question of natural versus synthetic vitamins.*

In contrast to Deutsch's point of view, Richard Passwater in *Selection 18* un-reservedly supports megavitamin therapy. He demonstrates why it seems needed and documents evidence of its success in treating people with mental and emotional disorders. Passwater does not recommend simply dropping the talk and tranquilizers of conventional psychiatry in favor of megavitamin therapy, but instead suggests a dual approach. Carlton Fredericks, a vociferous advocate of megavitamins for troubled patients, has pointed out that "every effort is being made to persuade physicians to remember that this is not a war in which all truth is on one side. It is, rather, the classical confrontation in the arena of science, on the basis of which most progress is made."[12]

Richard Mackarness, a British psychiatrist, believes that instead of mental illness causing physical illness, it is physical disorders (specifically, food aller-

---

*Although the consensus is that there is no difference between natural and synthetic vitamins, there does occasionally appear to be a difference in their effect. To account for this, some biochemists have suggested that (1) other micronutrients in the natural sources may maximize a vitamin's effect; (2) the body's enzyme system utilizes levorotatory natural vitamins more efficiently than dextrorotatory synthetic ones; and (3) natural vitamins that are in a colloidal state are assimilated more readily than synthetic vitamins that are in a crystalline form. (Kathy Dinaburg and D'Ann Ausherman Akel, *Nutrition Survival Kit* [San Francisco: Panjandrum Press and MidPress Productions, 1976], p. 134; and H. Curtis Wood, Jr., *Overfed but Undernourished* [New York: Tower Publications, 1971], pp. 33–34.)

gies) that cause as much as one-third of all mental disorders. This, of course, turns the orthodox concept of psychosomatic medicine on its head. But Mackarness reasons that, just as allergies affect the stomach and the skin and result in indigestion and rashes, they can affect the brain and produce mental problems.[13]

The theories of Mackarness jibe with the findings of Dr. Ben Feingold, an American allergist who maintains that certain chemicals in both natural and processed foods lead to a syndrome called hyperactivity. Dr. Feingold's particular concern is hyperactivity in children. His disciples are so impressed with the results of the therapeutic diet he has worked out that some 80 parent associations have sprung up in various parts of the country to spread the word. Of his detractors Feingold says: "The continuing thousands of successful responses of children throughout the world to the . . . diet outweigh the attempts of industry and industry-supported research to discredit my hypothesis."[14]

Feingold's work is challenged in Selection 19 by members of the Institute of Food Technologists. They define hyperactivity; describe, evaluate, and question Feingold's hypothesis and regimen; report on control studies; and conclude that further study is warranted.

How does alcohol consumption affect an individual's state of health and nutrition? Among the untoward effects of alcoholism, as Dr. Charles Lieber reports in Selection 20, are malnutrition and deficiency diseases. Alcohol, high in calories, not only displaces nutrient-rich food but also interferes with normal digestion and absorption. But Lieber warns: liver disorders in chronic drinkers are the result of the direct toxic effect of alcohol, and even the correction or prevention of nutritional deficiencies cannot guarantee protection against liver damage.

A widespread misconception, centuries old, is that alcohol is a heart "stimulant." There is now considerable evidence that it is, in fact, a myocardial depressant and that chronic drinking can lead to congestive heart failure. This is apparently not linked with dietary deficiencies; nor does it resemble heart disease stemming from thiamin deficiency, where a high-output failure is evident. If alcohol alleviates angina pectoris, it may well be because the sedative effect alters the individual's threshold for pain perception. Owing to these findings, some specialists have concluded that persons with chronic congestive heart failure and severe myocardial damage probably should not indulge in liquor at all. Other cardiac patients should restrict themselves to one shot (1.5 ounces) of whiskey, one can (12 ounces) of beer, or one 6-ounce glass of wine a day.[15]

For those who are not victims of heart disease or of alcoholism, recent findings reveal that a moderate intake of alcohol may not be a bad thing; it may even be beneficial. Alcohol does not appear to increase total cholesterol in the blood, and it may even shift the blood's lipoprotein balance so that there is an increase in the lipoproteins that have been linked with heart-disease resistance (see Selection 27). But alcohol can as yet hardly be endorsed as a heart-disease preventive: it is not known whether the levels of cholesterol or of the lipoproteins might be altered by decreasing or increasing alcohol consumption, or whether such alterations might in turn decrease or increase the risk of heart disease.[16]

In *Selection 21*, John Henahan presents several reasons why scientists are now claiming that some alcohol—specifically, wine and cognac—may be good for you. Wine is recommended as a fine tranquilizer, an appetite booster, a relief for frail hearts, an aid for diabetics, and a means of deriving more nutritional benefit out of any food consumed. Cognac is touted as, among other things, an effective remedy for cardiac disorders and the common cold. Henahan moderates his optimistic report by noting some of the hazards and imponderable consequences of alcohol consumption.

In *Selection 22*, Myron Brin probes the interrelations of drugs and vitamins: vitamin insufficiency can reduce the body's capacity to metabolize drugs; drugs, in turn, can cause vitamin insufficiency. Brin illustrates why it is advisable to increase vitamin intake in cases of drug and/or environmental chemical exposure.

Sugar has, at one extreme, been regarded as a scourge and, at the other, been lauded as a blessing that makes food—and sometimes even life itself—palatable. A few die-hard nutritionists and the sugar industry continue to insist that refined sugar is a splendid source of energy. Yet from the time of the caveman until a couple of centuries ago, human beings managed to live without this refinement and somehow work up enough energy to survive in exceedingly harsh environments, build empires, and spread their progeny the world around.[17]

The digestive system of the human being was designed to handle sugar in its natural state—that is, as a mixture of sucrose, lactose, fructose, glucose, and other simple molecules—in combination with the starch and other complex molecules of whole foods like fruits and vegetables. Only recently has the body been expected to cope with sugar in a chemically pure state—that is, as sucrose—and in large doses.

During the last few decades sugar consumption in this country has become a mania and, it is widely conceded, a menace to health. Almost everything we put in our mouths, including such nonfood items as medicine and tobacco, contains sugar in some form. At least three-fourths of the sugar we consume is hidden in processed foods, the labels of which often cover up the high proportion of sweetening by listing it variously as sugar, glucose, dextrose, or corn syrup. Recently a panel of gourmets, when asked to try to identify the *secret* ingredients lurking in some of the most popular American foods, concluded that in the majority of foods sampled one of the mysterious ingredients was sugar. (Specifically, the panel singled out McDonald's Big Mac Sauce, Underwood's Deviled Ham, Colonel Sanders' Kentucky Fried Chicken, Hellmann's Family French Dressing, Tabasco Sauce, and Miracle Whip.)[18]

Our average daily consumption of 500 "naked" calories of sugar, which accounts for up to half of our carbohydrate intake, is deemed okay by some writers of nutrition textbooks, who add that of course the rest of the diet should contain proper amounts of all required nutrients and that the total calorie content should not be excessive. Dr. Fredrick Stare says, on the one hand, that sugar is important to our diet "when used in moderation" and, on the other, that we "could healthily double" our consumption.[19] How helpful is all such advice? Those daily 500 calories can add up to 50 pounds of fat each year; and even if you are not worried about gaining weight, it will be difficult to squeeze in all the nutrients required for an adequate diet and all the harder for an optimum one. Moreover, according to Jean Mayer, the calories from sugar

> increase the requirement for certain vitamins, such as thiamine, which are needed to metabolize carbohydrates. They may increase the need for the trace mineral chromium as well. Thus, a greater burden is placed on the other components of the diet to contribute all the necessary nutrients—other foods need to show extraordinary "nutrient density" to compensate for the emptiness of the sugar calories.[20]

Refined sugar is generally acknowledged as the chief cause of dental decay. Is it also implicated in the higher incidence of heart disease and diabetes? In *Selection 23*, John Pekkanen and Mathea Falco report on both sides of the evidence linking sugar to these diseases. In addition, they review the extent to which the American public gratifies, and is tempted to gratify, its sweet tooth, and they consider the weak possibility of turning this tide.

Refined sugar, along with other processed carbohydrates, has been vilified in some quarters as the chief cause of hypoglycemia, a condition of low blood sugar in which an excessive quality of insulin is secreted into the blood. Not definitely a disease but rather a collection of symptoms that can appear for various reasons, hypoglycemia has been the focus of so much controversy that it has become a social issue. Orthodox physicians tend to regard it as a rare occurrence, a "fad disease"; unorthodox physicians, psychiatrists, and nutritionists of orthomolecular persuasion generally consider it to be epidemic.[21]

In *Selection 24,* Dr. Sydney Walker asks for some straight thinking on the subject. He demonstrates how hypoglycemia can be misdiagnosed and treated symptomatically as a psychiatric disturbance or an emotional upset, although psychotherapy alone will not cure a blood-sugar imbalance. He also shows how a physician who reaches a facile diagnosis of hypoglycemia can miss endocrine and neurological diseases that produce the same symptoms as low blood sugar. Carbohydrate problems are so subtle, he points out, that taking a pro or con position on hypoglycemia is hardly sensible.

Probably no word in the nutrition lexicon has received such a bad press as "cholesterol." The refrain "Cut down on cholesterol" is repeated like a broken record by physicians, nutritionists, and laypersons alike. Despite increasing evidence that it is unjustified, the vilification of cholesterol as the sole or primary cause of atherosclerosis and coronary heart disease continues. As noted in Selection 23, high triglyceride levels induced by excessive intake of sugar may prove to be more reliable predictors of heart disease risk than elevated cholesterol levels. (Whereas the per capita consumption of saturated fatty acids has remained nearly constant since the turn of the century, sugar consumption has increased more than 100 percent.) Too often forgotten, too, are other factors associated with the risk of heart disease—for example, hypertension, sedentariness, smoking, overweight, reaction to stress, lack of dietary fiber, diabetes, and, not the least, genetic variations in the ability to metabolize cholesterol and fatty acids from any source.

Cholesterol has served as a neat scapegoat because it appeals to our futile desire for every effect to be the result of a single cause. Statistically, the risk of coronary disease rises exponentially with an increase in cholesterol levels. The question is whether cholesterol is a cause or a symptom and whether the correlation is anything more than statistical.[22] Though frequently disregarded, exceptions to the statistical norm are countless, emphasizing the need to investigate multiple causes. For example, dairy products, including the much-maligned egg, are high in cholesterol, yet lacto-ovo-vegetarians have lower serum cholesterol levels and, statistically, their initial heart attacks (if they have any) occur a decade later than the national average. In Yemen, men who drink 10 pints daily of camel's milk, which is 10 times richer than cow's milk, show no evidence of high coronary risk. Moran warriors among the Masai people of East Africa live almost exclusively on the milk, blood, and meat of their cattle and have virtually no heart disease; neither do those Eskimos who stick to their primitive high-fat diet and don't succumb to our refined, "civilized" diet. (It has been suggested that most of these peoples do not live long enough to develop heart disease and that they may have an inherited ability to metabolize saturated fats more efficiently than other populations. They also get plenty of exercise.)

Heart-transplant surgeon Dr. Michael DeBakey once commented: "About 80% of my 1,700 patients with severe atherosclerosis requiring surgery have cholesterol levels of normal people."[23] And Dr. George V. Mann of Vanderbilt University's School of Medicine asserts:

> The evidence that our high-fat diet causes coronary heart disease is trivial despite the whooping of the American Heart Association. They have committed the nutritional disaster of the century by confusing association with causation, to the endless delight and profit of food companies that employ cholesterol-scare tactics in their advertising.[24]

In a similar vein, biochemist Ross Hume Hall comments:

> The dietary-fat heart disease correlation has been sanctified by the scientific establishment, whereas the correlation with refined carbohydrates has been ostracized. . . .
> . . . Medical scientists recognize that dietary factors are important, but they seek a solution to heart disease that does not disturb the basic technologic dietary patterns, a solution that conforms to the objectives of the technologic food system.[25]

Now that the egg, once called "the perfect protein" and even "the perfect food," has been so strongly (but perhaps not sagely) condemned, food processors have a "valid" excuse to market egg substitutes. Meanwhile, the egg industry (which Jean Mayer has called "the heart disease Mafia") continues its battle with the American Heart Association. Which side will win? Disentangling the evidence in the cholesterol controversy seems as hopeless as trying to unscramble one of those eggs. The correlation between dietary fat and heart disease has been neither proved nor disproved; statistics lead only to a qualified association. Until conclusive evidence appears, what is the prudent path to follow?

In *Selection 25*, David Kritchevsky explains the meaning of the serum cholesterol level and illustrates why a high level points to increased risk of coronary disease. Recommending concern and care about dietary cholesterol, he cautions against hysteria.

Raymond Reiser, in *Selection 26*, challenges the theory that foods high in cholesterol and saturated fats increase the risk of coronary disease. He discusses why he believes that few benefit from a low-cholesterol diet, and why conflicting data and interpretations of experiments and studies may be the result of failure to distinguish between normal and pathological variations in serum cholesterol levels. In concluding, Reiser disapproves of the recommendation that infants be put on low-fat milk and low-cholesterol diets.

In *Selection 27*, Mark Bricklin reports on new findings indicating that cholesterol levels are often misinterpreted. Apparently there is both "good" and "bad" cholesterol: the high-density lipoproteins (HDL) are protective, and the low-density lipoproteins (LDL) are dangerous. Someone with a low level of LDL and a high level of HDL would therefore not be a likely candidate for a heart attack. Bricklin also discusses the role of lecithin, soybeans, pectin, and calcium in lowering cholesterol levels.

It has been reported that middle-aged male runners have HDL levels almost 50 percent higher than those of their peers; their levels are much like those of young women, who, being naturally endowed with more HDL, rarely suffer heart attacks. Shedding excess weight and eating a diet that is rich in vegetables and vegetable oil, skimps on red meat and dairy products, and includes a moderate amount of alcohol (perhaps a daily cocktail or two) can also apparently elevate the HDL level.[26]

"After 26 years of continuous practice in East Africa," writes Dr. Hugh Trowell, "a colleague and I recorded the first case of coronary heart disease in the 15 million inhabitants of those countries; the patient was an obese East African judge consuming a partially Westernized diet."[27] Trowell is one of the physician-scientists who discovered the importance of dietary fiber. He and other researchers have found that cholesterol levels usually remain low on a high-fiber diet, even if the diet includes moderate amounts of animal fats, because fiber apparently affects the metabolism of cholesterol and/or bile salts. The primary value of dietary fiber lies in its "bulking" properties, which allow waste materials to be discarded rapidly by the body. Since the early 1970s, researchers have put together a strong case for the relation of fiber-depleted diets to a host of diseases and ailments besides heart disease: cancer of the colon and rectum, polyps of the colon, diverticulosis, diabetes, chronic constipation, hemorrhoids, appendicitis, gallstones, obesity, hiatus hernia, and varicose veins.[28]

Critics of the fiber theory contend that dietary fiber has now been exalted to a miracle status, that data on its preventive role are based on inconclusive experimental studies, and that a diet strewn with bran could cause more harm than good. The low incidence of colon cancer among people eating high-fiber foods, many nutritionists argue, could be the result of something other than fiber or of something that is *not* eaten.

The sudden publicity accorded dietary fiber has been accompanied by numerous distortions of the original theory. As Lawrence Galton shows in *Selection 28*, proponents of the theory do not declare that a fiber-depleted diet is unquestionably the sole or major cause of the diseases common to all economically developed countries. (The average American diet today contains less than half the dietary fiber that it did 75 years ago.) Yet the theory does offer a possible explanation of the epidemiology and interrelations of these diseases, and there is presently no alternative hypothesis. Galton also points out why bran, contrary to popular belief, is not a panacea; discusses the different components of dietary fiber; and offers basic guidelines for restoring fiber to the diet by eating unrefined carbohydrates and avoiding refined foods.

References

1   Senate Select Committee, quoted in "Digging Our Graves with Our Teeth," *San Francisco Examiner*, January 14, 1977, p. 11.
2   "American Nutrition: Ignorance in Abundance," *Medical World News*, January 5, 1973, p. 6.
3   Roger J. Williams, *Nutrition against Disease: Environmental Prevention* (New York: Pitman Publishing Corp., 1971), p. 13.
4   Ibid., p. 11.
5   Robert C. Atkins and Shirley Linde, *Dr. Atkins' Superenergy Diet* (New York: Crown Publishers, 1977), p. 139.
6   Ronald M. Deutsch, *The New Nuts among the Berries* (Palo Alto, Calif.: Bull Publishing Co., 1977), pp. 288–289.
7   Elizabeth M. Whelan and Fredrick J. Stare, *Panic in the Pantry: Food Facts, Fads and Fallacies* (New York: Atheneum, 1975), pp. 78–79.
8   "Talk of the Town," *The New Yorker*, August 9, 1976, p. 20; and Gerri Hirshey, "Barbara Cartland, the Queen of Hearts," *Family Circle*, April 5, 1977, p. 190.
9   "Overdosing on Water," *Newsweek*, March 14, 1977, p. 46.
10 E. Cheraskin and W. M. Ringsdorf, Jr., with Arline Brecher, *Psychodietetics: Food as the Key to Emotional Health* (New York: Bantam Books, 1974), p. 183.
11 Jean Mayer, *A Diet for Living*, Consumers Union ed. (New York: David McKay Co., 1975), pp. 46, 59.
12 Carlton Fredericks, *Psycho-Nutrition* (New York: Grosset and Dunlap, 1976), p. 146. See also Roger J. Williams and Dwight K. Kalita, eds., *A Physician's Handbook on Orthomolecular Medicine* (New York: Pergamon Press, 1977).
13 See Richard Mackarness, *Eating Dangerously: The Hazards of Allergies* (New York: Harcourt Brace Jovanovich, 1976).

14 Ben Feingold, quoted in Betty Franklin, "The Feingold Diet Works Wonders for Problem Kids—Even Pets," *Let's Live,* August 1977, p. 125.

15 Lawrence D. Horwitz, "Alcohol and Heart Disease," *Journal of the American Medical Association* 232 (June 2, 1975), pp. 959–960.

16 "Alcohol: A Heart Disease Preventive?" *Science News* 112 (August 13, 1977), pp. 102–103.

17 For a history and bitter indictment of refined sugar written from the viewpoint of an ex-sugar junkie, see William Dufty, *Sugar Blues* (New York: Warner Books, 1976).

18 "What's in This Stuff?" *Esquire,* June 1974, pp. 92–95, 200.

19 See Whelan and Stare, *Panic in the Pantry,* pp. 180–183; and Dufty, *Sugar Blues,* pp. 156–157.

20 Jean Mayer, "The Bitter Truth about Sugar," *New York Times Magazine,* June 20, 1976, p. 31.

21 In Whelan and Stare, *Panic in the Pantry,* pp. 182–183, it is suggested not only that very low blood sugar is a rare event, but that hypoglycemia is not caused by starch and sugars like sucrose. For a discussion of hypoglycemia as a common problem, see Fredericks, *Psycho-Nutrition,* passim. For recent research pointing to various foods (in addition to refined sugar and other processed carbohydrates), chemicals, and inhalants as culprits in hypoglycemia, see Carl A. Hyland, "Down the Rocky Road to Hypoglycemia," *Let's Live,* September 1977, pp. 105, 107–109.

22 See, for instance, Ross Hume Hall, *Food for Nought: The Decline in Nutrition* (New York: Vintage Books, 1976), pp. 219–258; Carl C. Pfeiffer and the Publications Committee of the Brain Bio Center, *Mental and Elemental Nutrients: A Physician's Guide to Nutrition and Health Care* (New Canaan, Conn.: Keats Publishing, 1975), pp. 71–87; James Trager, *The Bellybook* (New York: Grossman Publishers, 1972), pp. 433–462; and Edward R. Pinckney and Cathey Pinckney, *The Cholesterol Controversy* (Los Angeles: Sherbourne Press, 1973).

23 Michael DeBakey, quoted in Richard A. Passwater, *Supernutrition* (New York: Pocket Books, 1976), p. 100.

24 George V. Mann, quoted in ibid., p. 105.

25 Hall, *Food for Nought,* pp. 228, 229.

26 "'Good' v. 'Bad' Cholesterol," *Time,* November 21, 1977, p. 119.

27 Hugh Trowell, letter in *American Journal of Clinical Nutrition* 28 (August 1975), p. 799.

28 For a detailed discussion, see Genell Subak-Sharpe, *The Natural High-Fiber Life Saving Diet* (New York: Grosset and Dunlap, 1976), esp. pp. 41–74; and D. P. Burkitt, A. R. P. Walker, and N. S. Painter, "Dietary Fiber and Disease," *Journal of the American Medical Association* 29 (August, 19, 1974), pp. 1068–1074.

|15| Nutrition as Preventive Medicine

CARL C. PFEIFFER and the
PUBLICATIONS COMMITTEE OF THE BRAIN BIO CENTER

Dr. Carl Pfeiffer and his clinical and research colleagues at the Brain Bio Center (Princeton, N.J.) are pioneers and leaders in the field of orthomolecular psychiatric research.

From *Mental and Elemental Nutrients: A Physician's Guide to Nutrition and Health Care*, by Carl C. Pfeiffer and the Publications Committee of the Brain Bio Center (New Canaan, Conn.: Keats Publishing, 1975). Copyright © 1975 by Carl Pfeiffer, Ph.D., M.D. Reprinted by permission.

The well-nourished American is a myth. Despite the high level of education and the abundance of available food, many people make poor food choices and are badly nourished. Advanced stages of vitamin deficiency diseases still occur in America. Scurvy, beriberi, pellagra, rickets, and other deficiency diseases are found in large city hospitals. Recent evidence has shown that these classic syndromes constitute only a small segment of the total results of malnutrition. Undiagnosed subclinical malnutrition of trace elements and protein may exist and subtly cause such significant physiological damage to body and brain as stunted growth, premature aging, and early death. Using nutrition as preventive medicine, we can check the destructive course of malnutrition.

MALNUTRITION—A PRESENT-DAY PROBLEM

Malnutrition (or bad nutrition) may afflict up to 80 percent of the nation's population, according to Drs. E. Cheraskin and W. M. Ringsdorf. National nutritional surveys have indicated that most people have low levels of one or more essential nutrients, relative to the traditionally recommended levels. A study at Jersey City Medical Center showed that 83 percent of patients admitted to the hospital have at least one vitamin deficiency and 68 percent have two or more deficiencies. Malnutrition is not new, yet many were shocked by the CBS documentary called "Hunger in America" and by *Hunger USA*, published [in 1968] by the Citizens' Board of Inquiry [into Hunger and Malnutrition in the United States].

What exactly is malnutrition? In the report "Malnutrition and Hunger in the United States," by the American Medical Association's Council on Foods and Nutrition, malnutrition was defined as:

a state of impaired functional ability or deficient structural integrity or development brought about by a discrepancy between the supply to the body tissues of essential nutrients and calories, and the biologic demand for them.

The etiology of malnutrition may be divided into two categories, primary and secondary. Primary malnutrition results from the faulty or inadequate

BASIC CAUSES OF MALNUTRITION

FOOD CROP FAILURE

Lack of water
Poisoned soil
Inadequate soil

Inadequate sun
Floods

MANURE FAILURE

Only nitrogen, potassium, and
  phosphate
No trace elements

Too much copper, phosphate, nitrate,
  selenium, acid, or alkali

POVERTY

Overpopulation with inadequate arable
  land
Farming ignorance
Wage-earner illness

Unemployment
Inadequate protein
Neglect of children

MEDICAL FACTORS

Diarrhea
Nausea
Operations
Parasites
Food allergy
Prematurity
Vitamin dependence
Chronic infection
Pregnancy
Lactation

Malabsorption
Crash diets
Bad eating habits
Medications
Individual variation
Infirmities
Vitamins *plus minerals*
Loss of taste
Cancer
Anorexia nervosa

intake of nutrients caused by faulty food selection, lack of money, poisoned and contaminated foods, insufficient soil nutrients, or food shortages. Secondary malnutrition is due to factors interfering with the ingestion, absorption, or utilization of essential nutrients, or to stress factors that increase their requirement, destruction, or excretion. (See list below for causes of malnutrition.) Primary and secondary malnutrition may exist together, and great care must be taken to separate and correct the interrelated factors for each individual.

IMPROPER FOOD STORAGE

Potato carcinogen
Wheat and peanut fungus

Bacterial growth

CONTAMINATED FOOD

Swordfish with mercury
Seed grain with organic mercury
Pigs with methyl mercury
Rice with cadmium

Wheat with selenium
Oils with antiknock
Ginger Jake paralysis
Milk with Tremitol

FOOD PROCESSING

Milling of grain that removes vitamins
  and trace elements
Boric acid
Technical mistakes
Flame-retardant chemical
Freezing (with chelators) that reduces
  trace elements in commercial green
  vegetables

Sterilization in cans—may remove
  vitamin C and pyridoxine (B-6)
Canning—adds tin and may add lead
  and cadmium to foods
Aluminum added to food in cooking—
  needs investigation by modern
  methods

POISONED WATER

Excess copper, cadmium, or lead with
  acid well water
Bacterial contaminated water

Inadequate calcium and magnesium to
  lime the pipes
Nitrates from surface drainage

Both primary and secondary malnutrition contribute to the disorders already discussed. . . .

Malnutrition is a very real and insidious problem, and the effects may be severe and lasting. Adequate nutrition is essential for proper and optimal growth. David Kallen, Ph.D., asserts that malnutrition during development leads to high infant mortality and smaller physical size. Severe malnutrition may lead to intellectual impairment. However, the relationship between moderate malnutrition and intelligence is still unclear. Winick had illustrated a critical period of the first six months of development in animals and in man, during which time cell division takes place and malnutrition will produce irreversible damage. The late Professor B. S. Platt, of London's School of Tropical Medicine, found that protein-calorie deficiency during pregnancy in dogs caused neurological dysfunction simulating that of central nervous system (CNS) damage in human infants. The negative effects of malnutrition on intellectual capacity and on physiological development result in reduction in growth rate, delayed physical maturation, and decreased learning ability.

Furthermore, a synergistic interrelationship exists between malnutrition and infectious disease, the two largest world health problems. Malnutrition results in loss of productivity, disease creates metabolic demands, and this cycle is further complicated by parasitic infestations. Infections may be associated with pregnancy and the post-partum (after birth) state and diabetes. Perinatal mortality is high: over 45 per 1,000 in 1972 for "staff" deliveries at Wayne State University School of Medicine in Detroit; over 40 per 1,000 for nonwhites in the entire state of North Carolina in 1972. Obviously, little help stems from monitoring mother and fetus during the last few days of pregnancy when both have suffered months of malnutrition. Pregnancy is a severe nutritional stress. Good nutrition should begin many years before pregnancy.

MALNUTRITION AND PREVENTIVE MEDICINE

These statistics show the need for preventive nutrition. A lifetime of better nutrition can contribute significantly to modifying the development of many diseases. According to Dr. Edith Weir, assistant director of the U.S. Department of Agriculture's human nutrition research division, diet has played an important role in recent decades in reducing the number of infant and maternal deaths and deaths from infectious diseases, especially among children, and in extending the productive life span and life expectancy. A team of scientists at the University of Alabama Medical Center believes that Americans suffer from varied ailments, insomnia to cancer, largely because of improper diet. Overweight is linked to heart disease, hypertension, rheumatic disease, and other conditions. Some specialists are of the opinion that better diet would result in reduced incidence of respiratory, infectious, and heart diseases. They project a 25 percent reduction of heart disease in people under 65 as a result of improved nutrition.

Because of human biochemical individuality, each person must find out which nutrients are individually needed; that is, some may need minimum attention to some vitamins or trace elements while others may need much attention to stay well. Many scientists, such as Dr. Roger Williams and his colleagues of the University of Texas, argue that because of individual variability in nutritional requirements, essentially no one can be fed adequately on an average American diet. Although this is far from proven, many people—some schizophrenics, drug addicts, alcoholics, and others on the upper end of the spectrum of biochemical need—have shown particular deficiencies in some nutrients.

Emphasis should be placed on a preventive approach to disease rather than on the role of diet in treating health problems after they develop. Most doctors and hospitals are not nutritionally oriented and rarely advise patients about dietary needs. Many physicians still state that three square meals a day is all anyone needs. Among them are the surgeons who believe their post-operative patient can live for five days on intravenous saline alone, and the obstetricians who tell the zinc- and B-6-deficient mother with nausea of early pregnancy to "eat later in the day but don't gain weight." Or the doctor who doesn't believe in vitamins or trace elements at all!

Nutrition receives little attention in the medical school curriculum, and most American physicians have not yet recognized that nutrition is an essential part of good medicine. Nutrition is a young science, and our present knowledge about human nutritional needs is limited, especially for conditions such as pregnancy and old age. The gaps in human nutritional knowledge aren't being filled fast enough. Some doctors now feel that nutrition should properly be a specialty within medicine, emphasizing biochemistry and clinical nutrition. (And we agree!)

Malnutrition may be prevalent among hospitalized patients. Despite sophisticated diagnostic procedures and drugs in hospitals, patients' nutritional status does not necessarily receive adequate attention. Basic principles of nutrition are being ignored in the care of hospitalized patients. Dr. Elizabeth Prevost, of the University of Alabama School of Medicine, has emphasized this point. Dr. Prevost conducted a study surveying the nutritional status of 100 medical surgical patients hospitalized for two weeks or more.

Very few test data or other basic information relating to general nutritional health (such as weight and height) were normally collected at the hospital. Dr. Prevost found that almost one-third of the patients had histories of nausea, decreased appetite, and weight loss, which are potential indicators of nutritional problems. Two-thirds of the patients who actually had been weighed lost weight while in the hospital. About half had low serum albumin levels (blood protein), but high-protein diets were prescribed for only about two-thirds of the patients with this condition. About one-third were anemic when admitted, and about one-fifth became anemic while staying at the hospital. Few tests were done to determine vitamin status, despite the known association of various conditions and drug therapies with vitamin depletion. Evidence of vitamin depletion was found in about one-quarter of the patients but no vitamin therapy had been prescribed. Dr. Prevost found further hospital procedures potentially detrimental to patient nutrition: withholding of meals, failure to observe food intake, and prolonged use of glucose infusions.

Further evidence for the slighting of nutritional needs by hospitals and doctors was offered by Dr. Charles E. Butterworth, Jr., director of the nutrition program at the University of Alabama, Birmingham, and chairman of the AMA's Council on Foods and Nutrition. He has charged that hospital diets are often inadequate to maintain health or, at times, so bad as to worsen health. From visits to several hospitals and an intensive study at one, he found surgery performed without first preparing the patient's internal environment for the stress, followed by oversight of adequate post-operative nutrition. Unfortunately, post-operative neglect led in some cases to advanced states of malnutrition and occasional death.

Furthermore, as the patient knows, hospital diets (as in other large institutions) are usually overcooked, stored in steam tables, unappetizing, flavorless, and not well varied. One patient is reported to have pushed back the dinner tray and asked for seconds on the intravenous drip! Obviously, the nutritional status and supervision of patients should be of utmost importance in hospital care. Unfortunately, most of our hospitals emphasize corrective, rather than preventive, medicine. Yet, many doctors are becoming aware of the essential importance of nutrition in medicine, as is indicated by the recent book *New Breed of Doctor* . . . by Alan Nittler.

Diet is important to virtually every facet of your life. Good nutrition is more than just avoiding bad health and disease, says Nicholas Johnson, of the Federal Communications Commission; it is one of the basic essentials to attain the more abundant life. As he said before the graduating class of the College of Arts and Sciences, American University, "Diet affects your physical appearance, your energy levels, your intellectual and creative abilities, your mental health and general feeling of well-being, even your ability to enjoy love and sexuality." Anthelme Brillat-Savarin, renowned writer on foods, said, "Tell me what you eat, and I will tell you what you are."

Learning and practicing intelligent nutritional habits and correct food combinations should be of primary concern, essential to physical, mental, and emotional health. We believe that nutrition education should begin early in schools to equip youngsters with some knowledge of what they eat and why they eat it. The brain is composed, as is the rest of the body, of cells which must be nourished by nutrient biochemicals to function properly. Malnutrition may result in impaired brain function. Logically, mental illness may be best prevented by vitamins, minerals, and other nutrients. George Watson, author of *Nutrition and Your Mind,* says that in most cases there is no motivation for abnormal behavior (as psychotherapy would have it), that this behavior is a result of an undernourished brain, an exhausted nervous system, or any of a number of other physical problems directly related to imperfect mind function. Strong psychological stress or sudden shock can exhaust tissues of certain chemicals necessary for normal functioning. If your senses play tricks on you, if you hear or see things you know aren't there, you are probably suffering from a vitamin deficiency, a block in utilization in your body, or an increased need for some nutrient. Simple insomnia can precipitate these symptoms and biochemical imbalance. This somatic base of mental disease has traditionally been neglected. The importance of malnutrition as a major cause of mental illness is now being more widely recognized and accepted.

Poor dietary habits often stem from emotional disturbances and follow back to them. Poor nutrition can be at the root of behavior which perfectly imitates that of neurotic or psychotic, sometimes with no overt physical evidence of nutritional deficiency. An example is pellagra or subclinical pellagra, the disease resulting from a deficiency of niacin, whose mental symptoms mimic those of schizophrenia. Pellagra is a vitamin *deficiency* condition, while some mental illnesses are vitamin *dependency* conditions. Pellagrins can relieve their disease promptly by small quantities of niacin, while those with certain types of mental disorders, notably schizophrenics, must remain on higher quantities of nutrients due to a greater need for those nutrients.

A study conducted by Irene Payne, Ph.D., and Mildred M. Hudson on the dietary histories and actual three-day eating habits of forty-nine first-admission mental hospital patients revealed nutrient deficiencies similar to those of other groups in the U.S. Why did these people become mentally ill and not others? The RDR [recommended daily requirements] of nutrients used to judge the adequacy of intake may not apply to mental patients, who may have increased the needs. The individual's requirements vary greatly, much more so than is traditionally believed. Individual differences must be taken into account in the treatment of emotional and mental disorders.

We know that by altering man's physical state in very slight ways, emotional and mental responses are altered. This can be seen in everyday life. This is also evident in the working of drugs. Nutrients work to correct a biochemical imbalance usually more slowly than drugs, although some vitamins, such as inositol, have drug-like action. Drugs can have unpleasant and sometimes damaging side effects, whereas nutrients are safer and cheaper. Wherever possible in medicine, nutrients should be used as the first choice; however, this does not obviate the use of drugs when needed.

Proper nutrition and nutrient therapy have helped many schizophrenics, some of whom have been given up as hopeless after both drug and psychotherapy treatments. Learning problems, senility, alcoholism, and suicidal tendencies have been affected. The psychological state of healthy individuals has also been improved on nutritional therapy. Some nervous and physical disorders do require more than proper nutrition, but the regenerative powers of the body, and mind, and emotions are greatly enhanced by proper nutrition. However, nutrient therapy does not work for everyone; for some it may be unnecessary. Self-treatment could be dangerous or even fatal. Some nutrients become toxic at high levels; and what is needed by one person may be too much for another. We stress that the patient should not attempt self-diagnosis; proper clinical biochemical testing may be needed.

Biochemical treatment, or orthomolecular medicine, is the correction of faulty biochemistry. Linus Pauling coined the term "Orthomolecular Medicine," which involves the provision of the proper quantities of nutrients for the individual, not huge mega or pharmacologic doses. Pauling defines Orthomolecular Medicine as:

the preservation of good health and the prevention and treatment of disease by varying the concentrations in the human body of the molecules of substances that are normally present, many of them required for life, such as the vitamins, essential amino acids, essential fats, and minerals.

He states that in two years of experience with more than 1,000 schizophrenics, 60 percent treated with megavitamins either improved considerably or had complete relief of symptoms. Now, after further experience and research, higher recovery rates are obtained. The Canadian Schizophrenia Foundation found an 85 percent recovery rate using the original megavitamin therapy. Here at the Brain Bio Center . . . the estimated improvement rate is 90 percent using the biochemical approach. These figures are relative to a 35 percent complete spontaneous recovery rate, and an approximate 50 percent recovery rate for other more traditional therapies such as psychotherapy (however, this 50 percent may include the masked 35 percent of spontaneous recovery).

The North Nassau Mental Health Center compared its five years of experience using the orthomolecular approach with its previous five years using traditional psychiatric approaches. They found the orthomolecular approach to be more effective, shorter in duration, and cheaper. Also, the orthomolecular approach required less professional manpower and allowed the treatment of more patients with greater efficiency.

Dr. John Blass, physician and biochemist at the Neuropsychiatric Institute at UCLA, believes that megavitamins are a useful treatment which will eventually benefit 20 million Americans. The combination of good natural foods plus the correct nutritional supplements could eliminate most of the mental health problems (as well as physical illness) and is inexpensive when compared to drugs and doctor bills. Pauling pointedly states:

A psychiatrist who refuses to try the methods of Orthomolecular Psychiatry (nutrition as related to mental health) in addition to his usual therapy in the treatment of his patients is failing in his duty as a physician.

References

American nutrition: ignorance in abundance. *Med. World News* p. 6, 5 January 1973.
Brewer, T. Total blackout on role of malnutrition. *Medicine.* 24 October 1973.
Deadly hospital food? *Time,* 22 July 1974.

Hawkins, D. R., and Pauling L. (eds.). *Orthomolecular Psychiatry*. San Francisco: W. H. Freeman, 1973. [Added by editor.]

Kallen, D. J. Nutrition and society. *JAMA* 215:1:94, 1971.

Moser, R. Mango malnutrition déjà vu. *Med. Opin.* p. 72, November 1971.

National nutrition. *Science* 183: 1062, 1974.

Nittler, A. *A new breed of doctor*. New York: Pyramid Publications, 1974.

Nutrition held overlooked in care of patients in hospitals. *Intern. Med. News*, 1 July 1974.

Pauling, L. *Vitamin C and the Common Cold*. San Francisco: W. H. Freeman, 1970. [Added by editor.]

Payne, I., and Hudson, M. Dietary intakes of mental patients. *AJPH* 62:9:120, 1972.

Sackler, A. One man . . . and medicine: is nothing known? *Med. Trib.* 10 July 1974.

VITAMIN AND MINERAL SUPPLEMENTS

| 16 | ## Nutrition Medicine: A Vitamin and Mineral Program

ROBERT C. ATKINS and SHIRLEY LINDE

Robert C. Atkins, M.D., is author of the best-selling and controversial *Dr. Atkins' Diet Revolution: The High Calorie Way to Stay
Thin Forever.* He has his own radio program, "The Diet Revolution and You," has been featured on dozens of radio and
television shows and in many magazines, and is a frequent
lecturer on metabolism and nutrition at medical meetings and
conventions. Shirley Linde is an award-winning medical author
with a dozen books and hundreds of magazine and newspaper
features among her credits. Her recent books include *Sickle
Cell: A Complete Guide; The Complete Allergy Guide;* and
The Sleep Book.

Taken from *Dr. Atkins' Superenergy Diet* by Robert C. Atkins
and Shirley Linde. Copyright © 1977 Robert C. Atkins, M.D.
and Shirley Linde. Used by permission of Crown Publishers,
Inc. (References have been omitted.)

... In newspapers and magazines you have been ex-
posed to a bewildering barrage of claims about the benefits of vitamin
therapy and counterclaims that we don't need any surplus vitamins at all.
The counterclaimers seem to be more numerous; so most people, hearing
the frequent statements that vitamins aren't necessary, don't even try them.

One of the questions I ask new patients is whether they take vitamins
and, if so, which ones. The majority either take no vitamins regularly or

follow regimens which are woefully inadequate in several major nutrients. When these dietary histories are cross-indexed with existing medical problems it shows that *those who need vitamins most are the ones least likely to be taking them.*

. . . What about studies showing that certain vitamins don't work? To a person with a nutritional background, these studies seem incredibly naive. Usually they involve administering a vitamin just as a drug is given—merely giving it alone. No other nutrients except the one in question are given, and no attention is paid to the patient's diet. But vitamins can work only as part of a nutritional team. They cannot work alone. Nor can vitamins work against the obstacle of an improper diet. For example, vitamin therapy cannot work when an underlying hypoglycemia is not controlled. This could be the hidden factor in whatever studies with vitamins have shown negative results. The studies did not disprove the value of vitamins, but only proved that in addition to the vitamin supplements, the diet also needed to be modified to make it possible for those vitamins to be effective. . . .

An example is the scathing attack by the American Psychiatric Association upon niacinamide therapy for schizophrenia after a series of studies showed that this remarkable vitamin, *when used alone without a dietary change,* had very little effect on most mental disease patients. The Association ignored the studies in which the vitamin was used successfully in conjunction with dietary improvements. . . .

Vitamins, even when they are desperately needed, when used without the proper diet, rarely produce much tangible benefit. . . .

Vitamins were first discovered, in a way similar to bacteria, as a result of the "one cause—one cure" theory. Scurvy, beriberi, pellagra were caused by deficiencies of certain vitamins. Thus developed the corollary concept: if the absence of a vitamin does not cause a disease, then that vitamin is not required. . . .

Further confusion arises from failure to recognize that a vitamin can have more than one use, and that a biological function can be served by more than one vitamin. . . .

. . . Those who say that we get enough vitamins and minerals in our everyday diet don't take into account that so many things in our modern-day life destroy the vitamins and minerals that we should be getting: the processing and storing of foods; the vitamin-stripping refining of flour and sugar; "TV-dinners" that mean you cook food twice, increasing vitamin loss; additives that prevent the absorption of nutrients so your body can't even use them when they are there. Increased intake of polyunsaturated fats can produce vitamin E deficiency. Cigarette smoking destroys vitamin C. Many medicines cause vitamin deficiencies. Antibiotics change normal intestinal bacteria which ordinarily synthesize certain vitamins. Diuretics can wash out potassium, sodium, and other minerals. Environmental pollutants increase the need for vitamins C and E. And our soil is depleted of certain key trace minerals. All this translates into deficiencies in our diet that weren't there in "the good old days."

. . . [In addition], our metabolic responses vary greatly, and so do our needs for vitamins and minerals. The activity of certain enzymes has been found to differ by as much as fifty times from one person to another.

The needs for vitamins differ just as greatly. What is a satisfactory amount for one person may not be nearly enough to supply the body needs of another.

As we study specific vitamins and minerals, we find example after example of ways in which dosages above those recommended by the FDA play a role in nutrition medicine. (Nutrition medicine is the diagnosis, treatment, and prevention of disease with nutrition techniques: vitamins, minerals, and a change in diet.)

We'll discuss the vitamins and minerals in the following sequence: first the water-soluble vitamins, C and the B's; then the fat-soluble vitamins, E, A, D, and K; and then the minerals and other nutrients.

VITAMIN C

The need for extra vitamin C in man is quite logical. Most animals have the enzymes to synthesize their own vitamin C. Man and apes do not. The animals that do manufacture vitamin C seem to produce it in quantities at the tissue saturation level. This led Dr. Irving Stone and Dr. Linus Pauling to speculate that the proper dose for man would be in the 2,000 mg. or more range, and led to their recommendations of vitamin C in high doses to treat colds. . . .

Will vitamin C help in other illnesses? There is evidence that it will. The latest report from Japan shows that in doses of 3 to 6 grams daily it is effective in preventing viral hepatitis. In test tubes it has been shown to inactivate viruses of poliomyelitis, herpes simplex, and rabies. . . .

Vitamin C has long been recognized as essential to the formation of the connective tissue called collagen. In this role, it protects the gums from bleeding and the blood vessels from easy bruising, and it improves the healing of wounds.

As a detoxifying agent it has been found useful to treat several kinds of poisoning. It also helps remove accumulations of toxic heavy metals, copper, lead, and mercury, and has even prolonged life in terminal cancer patients.

... Vitamin C also seems to neutralize some of the effects of cigarette smoking. One estimate is that one cigarette uses up 25 mg. of vitamin C. A heavy smoker who does not take supplements of vitamin C will be deficient in that vitamin. A one-pack-a-day smoker must take 1 to 3 grams of ascorbic acid to maintain blood levels of that vitamin.

. Vitamin C is an integral part of the anti-schizophrenia program of orthomolecular psychiatry. When a very large dose of vitamin C is given to schizophrenic patients, they do not excrete the extra vitamin C as completely as do normal people. Their tissues take it up to correct the deficiency state, as much as 3 to 40 grams being necessary to cause spillage in the urine. With vitamin C there is usually a significant improvement in the impaired perception that characterizes schizophrenia.

... Like so many other nutrients, vitamin C is developing quite a track record in reducing serum cholesterol and triglycerides. At the Institute of Human Research in Czechoslovakia, Dr. Emil Ginter gave vitamin C daily to middle-aged men and women and found that in those with high serum cholesterol readings the cholesterol dropped; triglyceride values decreased to almost one-half their previous level.

Many studies have confirmed the beneficial effect of vitamin C in atherosclerosis. Its effectiveness may be due to the fact that it is essential for the conversion of cholesterol into bile, which can be excreted. Or it may be effective because it increases the concentration of substances called chondroitin-4-sulfates, as Dr. Anthony Verangieri of Rutgers University has demonstrated. These same substances have been used experimentally to treat coronary atherosclerosis and were reported to produce an 80 percent decrease in the death rate.

... The need for vitamin C is increased during and following serious illnesses, injury, intestinal bleeding, burns, or surgery; and in severe burns or extensive surface injuries vitamin C levels may fall rapidly to zero. Wound problems occurred eight times more often in patients with vitamin C deficiencies than in those with adequate vitamin levels. Giving vitamin C shortens convalescence time.

Dr. Richard Passwater, author of *Supernutrition,* postulates that vitamin C can protect us against carcinogens (cancer-inducing chemicals). He has been able experimentally to reduce the incidence of carcinogen-induced cancers in mice by 90 percent if he simultaneously administers vitamins C and E, plus the trace mineral selenium. And Tulane urologist Dr. Jorgen E. Schlegel has been using vitamin C effectively to prevent recurrences of bladder cancer. Vitamin C can also prevent the formation of nitrosamine, the cancer-causing chemical our body produces after we eat foods preserved in nitrates, such as bacon. . . .

In my own experience, vitamin C has served as a fatigue fighter, fatigue tending to reappear whenever a patient has neglected to take his usual dose. I also find it useful sometimes in the treatment of allergic conditions such as asthma and hay fever.

THE B COMPLEX

B₃ (niacin) . . . Orthomolecular medicine, the medical treatment of the future, began quietly. Drs. Abram Hoffer and Humphrey Osmond in Saskatchewan, Canada, could not shake from their minds the similarity between the psychosis of pellagra, the niacin-deficiency disease, and schizophrenia. In 1952, they treated their first schizophrenic patient with vitamin B_3 and . . . their results were dramatically successful. . . . The two pioneers persisted, learned the efficacy of this vitamin, then of other vitamins given in conjunction, first in schizophrenia, then in other psychiatric problems. They enlisted the interest of a few other psychiatrists, then a few more, who in turn performed other studies, all expanding upon the role of vitamin therapy in a variety of conditions. In 1968, Linus Pauling coined the term "orthomolecular psychiatry," and later he and Dr. David Hawkins coedited a book with that name, a landmark for the new science. . . .

Niacin was the cornerstone of this movement based on megavitamin therapy. It was administered in doses of 3 to 20 grams, which is 150 to 1,000 times greater than the 20 mg. RDA. . . .

B_3 has also been used to help smokers reduce their dependency on nicotine, to allow reduced dosages of tranquilizers, and even to help some arthritic conditions. . . . This fatigue-fighting vitamin also raises the blood sugar levels in the hypoglycemic person. In addition, dietary sugar consumes niacinamide, thus increasing its requirements. . . .

There are a few precautions. Large doses of niacin can produce an uncomfortable warm itchy "flush" [within] an hour after taking it. Niacinamide avoids this, but occasionally worsens a depression. Peptic ulcer, hyperacidity, and diabetes can be aggravated. An occasional patient may experience headache or nausea.* In all these cases, the dosage should be reduced. . . .

Vitamin B₆. Pyridoxine—B_6—has long been known by the megavitamin therapists to be one of the most effective agents in their arsenal. And for me, it has been one of the most important additions in the fight for Superenergy.

There are reasons for this. First, the pyridoxal structure governs dozens of chemical reactions, especially those involved in the metabolism of protein. Second, deficiencies are widespread because B_6 is removed from flour in the milling process, but is *not* included in the mandatory enrichment program. To make matters worse, there are many best-selling vitamin preparations almost fraudulently labeled "high potency" which are very low in B_6 content, some containing less than one milligram. In addition, B_6 is easily destroyed by cooking, food processing, and refining. Its level is lowered by The Pill and by the estrogens used to treat menopause. It is wrong to stay on those medications without significant B_6 supplements.

Pyridoxine has been used to treat nausea (including that which follows surgery), edema, toxemia in pregnancy, and premenstrual edema, and it is perhaps the most useful vitamin-diuretic; I have confirmed its ability to combat water retention many times, circumventing the need for diuretic medicines.

Pyridoxine plays an important role in fat and cholesterol metabolism. It can correct a common type of nutritional anemia. It is used to prevent kidney stones. Dr. Platon J. Collipp and his associates showed it can improve asthmatic children significantly. . . .

Scientific papers have also been written describing its use in Parkinsonism, peripheral neuritis, acne, psoriasis, hair loss, ulcers, [childhood epilepsy], and a variety of psychiatric problems. . . .

Vitamin B₁—thiamine. This was the first B vitamin discovered, being isolated in 1911 from the rice polishings that prevent beriberi. It is essential to the functioning of the central nervous system. When it is deficient, there can be numbness in the arms and legs, or a tingling or burning sensation. Powers of concentration, memory, mood, and perception may be affected. Fatigue and depression can be caused.

---

*EDITOR'S NOTE: Niacin can sometimes *alleviate* a migraine headache if taken at the very first symptoms. The procedure here is to take a 50-mg. tablet of niacin immediately. If a flush ensues within 10 minutes, the dose is sufficient to relieve the constricted cerebral blood vessels and end the pain. If there is no flush, a tablet can be taken every 10 minutes until a flush is produced.

Like other B vitamins, thiamine is lost in the milling of wheat or the polishing of rice. And thiamine requirements are much higher among people who consume sugar or significant amounts of alcohol. The government's RDAs fail to take this into account.

Five hundred to 2,000 mg. daily will provide the key to fatigue problems in some patients.

Deficiencies of thiamine are somewhat less prevalent than others of the B complex, probably because thiamine is included in the enrichment program and stressed in multiple vitamin preparations, but it has been used to treat hundreds of conditions and must be included in any program involving the B complex.

Vitamin B_2—riboflavin. Cracking and inflammation at the edges of the lips, a reddened inflamed tongue, and bloodshot, burning, tearing, and light-sensitive eyes are signs of B_2 deficiency.

Riboflavin levels were found to be low in the plasma of many rheumatoid arthritis patients. Another study links B_2 deficiency to mental depression, and recent work suggests it may play a role in the prevention and cure of cataracts.

B_2 is replaced in enrichment programs and has not been widely used in megavitamin regimens.

It should, of course, be included in quantities proprotionate to the B_1 and the rest of the B complex.

. . . *Pantothenic acid.* This B vitamin has a key role in energy metabolism because it is part of coenzyme A which helps form the most pivotal of all metabolic compounds—acetyl coenzyme A. Acetyl Co A, as it is called, is the common end point of the metabolism of protein, fat, and carbohydrate, and it can break down to form energy or can be used to manufacture cholesterol, the steroid or sex hormones, or antibodies.

Pantothenic acid. . . is used in megavitamin therapy and has been safe at any dose tried up to this point.

Pantothenic acid is a biochemical precursor of the adrenal hormones and is found in great quantities within the adrenal gland tissues, so nutrition pioneers have tried it in those conditions where adrenal hormone therapies might be used—arthritis, allergies, asthma, stress reactions, and hypo-glycemia. . . . I have confirmed all of these applications in numerous patients; it is safer than cortisone or other steroids and should be tried first, reserving the stronger therapy for those cases where pantothenic acid (and the other vitamins that must accompany it) does not do the trick. Dosages must be in the 500—1500 mg. range. Note that when given in the form of calcium pantothenate, it can induce drowsiness. This quality can make it valuable as a "sleep" vitamin.

Inositol. This is a B vitamin which I personally have found to be invaluable. No one has yet proved any clearcut deficiency state and so the FDA carries it under the heading "Need in human nutrition has not been established."

But inositol is one of those nutrients that is lost when whole wheat, which was its major source, is refined into flour, some 87 percent of it being lost in the process; and it is not restored through enrichment.

Inositol is a constituent of an important class of body chemicals called phospholipids, which are important in atherosclerosis prevention and in brain metabolism. Both cholesterol and total lipid levels have been reduced by giving 3 grams of inositol daily to older patients.

Inositol's effect on the brain is similar to that of a moderate-to-mild tranquilizer-sedative. Dr. [Carl] Pfeiffer finds 2,000 mg. per day to be an effective treatment for high blood pressure. I have found 2,000 mg. of inositol taken at bedtime to be a remarkable sleeping medication in many patients; and 650 mg. makes an effective daytime sedative. And how much safer it is than sleeping pills!

Choline. This B vitamin is a provider of the methyl group which is needed for an endless variety of biochemical reactions, but it is not essential because other nutrients—methionine, betaine, vitamin B_{15}, folic acid, and B_{12}—can serve the same function. However, all these nutrients are often in short supply and methyl groups must be provided through some means. . . .

Biotin. Like the rest of the B complex, biotin serves as a coenzyme for a large number of enzymes. Eating too many raw egg whites will destroy biotin. But biotin is readily made by intestinal bacteria; and so little is needed that deficiencies are unlikely.

PABA. Para-aminobenzoic acid plays several roles in the body, and for a very high number of my patients is a key to Superenergy. . . .

In a Soviet study, 450 mg. of PABA was shown to lower cholesterol in one-half of the patients tested.

PABA is known to act as an effective sun protectant. It has been used with benefit in a variety of skin conditions. I have found it to be dramatically effective in some of my patients with bone and joint disorders.

Since a 1941 study by Dr. Benjamin Sieve, several studies report that PABA is effective against graying of the hair, but the majority opinion is that PABA is not effective in combating gray hair. . . .

Folic acid—a key to vitamin therapy. How often have you heard people say: "I've taken a lot of vitamins, but I don't feel any better"? The . . . majority of those people for whom vitamin therapy does not seem to work either do not follow a careful enough *diet* along with their vitamins, or have a vitamin regimen that does not contain enough folic acid.

Folic acid deficiencies are widespread. The Ten-State Survey [a 1968–1970 government survey] showed low levels of folate in the red blood cells, a rather far advanced deficiency finding, in over half the population of Michigan. A Canada survey found it to be the single most prevalent deficiency among the nutrients tested.

The reasons for folate deficiencies are clear. Folic acid is easily destroyed by cooking or canning; 50 to 95 percent may be destroyed by these processes. Alcohol intake interferes with its use also. Alcoholics, in fact, are almost all severely deficient in folic acid. They cannot absorb it or vitamin B_1 or B_6 from food even a week after they stop drinking.

The Pill, as well as estrogen and pregnancy, causes a major loss of folic acid. Vitamin C increases urinary excretion of folic acid and therefore the body's demands increase. . . .

The FDA has placed an exceedingly low restriction on the folic acid content of multivitamin pills—just one-tenth of a milligram—and reduced the largest dose available with a doctor's prescription to just one milligram. Contrast this with the Canadian regulations, which quite properly allow for the over-the-counter sale of a 5 mg. preparation.

Nature put folic acid in the B complex, but the FDA took it out.

Folic deficiency is a well-known cause of megaloblastic anemia, but the earlier stages are much more prevalent than the late anemic stage. According to folic acid expert Dr. Victor Herbert, the symptoms may include irritability, forgetfulness, weakness, tiredness, diarrhea, headache, palpitations, and shortness of breath. To this list Dr. Carl Pfeiffer adds: agitation, moodiness, depression, delusions, hallucinations, and paranoia. I will personally confirm its great value in correcting these symptoms, and add one more— the decreased sex drive seen in heavy drinkers. One alcoholic relabeled it "frolic acid."

It should be given with caution in patients with seizure disorders, and always with vitamin B_{12}. Not all patients feel better in high doses of folic acid. Some will feel worse. I'm sure this correlates with Dr. Pfeiffer's work showing that many patients have low levels of histamine, which is raised to normal with folic acid. However, a small number of patients have histamine levels which are too high, and they get worse on folic acid.

Vitamin B_{12}. May the Lord forgive me for all the times in my early career when I thought that doctors who gave their patients B_{12} shots were quacks. I have since learned how often that type of therapy works as a fatigue fighter.

Much of what was said about folic acid can be said about B_{12}. It, too, is corrective of an anemia, pernicious anemia. But all too often the thinking of the medical profession goes sometimes like this. "B_{12} is used in the treatment of pernicious anemia, so using it for any other condition is quackery." Scientifically nothing could be further from the truth.

B_{12}, the cobalt-containing vitamin, is part of a coenzyme involved in the metabolism of proteins, fats, and carbohydrates. It is involved in the formation of the sheaths of nerve fibers and its deficiency produces a well-recognized form of neuritis. Poor growth, a sore tongue, and most of the symptoms of folate deficiency are seen in B_{12} deficiency.

B_{12} is sometimes difficult to absorb when taken by mouth. Therefore, it is customarily given by injection.

Actually, it is not easy to become *deficient* in B_{12} because it is stored rather well in the body. However, it is not readily available in vegetable foods, being found mainly in animal protein foods, and vegetarians often have a B_{12} deficiency. B_{12} is lost in women on The Pill, people taking . . . the drug dilantin, or those who consume alcohol in large quantities.

Pangamic acid—vitamin B_{15}. This vitamin is recognized in many nations, but not in the United States, even though it was discovered by an American, Dr. Ernst T. Krebs, Jr.

Pangamic acid, an important methyl donor, is used widely in Russia. During a 1964 Moscow symposium, thirty-four papers were read, all indicating a consistently reproducible benefit in heart disease. B_{15} tends to lower the cholesterol level and provides oxygenation to the heart muscle. It is valuable in combating alcoholism and alcohol intoxication. It reduces sugar levels in mild diabetes. And all without side effects. . . .

The distressing fact is that even though this international meeting was held in 1964, no one in the United States has picked up this valuable lead and evaluated it. The fact that the best of Soviet cardiologists participated in these studies involving more than one thousand patients has apparently not created a dent in American medicine.

I have used this remarkable vitamin, and there is no doubt in my mind that it works extremely well and should be allowed to take its place with the other members of the B complex.

Vitamin B_{17}—also called amygdalin or laetrile. This vitamin too was developed by Dr. Krebs, being extractable from seeds of many fruits, especially the apricot kernel. It seems to be a good treatment for sickle cell anemia.

Laetrile is the center of a furor over the fact that it has been used in over twenty-thousand cancer victims as a palliative. It is quite legal in at least twenty-three medically sophisticated nations.* Among many researchers, Dr. Hans Nieper of Hannover, West Germany, and Ernesto Contreras of Tijuana, Mexico, have reported many successes with a combination of non-toxic cancer chemotherapy based in part upon this vitamin's effect on the dividing cancer cell.

The closed-mindedness directed against this vitamin, which seems to prolong life, or at least relieve suffering, in otherwise hopeless cancer patients, will surely go down as one of the blackest pages in our medical history. . . .

The pertinence of this discussion in this context is not to tell you that B_{17} fights cancer or that it's good for your fatigue, but to show you the extent to which some medical leaders will go to suppress medical advances. . . .

THE FAT-SOLUBLE VITAMINS

The fat-soluble vitamins pose a problem that does not have to be faced with vitamins B and C; namely, they can accumulate in the body. In this group, overdosage can be a problem.

Vitamin E—tocopherol. In no case are the battle lines against vitamins more clearly drawn than in the case of vitamin E. Doctors think it's either worthless or the greatest.

I'm in the latter group . . . I think vitamin E can be of extreme value. It is one of the nutrients removed from wheat and not replaced; accordingly, the national intake is rather low, and deficiencies are quite possible.

Vitamin E seems to have a beneficial effect on wound-healing and scar formations. Widely heralded as treatment for heart disease, its use to diminish the cardiac pain called angina pectoris has proved "mixed reviews." But doctors have found benefit in peripheral artery disease, in easing pain of blood vessel spasms, and in preventing blood clots after surgery.

---

*EDITOR'S NOTE: In 1977, laetrile became legal in 12 states in this country and was being given proper clinical testing. As this book goes to press, new reports on its cancer-fighting propensities are negative. Incidentally, laetrile hardly qualifies as a vitamin: there is no indication that it is essential for any body function, and sources of laetrile are uncommon in the diets of most of the world's people.

It has also been successful in treating hemolytic anemia, chronic cysts in women's breasts, leg cramps that occur at night, and various skin conditions.

Also heralded as a sex vitamin, it occasionally will improve male impotence. And I have confirmed in hundreds of patients that it effectively combats the distressing hot flushes of the menopause. When vitamin E is given early in the menopause, the menstrual cycle frequently returns and endometrial smears indicate a higher degree of estrogen activity.

I am convinced, too, of the usefulness of vitamin E in preventing some pregnancy complications, such as repeated miscarriages. It also combats the toxic effects of industrial pollutants, cigarette smoke, and polyunsaturated fatty acids.

There are many complex biochemical reasons that vitamin E might ultimately prove to help slow the aging process, one reason why I make sure to take at least 800 units daily. . . .

Vitamin E should be used with caution if you have a tendency to high blood pressure or a history of rheumatic fever. But very little in the way of vitamin E toxicity has been reported even in large groups of subjects taking more than 2,000 units daily. If one starts with 200 units and gradually builds to 600 to 1,200 units, most toxicity problems are avoided.

Vitamin A. The chances of your having a vitamin A deficiency are fairly great. . . .

Vitamin A is essential to normal growth and to the health of the mucous membranes and skin. It is necessary to prevent night blindness. In this regard its dosage can be regulated with a do-it-yourself test. If you drive at night with oncoming traffic and can't distinguish the dividing line in your lane, it means you have night blindness and you need more vitamin A.

You should also suspect a vitamin A deficiency if you develop boils, acne, dryness, flakiness, skin rashes, itchy eyes, dry and brittle hair, loss of appetite, or increased susceptibility to infections.

In intriguing recent developments, vitamin A has been shown to have cancer-inhibiting effects in some animal tumors. It seems to protect body tissue against infection also; and at a recent American Chemical Society meeting, Dr. Eli Seifter of New York described it as a powerful agent against viruses, greatly enhancing the body's immune response. . . .

Since vitamin A increases the lubrication of mucous membranes, it is of benefit to such diverse problems as irritation from contact lenses and dryness of vaginal membranes in intercourse.

Despite all the publicity about dangers of vitamin A, there are only are only a few recorded cases of persons who took too much vitamin A and suffered distress, and these were people who had taken huge doses of 100,000 and 600,000 units a day for months or years before they had reactions. Overdose is, of course, to be avoided, but don't avoid taking supplements because of false fears.

The general rule: any time it's necessary to go over 10,000 units a day it should be done only under a physician's care.

Vitamin D. This vitamin can be considered a hormone. It regulates the metabolism of calcium and phosphorus. Too much is as bad as too little. Please avoid the pitfalls of too many amateur vitamin-takers—*don't* take three or more D-containing multivitamin pills daily without being aware of the risk.

Vitamin K. This is a clotting factor which can be risky in large doses; therefore it is rarely included in multiple vitamin preparations. It is plentiful in a diet consisting of dark green leafy vegetables, liver, and egg yolk.

MINERALS

. . . There are several groupings of minerals necessary to human nutrition. The soluble minerals, which are essential to life at the cellular level, include sodium, potassium, and chlorine. Then there are the minerals which are part of our bones: calcium, magnesium, and phosphorus. There are the other essential microminerals: iron, iodine, and sulfur. The rest are trace minerals—needed in only small amounts by the body, but vitally needed; they *must* be provided for the body to function because they cannot be synthesized.

Sodium, potassium, chlorine. Since these are present in all foods, it is virtually impossible to have a deficiency of these elements under ordinary circumstances. But shortages can occur with prolonged vomiting or diarrhea, sunstroke, burns, dehydration, kidney disease, hormonal imbalances, diuretic therapy, or sometimes when salt restriction used in the management of blood pressure or water retention is too effective. . . .

Potassium losses may occur in very strict effective diets such as fasting, or a low-carbohydrate diet in someone with low potassium reserves, so dieting can be a risk if done in conjunction with diuretics or sodium and potassium restriction.

Calcium—the body's most abundant element. We need approximately 1,000 mg. of calcium per day. If our diet is deficient in it, the body will rob the calcium out of the bones, and osteoporosis (porous bones) will result.

According to the U.S. Department of Agriculture's survey, three out of every ten families showed calcium intakes below the recommended minimum.

Milk is the best source of calcium. But for those who must avoid milk because of lactose intolerance or because they must adhere to a low-carbohydrate diet, cheese, particularly the harder kinds, can provide the minimum requirement with just four ounces . . .

Calcium, like cholesterol, is one of the substances found in the lining of the arteries in arteriosclerotic patches. This does not mean that calcium *causes* arteriosclerosis. Nonetheless, the removal of this calcium provides the basis of a very effective means of treatment, called chelation. Excessive calcium can cause tetany (spastic muscles) and kidney stones.

Magnesium. Like calcium, magnesium is involved in the structure of bone and the transmission of nerve and muscle impulses. Magnesium, in addition, plays a key role in enzymatic reactions used to provide energy.

And magnesium *can* be deficient. Those who avoid nuts, seeds, and dark green vegetables and those who drink heavily run a good risk of being magnesium deficient. So, too, is magnesium deficiency a possible consequence of long-term diuretic usage, malabsorption, intravenous feedings, or kidney or liver disease. High sugar intake has been implicated as a cause of magnesium loss, and 85 percent of the magnesium content of wheat is removed by milling it to flour. Levels are lowered further if you use estrogen pills, or have high intakes of vitamin D or fat.

Magnesium is essential for vitamins to be absorbed properly. Marginal deficiencies of magnesium can lead to atherosclerosis, depression, irritability, restlessness, convulsions, dizziness, muscle weakness, high blood pressure, sweating, painful cold hands and feet, and upsets in heart rhythm.

A proper amount of magnesium is tremendously important for a healthy heart, and death from heart attack is much less prevalent among people who live where there is hard water which has more magnesium. The death rate goes up if hard water is softened.

Dr. Roger Williams cites experiments showing that magnesium protects rats from atherosclerosis and brings about dramatic improvements in patients with angina. Excellent results are reported in South America, Europe, and Great Britain, where magnesium is used in treating angina and even in treating patients during heart attack where it is injected immediately, followed by regular injections during the entire recovery period, to improve the rate of survival.

Note: It is important for the magnesium you take to be balanced with calcium, about one part magnesium to two parts calcium, a proportion found in the naturally occurring mineral called dolomite, an excellent supplement. Many mineral supplements have the proper 1 to 2 balance.

Phosphorus. In the form of phosphate, phosphorus is essential in the chemical reactions involved with the liberation of energy fuel.

Phosphates should be in a balance with calcium, and this is regulated by the parathyroid hormone and by vitamin D. High-protein food, except for cheeses, tend to be high in phosphorus, but low in calcium, so a calcium supplement is recommended in conjunction with most diets. . . .

Sulfur. This mineral exists as a sulfate or sulfhydryl molecule of the structure of the important sulfur-containing amino acids. Nutritional deficiencies of sulfur are not known to occur, but the sulfur-containing amino acids are quite essential to nutrition, and eggs provide one of the best sources.

Iron—the most important of the microminerals. Iron is essential to the formation of hemoglobin, which carries the oxygen in red blood cells. Iron has been well promoted as a dietary supplement, yet deficiencies are quite common.

Fatigue frequently is caused by iron-deficiency anemia, either when dietary intake of iron is inadequate or when there is a chronic loss of blood such as from heavy menstrual periods or from a silently bleeding ulcer.

Common symptoms of iron deficiency are: weakness, depression, dizziness, and fatigue.

It is difficult to get enough iron in food. Even the Food and Nutrition Board notes that the RDAs "cannot be met by ordinary food products in respect to iron," and it says that there is iron deficiency in two-thirds of menstruating women and in most pregnant women. Millions of men have it too.

I do not recommend megadoses of iron because it can be deposited in tissues and cause side effects when taken in large amounts. I try to ensure that the iron content of supplements falls into the 12- to 18-mg. per day range. When treating a nutritional anemia, I make sure to provide vitamin C, zinc, B_6, and vitamin E as well as iron.

Note: It's best to take iron between meals rather than at meals, and it is best to take it in the form of ferrous sulfate and not in time-release capsules which cause late absorption too far down in the intestine. Don't take vitamin E and iron at the same time of day since they compete.

If you have thalassemia or sickle cell disease or a blood disease called hemochromatosis, iron should not be taken because it causes an iron overload.

Anyone who has an iron-deficiency anemia should work with a physician to find the underlying causes, since an ulcer, or even cancer of the lower intestine, can cause bleeding.

Zinc—most critical of the trace minerals. Zinc is a part of some two dozen enzymes, including one which releases carbon dioxide from the blood and one closely related to insulin.

Because so much zinc is removed in the milling, refining, and canning processes, probabilities of zinc deficiency are very real. And since zinc is an important constituent of egg yolk, those who have bought the "avoid eggs" propaganda are further subject to zinc deficits. Low zinc levels are often found in patients with leg ulcers, diabetes, alcoholic cirrhosis, schizophrenia, cystic fibrosis, and chronic infections.

Zinc is necessary for the uptake of vitamins B_{12} and A. It is a specific therapy for an impaired sense of taste. More than four thousand patients with this problem have been treated by Dr. R. I. Henkin and P. J. Schechter at the National Institutes of Health.

Zinc supplements do wonders at speeding up healing of wounds, skin ulcers, sores, burns, and surgical incisions. A U.S. Air Force study showed that men with standard treatment after serious operations took sixty-two days for healing, but men taking a zinc capsule every day healed in forty-five days.

And latest animal research at the Human Nutrition Laboratory in North Dakota shows that if the mother has a zinc deficiency during pregnancy, the *offspring* are abnormally aggressive, are less tolerant of stress, and have decreased learning ability and smaller brains. . . .

Low zinc levels should be suspected if you have white spots on your fingernails.

Manganese. Like several other trace minerals, manganese is a factor in many coenzymes, in this case, involving the thyroid function and acetylcholine formation. It is almost completely removed from milled wheat. Deficiencies have been demonstrated in many kinds of animals, causing defects in brain function, fat and sugar metabolism, bone formation, growth, and reproduction.

It is obviously essential in man and must be provided for. It has been shown to work in conjunction with zinc in many of its reactions. It is absorbed rather poorly from the digestive tract.

Copper—a good-bad mineral. Copper is essential to many enzyme reactions, but a problem occurs when levels get too high. Nutrition psychiatrists have found high copper levels in many schizophrenic patients. When these levels are lowered by increasing the intake of zinc and manganese, there can be a major clinical improvement.

Copper excess can produce everyday problems too, such as insomnia, depression, headaches, stretch marks, gray hair, and hair loss. And high serum copper levels are found in conditions such as viral and bacterial infections, rheumatoid arthritis, heart attacks, malignancies, cirrhosis, and leukemia. Even the copper from copper water pipes can cause a problem. In view of these findings, I now consider it wise to switch to vitamin and mineral preparations that contain zinc with very little or no copper.

Iodine. Iodine provides the thyroid gland with an essential building block for thyroid hormone. Iodine deficiency leads to a goiter; excess iodine is mostly excreted. This does not mean that large doses of kelp, the iodine-containing seaweed, can be taken with complete safety, since both under- and overactivity of the thyroid can result from excess iodine intake. But at least enough kelp or seafood or iodized salt should be included in your diet to provide one-tenth of a milligram of iodine per day.

Cobalt. The prime function of cobalt is to be a part of vitamin B_{12}. In animals, there is a need for cobalt beyond that in B_{12}, but this has not been demonstrated in humans.

Selenium—as important as vitamin E. This is because many of their functions overlap. Selenium has effects as an antioxidant of fats and scavenger of free radicals, much the same way as vitamin E. It is important in the prevention of heart disease. High-selenium soil areas seem to have a decreased incidence of cancer and of heart disease.

Not enough is known about selenium to state whether deficiencies are prevalent, or even possible. It is sparsely distributed in the vegetable kingdom, although adequately represented in meat.

Chromium—the one most important mineral to provide for. Almost everyone on the American diet probably fails to get enough chromium. Although levels of minerals almost always increase with age, chromium does not. Dr. Henry Schroeder in his important book *The Trace Elements and Man* [1973] points out that chromium was undetectable in the major artery of "almost every person dying of coronary artery disease . . . and was present in almost every aorta of persons dying accidentally." And he calculated that the 150 grams of sugar we consume daily leads to a net loss of 8.75

mg. of chromium per year, more than the body's total content! Until very recently, there was no way to take chromium in pill form so that it could be adequately absorbed. . . .

You can obtain chromium in the diet through brewers' yeast and some [kinds of] nuts. . . .

OTHER NUTRIENTS

There are many compounds found in the body that are considered nutrients but are not vitamins or minerals. They can sometimes give therapeutic effects. Examples: the orotates, aspartates, deanol, betaine, and lecithin.

Individual amino acids, the building blocks of protein, can be of extreme value in medicine. For example, tryptophan, given in doses greater than 1,500 mg., makes a remarkable sleep-inducing sedative and antidepressant. Another, glutamine, has proved useful in reducing cravings for alcohol in heavy drinkers.

Then there are food sources which contain many nutrients, some of which may be as yet undiscovered. Therefore, their inclusion in the diet may provide benefits beyond taking all the *known* vitamins and minerals. The classic examples are brewers' yeast and liver extract. In this category I would also place ginseng, wheat germ, bran, kelp, and bee pollen.

TAILORING YOUR OWN VITAMIN AND MINERAL PROGRAM

Now that you have a thumbnail knowledge of the philosophy behind vitamin and mineral therapy, how can you put it into practice so that it makes sense for you?

No two people's needs are alike; and neither are their responses to vitamins. . . .

There are four phases of vitamin therapy:

1 Basic formula
2 Experimentation (building up)
3 Tapering down
4 Maintenance

Your basic formula. The nucleus of the basic formula is a good multiple vitamin-mineral formula. There are several formulations that I find suitable. Most are obtainable from a health food store or a drugstore that carries some of the vitamins distributed by vitamin specialists rather than pharmaceutical houses. Many of the ethical drug companies' formulations are based on older formulas and tend to be pitifully low in B_6, zinc, and magnesium and too high in copper. Nor do they often contain significant amounts of the important nutrients PABA, choline, inositol, bioflavonoids, or biotin.

One typical multiple vitamin supplement I use has twenty-eight different vitamins and minerals, but I use it primarily for content of vitamins A (10,000 units) and D (400 units). (The remainder of the formula is of less importance as long as it will be supplemented by additions of B complex, C complex, E, folic acid, and trace minerals.) Take one of these each day to provide the base line. . . .

The experimentation phase. If you're not yet at your best, it is appropriate to see what benefits you can derive from increasing dosages of certain vitamins and minerals.

There are several nutrients which you can take in what I call "step-out" doses. The idea is to try each new dose for a week and decide whether it has benefited you. Vitamins may have functions beyond those involved in being a part of an enzyme system. Oxidizers, antioxidants, methyl donors, hydrogen acceptors, free radical deactivators—all these are biochemical terms describing the other important nutritional roles that vitamins play. . . .

The next phase—tapering down. None of us wants to spend the rest of his life taking unnecessarily large quantities of vitamins, so the next phase is a very important one—decreasing doses where possible. This can be done after a while because needs diminish as the overall nutrition picture improves. The removal of the sugar, or the alcohol, or The Pill, or diet pills, or diuretics serves to normalize a previously excessive need for some vitamins and minerals.

The tapering-down experiment is the same principle as stepping out, only in reverse. You cut back one at a time on those vitamins that are being consumed in especially high doses (or those that are particularly expensive). Reduce them 25 to 30 percent each week, one at a time. Continue to record your symptom score; if you notice any worsening, you may have confirmed that you do need the vitamin in question in the dosage you *were* taking. Repeat the maneuver somewhat later to be sure. Otherwise you will successively reduce your dose until you are down to what will be your maintenance formula.

For maintenance. It's hard to recommend much less than the basic multiple vitamin and trace mineral supplements plus some extra E, C, and folic acid. More often, if you are keeping close tabs on your symptoms, you will find that many of the vitamins you have used do provide a noticeable effect, and you will decide to maintain their usage.

Make your judgment based on the results of your tapering-down experiments. You don't want to take more vitamins than you need to, but you want to keep those optimum dosages that truly keep you feeling your best.

| 17 | Do We Need Extra Vitamins?

RONALD M. DEUTSCH

Ronald M. Deutsch is the author of books and articles dealing primarily with public health matters; he also serves as a lecturer and educator, especially in nutrition, his particular concern being fads and fallacies. Mr. Deutsch has written two best sellers on nutrition, *The Nuts among the Berries* and *The Family Guide to Better Food and Better Health*. Among his recent books are *The New Nuts among the Berries* and (with the National Nutrition Consortium) *Nutrition Labeling*.

Abridged from *Realities of Nutrition*, by Ronald M. Deutsch (Palo Alto, Calif.: Bull Publishing Co., 1976). © Copyright 1976, Bull Publishing Co Reprinted by permission.

In 1915, at least 200,000 Southerners were suffering, and in many cases dying, from *pellagra*. The name came from Italy, where it meant "rough skin," and referred to the fact that the first signs were rashes on exposed parts of the body, which fissured and developed into sores. As the disease progressed, the sores and cracks spread to the mouth. Then diarrhea began, with back pains and general exhaustion. Victims became sleepless and irritable, and in the end there was dementia and death.

In 1913, Dr. Joseph Goldberger was sent to the South by the U.S. Public Health Service to seek the cause and cure of pellagra. Most physicians believed that he should look for a microbe—that pellagra was an infection. But after preliminary research, Goldberger began to look for something else. . . .

For Goldberger was sure that pellagra was not contagious but rather a nutritional deficiency problem. And soon he proved that, with dietary changes, he could cure the disease.

WHAT IS A VITAMIN?

It is hard for many people to realize that when the first guns of World War I were fired, and Goldberger was patiently asking questions through the orphanages of Georgia and Mississippi, the scientific concepts of vitamins were just beginning to take shape.

A decade before, [British biochemist F. G.] Hopkins had said that there was something more to nutrition than protein and carbohydrate and fat, some sort of tiny essence needed for life. Until that time, scientists had merely sought the correct proportions of the three macronutrients. When Hopkins fed only these nutrients in rather pure form to rats, they sickened. When he added small amounts of certain foods—a teaspoon of milk, for example—they thrived.

In 1913, when Casimir Funk, working in London, found a substance that would cure *beriberi* in pigeons, he was sure that it was *the* missing chemical. He knew that the stuff was an amine, and that it was essential to life (in Latin, *vita*). So he called it the *vita-amine*. . . .

OF VITAMIN DEFICIENCIES AND NARROW DIETS

But by 1916, the Americans [E. V.] McCollum and [Cornelia] Kennedy had opined that there must be not one *vitamine,* but two—one soluble in water and one in fats.

Goldberger and his team did not suspect that the cause of pellagra was an absent "vitamine." They were sure that the cause was related to a protein deficiency. True, their disease, like beriberi, resulted from a narrow diet. But they found that they could overcome pellagra by giving patients more protein to eat.

The Southern pellagra victims often had enough food, but it was limited mainly to corn. Added to the corn were greens and rice, gravy and sweet syrup, and sweet potatoes. In one orphanage Goldberger used Federal funds to improve the diets of the pellagrous group. The babies had been all right; they got milk. And the youngsters of 12 or more were not ill; they did work, and so for strength they got some beans and meat. It was the children in between who got only what little was left over, and many were sick with pellagra. Goldberger made sure that they ate meat four times a week, peas and beans all winter, and an egg a day. And the pellagra disappeared.

By 1921 Goldberger's team had found that they could cure pellagra with a single amino acid, *tryptophan,* in its pure form. And they had seen that the principal foods eaten by those with pellagra were low in tryptophan.

Then came a blow—evidence that others had cured pellagra with an extract of yeast, an extract that contained no nitrogen from amino acids. The puzzle became bewildering. For if pellagra could be cured by this yeast extract, how could the cause of the disease be a shortage of an amino acid? And why should tryptophan cure pellagra? All that the scientists knew for sure was that there was something wrong with a diet composed mainly of corn.

The solution? The main protein of corn is *zein*. Zein is a limited protein, limited chiefly in two amino acids, *lysine* and *tryptophan*. The missing nutrient which led to pellagra was not lysine or tryptophan, however; it was the vitamin *niacin* (which was not to be isolated until 1937). The yeast extract which had cured pellagra had contained niacin.

Then why should tryptophan have cured pellagra, too? Because the body can convert tryptophan to niacin. Each 60 extra milligrams of tryptophan can furnish a milligram of niacin. And high-quality proteins have considerable tryptophan.

WHEN IS A VITAMIN SUPPLEMENT NECESSARY?

If we look at the realities of niacin, we can see why deficiencies of this vitamin are practically nonexistent in America today, and why special supplements are pointless.

First, look at the best sources of niacin. Usually these are the richest sources of protein—foods such as meats, poultry, fish, eggs,and legumes. And the same foods which are good sources of niacin tend also to be good sources of the amino acid which can be converted to the vitamin. So among a protein-eating people, a niacin shortage is hard to imagine.

. . . The U.S. per capita consumption of tryptophan is some 1,200 mg. a day. The need for this amino acid is about 200 mg. So almost 1,000 mg. are left over to yield niacin. At the 60-to-1 conversion rate (60 mg. of tryptophan yielding 1 mg. of niacin), we can each get an average of some 17 milligrams of converted niacin from our food each day. This happens to equal the U.S. RDA. This then would supply our needs, even without allowing for the fact that the foods which contain generous amounts of tryptophan also supply much pure niacin.

It seems plain from this information—and from recent surveys which show no significant deficiencies of niacin in the U.S.—that adding extra niacin to our intake is pointless. According to the Food and Nutrition Board, Americans get between 50 and 300 percent more niacin than the U.S. RDA.

(And remember that the U.S. RDA is based upon the RDA, with its safety margins; and that the U.S. RDA is usually based on the highest recommendation for a normal adult, generally for the typical adult male.)

However, most breakfast cereals contain (mainly through additives) 25 percent of U.S. RDA for niacin. And most popular one-every-morning vitamin pills have large amounts of niacin, usually 100 percent of U.S. RDA. Niacin is even an ingredient of enriched flour, cornmeal, and the like.

HOW DO WE KNOW HOW MUCH OF A VITAMIN WE NEED?

In general, the basic understanding of vitamin needs comes from observations of deficiency signs. The minimal need is that which prevents deficiency symptoms. But the bare minimum is not used as the standard; one does not put health on a tightrope. To understand something of how science determines a healthful intake of vitamin, we we must know a little more about what vitamins do.

. . . The body breaks foods down into simple chemical building materials or fuels. . . . Proteins from foods are separated into their constituent amino acids, and . . . new proteins are built. . . . Carbohydrates [are] broken down into simple sugars [and] the sugars converted into glucose and then burned or stored. . . . Hydrolysis takes fats apart and puts them together again.

How did these reactions take place? In almost every case, *enzymes* did the work. The cells, with the blueprints provided by DNA, make the protein portion of these enzymes (the *apoenzymes*); but often, to function properly, enzymes require *coenzymes*.

The situation is a little like trying to open a tightly sealed jar with one hand. Apply all the force you like with one hand by itself, addressing the force to the lid, and nothing happens; the jar turns with it. We need two hands open the jar, one turning the lid and the other holding the jar. In effect, the coenzyme acts like a second hand, which holds the jar while the first hand turns the lid.

The role of coenzyme is the chief function of most vitamins, especially of the water-soluble vitamins in the B complex. The vitamin does not necessarily undertake this role alone; it generally acts as the essential active part of a larger total coenzyme. For example, niacin is a key part of two coenzymes.

. . . Similar basic chemical reactions, such as hydrolysis, are repeated in many different body processes. So it is not surprising to learn that the coenzymes as a group have chemical functions which can be used in a number of processes. In a sense, we might see them as tools with special capabilities, like certain sizes and shapes of wrench or screwdriver. Just as a specific wrench might be used for various jobs in the building of a house—here by a carpenter and there by an electrician or plumber—so vitamins may take part in a variety of jobs. Niacin's coenzymes, as examples, are important in breaking down carbohydrate for energy; they are crucial to the synthesis of triglycerides by the body; and they are essential in the supplying of oxygen to many tissues. In light of the wide variety of such work, it is not hard to see why a pellagra victim, short of niacin, feels weak, particularly when one remembers that glucose is the efficient fuel for the brain and nervous system.

This all suggests some other ways in which we can determine when vitamins are adequately supplied. For when we have enough of a vitamin which serves in a coenzyme, the chemical reactions which it fosters produce specific products. When the vitamin is in short supply, the reactions may not take place, or may take place only partially, and there will be less of the particular products. Commonly, the chemical products of complete or incomplete reactions can be identified in the blood or the body wastes. And this can indicate the adequacy of vitamin intake. For example, much of what we know about niacin needs was first learned by Dr. Grace Goldsmith and her colleagues, who found that up to a certain point, increasing tryptophan and niacin intake yielded more products of niacin-linked reactions in the urine.

Information about vitamin intakes can be gained in some cases by checking how much of the vitamin spills over into the urine because there is an excess—as in the case of vitamin C. Or certain levels of vitamin in the blood, as in the case of vitamin A, may indicate that more is available than the body can use.

DO EXTRA VITAMINS OFFER EXTRA HEALTH?

Again, let us look at niacin as an example. There is a popular belief that a kind of "super nutrition" is possible through the gulping of extra-large doses of vitamins. Consider niacin's role in making energy available from glucose. So far as science knows, no more can be helpful than the amount needed to deal with the available glucose.

It is partly because of this relationship of niacin to energy use that the need for niacin is related to the number of calories we take in. The RDA Committee, including its usual safety margins, recommends that we get 6.6 mg. of niacin for each 1,000 calories we eat. Is it sensible then, to do as many people do, and consume pills containing 50 mg. of niacin a day? Only if they are eating 7,570 calories a day, a reasonable intake for a 473-pound (or an extremely active) man. (And of course this assumes that among the 7,570 calories of food, there is no niacin, and no protein which contains any trypotophan.)

This example suggests why nutritionists say that rarely are supplemental nutrients needed by normal people who consume good, varied diets. In considering micronutrients, we should remember that the plan of life is awesomely well integrated. The chemicals which we need to make use of food are either produced by the body or available in our food. If human existence depends on a health-food store full of pills, how has mankind survived?

But, if niacin helps to supply the needed energy of our brains and nerves, can't we improve their function with more niacin? No more than supplying a machine with more and more fuel would make it run faster and faster without limit. If this were true, we could outfit the family station wagon with a very large gas tank and a huge fuel pump and enter it at Indianapolis. Obviously the design of the system sets a ceiling on how much fuel can be used.

WHEN WILL VITAMINS CURE DISEASE?

Not long ago, an issue of *Glamour* magazine offered its readers an article called "Vitamins—Do They Really Cure Everything from Colds to Menstrual Cramps to Schizophrenia?"[1]

A feature of the article was a two-page chart, entitled "Therapy Claims of Vitamin Enthusiasts." In the lefthand column of the chart was a long list of ailments. To the right were five columns for vitamins, with testimonials from the late Adelle Davis and others which had said they would prevent or relieve the ailments. Niacin, for example, was claimed as a preventative and cure for anxiety and schizophrenia, as well as skin problems.

Where did the enthusiasts get the idea that the vitamins would cure these illnesses? Simple. If one looks through the catalog of deficiency symptoms for various nutrients, one finds that virtually every organ of the body can be involved in *some* deficiency state. One also finds that when the deficient nutrient is restored to the diet, the symptoms are likely to abate. With niacin, for example, there are skin, brain, and nerve symptoms of deficiency, and if niacin is replaced in time, these ills will go away.

It is thus *easy* to *see* how some enthusiasts began to believe in curative links between particular vitamins and particular organs. If a shortage of the vitamin can injure the organ, they assumed, then whenever that organ is in trouble, vitamins will make it better. But as we see with niacin, vitamins are related less to organs than to chemical reactions. When a vitamin is missing, a whole spectrum of symptoms appears, ranging over the whole body, a fact enthusiasts often forget.

Seeing a tendency of the gums to bleed, certain dentists think of scurvy and prescribe vitamin C, forgetting that the bleeding gums are only one sign of the total bodily problem of scurvy. (There is also tenderness of the extremities and muscle weakness, hemorrhages under the skin, in the nose, and throughout the body, often quite painful; there is delayed healing of wounds and high risk of infections.) When one understands the well-documented fact that scurvy is now practically unknown in the U.S. it is not logical to prescribe vitamin C for every bleeding gum.

In extra doses, used essentially as medicines, vitamins and minerals cure scarcely anything except deficiencies of vitamins and minerals.

Not long ago, Dr. Alfred Harper, then chairman of the RDA Committee, wrote to Senator William Proxmire (relative to possible legislation regulating large doses of micronutrients). Said Harper: "When a nutrient is used to treat a disease that is NOT caused by an inadequate intake of that nutrient, the use is no longer nutritional, it is pharmaceutical. The nutrient is being used as a drug."[2]

There are few situations, although very few, in which nutrients are responsibly used as drugs. For example, Harper cites the use of vitamin C to treat certain bladder infections, by making the urine more acid. But note that in this use, vitamin C is not intended to function as a vitamin. It is being used primarily because it is a mild acid, because excesses of ascorbic acid are cleared by the kidneys and quickly dumped into the bladder, and because it is relatively nontoxic in the amounts needed to make the urine sufficiently acid.

On the other hand, there are some healers who become fascinated by the deficiency-symptom relationship, and prescribe massive doses of a vitamin. An example is the "orthomolecular psychiatrist," who gives "megavitamin" doses of niacin to people with schizophrenia—because niacin stops the dementia of pellagra.

One of the old names for a type of schizophrenia was dementia, especially dementia praecox, the lamentably common schizophrenia which emerges at the border of adolescence and adulthood. The origin of the disorder has not been explained, no reliable cure has been found, and there is often a spontaneous remission—characteristics which make it fertile ground for vitamin "cures."

An expert panel of the American Psychiatric Association reviewed the uses of megavitamin therapy, and concluded: "The results and claims of the advocates of megavitamin therapy have not been confirmed . . . their credibility is further diminished by a consistent refusal over the past decade to perform controlled experiments and to report their results in a scientifically acceptable fashion. . . . Under these circumstances this [panel] considers the massive publicity which they promulgate via radio, the lay press and popular books . . . to be deplorable."[3]

Nevertheless, the orthomolecular enthusiasts continue to treat virtually every variety of serious emotional illness with megavitamins, particularly with niacin. One popular book describes the supposed nutritional science behind such treatment, illustrating with the case of a girl called Joan, who supposedly took diet pills and ate very little for about a month.[4] "In the space of a month," write the authors, "the strain on her nutritional reserves was so severe that she developed pellagra—but apparently only the mental symptoms of the deficiency disease. This is confirmation of the theory behind 'orthomolecular psychiatry'" (the theory of Dr. Linus Pauling). Norman Cousins, editor of the Saturday Review, is reported to have been so impressed with Joan's story that he wrote an article about her pellagra of just the brain and nerves. Science, of course, knows that pellagra is an illness of the whole body.

How much niacin (among other things) is such a patient given? Dosages are commonly between 3,000 and 4,000 mg. daily—or the RDA for some 230 days at the highest level. At 6.6 mg. of niacin per 1,000 calories, we may compute that a megavitamin patient was being equipped to deal with some 600,000 calories of food a day. As a comparable example, we might note that Pauling's dosage of vitamin C for the common cold, 1,000 mg. per hour, would supply in about 12 hours the RDA of vitamin C for some nine months,[5] an amount which has no possible relation to vitamin function.

The chemical and physiologic thinking behind such doses is obscure to most scientists. But the hazards are often clear. We have noted examples even with water-soluble vitamins, where most of an excess is simply urinated away (but where injury can be caused in the process). But the hazards are especially notable in the case of fat-soluble vitamins, such as vitamin A, in which long-term doses of only five to ten times the U.S. RDA have had toxic effects. Yet in a recent issue of one health-food magazine, a columnist responds to a reader's letter by recommending 100,000 units daily, 20 times the U.S. RDA, and saying: "Any toxicity found from A and D vitamins has always been caused by the synthetic forms. The natural forms . . . can be taken with impunity."[6] This idea is quite untrue.

DEFINING VITAMINS—"NATURAL" AND SYNTHETIC

Are "natural" and synthetic forms of vitamins really different from one another? To answer this question, we ought first to define our terms. Because the family of vitamins is so large and various, any useful definition tends to be broad. An example of a definition for vitamins is:

Vitamins are organic substances in foods which are essential in small amounts for body processes.

This definition distinguishes vitamins from other nutrients in several ways. First, the fact that they are organic (made with a skeleton of carbons) separates them from minerals. Second, the fact that they are needed in very small amounts sets them apart from other organic nutrients—fats, proteins, carbohydrates. Third, they are food essentials, meaning that they must originate outside our cells. . . . (Some vitamins are made by bacteria in our intestines; however, they are thus still nutrients which originate outside our cells, although we may not be ingesting them in food.) Fourth, the fact that they are necessary for body processes tells us that the processes will be interfered with when vitamin supplies are inadequate and will usually be restored when deficiencies are made up.

Both "natural" vitamins—those which are extracted from foods—and synthetic vitamins made by the chemist, who assembles the proper atoms in the proper form, meet the tests of this definition. If synthetic vitamins (the term derives from the Greek for "put together") are given, no deficiency occurs; and if there are deficiency symptoms, they are relieved equally well by the man-made forms.

Those who market "natural" vitamins often maintain or imply that something extra comes with them. Obviously, this is true only if the vitamins come in foods (the "extra" being other ingredients of the foods), not if pure vitamin extracts are taken. . . .

. . . Why do many people become suspicious of a man-made vitamin? Possibly because the word synthetic is often slightly misused. *Synthetic* rubber, for example, is not a reproduction of rubber made from trees; it is something that merely looks and acts similarly. The term synthetic tends to be used loosely by some industry, but not in nutrition, where it means an exact reproduction of the molecule.

One particularly meaningless idea is that the source from which the vitamin was refined makes a difference. For example, "natural vitamin C from rose hips" is only vitamin C.* Milligram for milligram it is the same as the vitamin C from oranges, potatoes, or cabbage. However, it is not surprising that special "kinds" of vitamins are bought at premium prices in a land where people regularly pay more for sucrose refined from cane than for sucrose refined from beets. Sugar cane and beets are quite different; oranges and potatoes are different. But sucrose is sucrose and vitamin C is vitamin C. . . .

References

1   Berkman, R. *Vitamins: Do they really cure everything from cold to menstrual cramps to schizophrenia?* Glamour, Mar. 1971.

2   Harper, A. E. Letter to Sen. William Proxmire.

3   Task Force on Vitamin Therapy in Psychiatry, *Megavitamin and orthomolecular therapy in psychiatry,* in Nutr. Rev., July, 1974, p. 44.

4   Adams, R. and Murray, F. *Megavitamin Therapy,* Larchmont Books, New York, 1973, pp. 136–64.

5   Pauling, L. *Vitamin C and the Common Cold,* Bantam, New York, 1971.

6   Nittler, A. Column in Let's Live, Jan., 1974.

*In actual commerce, much of the vitamin C value in such products has sometimes been found to come from pure ascorbic acid powder which has never been near a rose.

NEUROPSYCHIATRY

|18| Megavitamin Therapy Cures Mental and Emotional Disorders

RICHARD A. PASSWATER

Richard A. Passwater is director of research, American Geron-
tological Research Laboratories. He had done pioneering research in selenium and vitamin E supplementation, and is also
the author of *Supernutrition for Healthy Hearts*.

The amazing success in curing the mentally confused
by using large doses of vitamins is [an] example of the Supernutrition principle. [Supernutrition is a program for good health based on foods supplemented by vitamins.] Megavitamin therapy, the popular name given to the
technique of Dr. Abram Hoffer (former director of psychiatric research, University Hospital, Saskatoon, Saskatchewan) and Dr. Humphrey Osmond
(New Jersey Neuro-Psychiatric Institute, Princeton, New Jersey), preceded
Dr. Pauling's orthomolecular medicine. In 1968 Dr. Pauling published his
initial article on orthomolecular psychiatry in *Science* magazine. Megavitamin therapy had suffered from great criticism and skepticism from its start in
Canada in 1952, but when Dr. Pauling championed the concept, it received
more respectful attention. Yet today, after more than twenty years' success
with more than thirty thousand schizophrenics, alcoholics, addicts, and autis-
tics, there are still those who denounce the concept.

Megavitamin therapy derives its name from *mega*, meaning great (as in
huge or "great" doses). Typical programs include 1 to 8 grams of

niacinamide, 1 to 3 grams of vitamin C, 200 mg of pantothenic acid, and 150 to 450 mg of vitamin B_6. How can these large doses of vitamins relieve mental and emotional disturbances, especially those caused, at least in part, by inherited chemical imbalance? To hear some psychiatrists talk, you have to be nuts to take large doses of vitamins in the first place.

MENTAL DISORIENTATION AND THE B-COMPLEX VITAMINS

Let's begin by examining the problems of mental disorientation and then look at the mode of action of the B-complex vitamins. Mental disorientation arises when an individual misinterprets the signals from his senses; the chemical reactions and electrical impulses produced by the senses go awry on the way to the brain or in the brain. People with healthy body chemistry interpret the senses correctly, but the mentally confused often see a distorted world with weird sounds. They have difficulty with time perception and logical thought processes; they may see others as having piercing eyes, strange pulsating faces, or glowing halos around them; when they close their eyes, they may continue to see strange things and hear sounds that aren't there; their minds occasionally go blank.

These events can all be explained chemically. The mentally confused usually have either been born deficient in some enzyme needed to carry out the proper chemical reaction, or have had poor nutrition and as a result cannot provide the chemicals to produce the necessary quantity of the required enzymes and hormones. A smaller number of mental illnesses are caused by physical injuries, tumors, emotional shock, syphilis, or poisons.

About 2 out of every 100 people have some schizophrenic reactions. Schizophrenia and depression, the two most prevalent mental disorders, affect more than 10 million Americans each year. In the past, schizophrenics constituted 20 percent of first admissions to public mental hospitals and 60 percent of their permanent residents. The condition usually develops in adolescence or early adult life, but onset can range from childhood to late middle life. Symptoms are often precipitated by a traumatic experience; the traumatic experience is not the cause of schizophrenia, only the "last straw." Previously, the disorder had been wholly blamed on personality stresses, lack of adaptability, or failure of the parents. Today, the biochemical basis is well documented.

Paranoia differs from schizophrenia in that the confusion is characterized by a persistent delusion of persecution or grandeur. Normally there are no hallucinations in paranoia. Manic-depressives alternate between two phases—overactivity and depression. Infantile autism is a condition best described as the presence of unusual learning difficulties unaccompanied by mental retardation. All these personality disorders can be appreciably helped by megavitamin therapy.

If you were born deficient in a critical enzyme, how can taking extra vitamins overcome your enzyme deficiency? The answer is in two parts: the first deals with the nature of the B-complex vitamins, and the second involves basic chemistry.

THE NATURE OF THE VITAMIN B COMPLEX

The B vitamins appear together in nature as a family and have similar chemical properties. They are water soluble and act as catalysts. The B-complex family consists of thiamine (B_1), riboflavin (B_2), niacin (B_3, also called niacinamide or nicotinic acid), pantothenic acid (B_5), pyridoxine (B_6), cyanocobalamin (B_{12}), pangamic acid (B_{15}), amygdalin (B_{17}), lipoic acid (or thioctic acid), biotin (H), folic acid (B_c or M), inositol, p-aminobenzoic acid (PABA), choline, and other, still unisolated vitamins. With the exception of choline, all function as coenzymes.

A coenzyme is a part of an enzyme, a large molecule that is a body-chemistry catalyst. Without enzymes, the chemical reactions that occur in the body would proceed too slowly to sustain life; enzymes speed these reactions and control their rate. Enzymes have two major portions, the coenzyme and the apoenzyme: the apoenzyme is the protein portion and the coenzyme is the nonprotein portion. The B-complex vitamins form major portions of many coenzymes. Without enough B-complex vitamins, sufficient enzymes cannot be formed to carry out many vital body reactions.

Niacinamide (B_3) is usually given in large doses in megavitamin therapy. It forms two important coenzymes, nicotinamide adenine dinucleotide (NAD) and nicotinamide adenine dinucleotide phosphate (NADP). More than fifty enzymes have NAD or NADP coenzymes in them. They metabolize carbohydrates (especially sugars), fats, and proteins. Without adequate NAD or NADP, these normal nutrients—especially the amino acid tryptophan—end up as poisons in the blood because they are improperly metabolized. The resulting poisons are believed to be the cause of hallucinations. The amino acid tryptophan can form serotonin, a mental stimulant similar to LSD. A similar chemical normally found in the brain, tryptamine, can be converted into a well-known hallucinogen called dimethyltryptamine, if the brain chemistry is abnormal.

Catecholamines (hormones affecting nerve-impulse trasmissions) are also abnormal in cases of schizophrenia, resulting in improper transmission of nerve impulses. They, too, are affected by enzyme levels. Sugar-restricted diets are used in megavitamin therapy for schizophrenia because sucrose unnecessarily consumes valuable nicotinamide during its metabolism. *A subclinical deficiency (one having no apparent clinical symptoms) of niacinamide produces depression; and a niacinamide-deficiency disease, pellagra, produces hallucinations and behavioral changes similar to schizophrenia; in fact, some physicians prefer to classify schizophrenia as subclinical pellagra.* Similar chemical alterations of normal nutrients can cause depression, and destruction of chemicals called monoamines can also cause depression. Pyridoxine (B_6) is also involved in tryptophan metabolism. One study showed that 9 of 16 patients had improper tryptophan metabolism and were helped by extra vitamin B_6. (The investigators were Drs. A. S. Heely and G. E. Roberta; the study was published in *Developmental Medicine of Child Neurology*, 1966.)

Pantothenic acid (B_5) is also used in megavitamin therapy. It is a constituent of coenzyme A, which is involved in a great many reactions, including sugar metabolism and hormone production. A pantothenic acid deficiency causes nerve degeneration and depression.

Thiamine (B_1) forms the coenzyme thiamine pyrophosphate, which in turn forms many different enzymes. A thiamine deficiency causes degeneration of peripheral nerves, deterioration in the hypothalamus, loss of appetite, mental depression, irritability, confusion, memory loss, and inability to concentrate. Thiamine supplementation restores normality.

Biotin deficiency produces hallucinations, depression, panic, and lassitude. Other vitamins aid circulation of blood in the brain, balance coenzyme formation, and balance the B-complex to avoid a deficiency.

VITAMINS CAN CORRECT ENZYME DEFICIENCIES

A person producing only half of the apoenzymes he needs can still have a normal level of active enzymes by doubling his coenzyme production. A person ordinarily producing only 1 percent of a required enzyme might be normalized with a hundredfold increase in B vitamins in the blood.

The same equilibrium principle holds true in coenzyme production. Taking more vitamins shifts the equilibrium toward the synthesis of more coenzyme. Therefore, taking large doses of the B-complex vitamins can restore proper enzyme activity and health, mental and physical. The old medical school adage that says taking extra vitamins is like trying to pour more coffee into a full cup is wrong. In the body, the cup is never full; although some spills over, more is used.

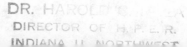

BODY CHEMISTRY INFLUENCES MENTAL ATTITUDE

The idea that mental attitude can influence the production of chemicals in the brain and that chemicals produced in the brain can influence mental attitude is relatively new. Scientists have learned more in the last 25 years about the chemistry of the brain and human behavior than in all the rest of history. I do not mean to suggest that psychiatrists and psychotherapists cannot cure emotional illness. These specialists have cured many, but not, I believe, as many as they *could* cure with psychotherapy or drug therapy and megavitamin therapy combined. All too often the psychiatrists or psychotherapists in mental institutions prefer electric shock, insulin shock, Metrazol shock, or lobotomies. Much evidence indicates that mental and emotional disorders are nutritional problems, triggered by a stress or shock that requires more than the body's reserves can handle. The stress or shock precipitates the mental illness; but teaching the patient to cope with the stress or shock or attempting to cure him by means of the above therapies will not alleviate the underlying problem of undernutrition or genetic defect. *Those treating emotional disturbance must also diagnose and treat the nutritional or genetic deficiency.*

With the evidence mounting on biochemical causes of mental disturbances, additional clinical tests can be added to the arsenal of the scientific psychiatrist. A simple urine test detects "mauve substance," which is present in high concentrations in 75 percent of acute and 50 percent of chronic schizophrenics. It is also high in 50 percent of the mentally retarded, 40 percent of alcholics, 20 percent of neurotics, and 10 percent of other physically sick persons. Rarely is it detected in mentally and physically healthy people. If the psychiatrist does not employ clinical tests and relies solely on the old teachings, he is practicing only the art, not the science of psychiatry.

If you want to learn more about the biochemical basis for emotional disturbance, read:

Mark Bricklin's article "Psychiatry Is a Sick Science" in the July 1973 *Prevention* magazine

Orthomolecular Psychiatry [edited] by David R. Hawkins and Linus Pauling [1973]

The article by Drs. William Philpott and Marshall Mandell in the February 1972 *Roche Image of Medicine and Research*

Dr. D. Vann in *Medical Journal of Australia* (November 11, 1972)

The June 27, 1959, issue of the *Journal of the American Medical Association*

Shrinks, Etc. [by Thomas Kiernan] (1974), which reveals more about the problems of psychotherapy

My point is that science must be added to psychiatric treatment.

PSYCHIATRISTS AND MEGAVITAMIN THERAPY

One proof that mental illness has a biochemical basis can be seen in the fact that symptoms can be switched off and on at will by adding or withdrawing megavitamin therapy—even when the patient is not aware of the change in treatment. Most of the mentally and emotionally ill are deficient in one or more of the B-complex vitamins or vitamin C. Stable people may have vitamin C deficiencies, but their bodies may have sufficient enzyme or catecholamine production to compensate. When catecholamine or enzyme production is meager, a vitamin C deficiency may trigger abnormality. British physician Dr. R. Shulman reported in 1967 in *the British Journal of Psychiatry* that 48 of 59 psychiatric cases had folic acid deficiencies. . . . Other evidence that mental illness has a biochemical basis: (1) the symptoms of mental disturbance can be mimicked in healthy people by the use of chemicals; (2) the presence of abnormal chemicals in mental patients' urine; (3) the hereditary nature of mental disorders; and (4) physical changes brought about by the disease. All four indicate chemical reactions rather than purely "psychological" factors.

Still further evidence is to be seen in the fact that normal people become depressed and experience other early symptoms of emotional disturbance when made niacin or folic-acid deficient. People born in the first three months of the year, when fresh vegetables are scarce, have nearly a 10 percent greater incidence of mental disturbances. Drs. Edward Hare, John Price, and Eliot Slater examined the records of all patients admitted to psychiatric units in England and Wales during 1970 and 1971. They noted that the birth rate of schizophrenics and manic depressives was 7 to 9 percent above normal during the first quarter of the year. No other mental disorders showed an abnormal relation to birth date. The researchers concluded in the *British Journal of Psychiatry* (Vol. 124) that "winter-born children are prone to nutritional deficiencies or infections which may damage the constitution and so facilitate the manifestation of a functional psychosis in those generally at risk."

The question arises then: Why don't more psychiatrists use megavitamin therapy? Is it because you can't teach old dogs new tricks? Is it because they would rather earn more money from long periods of treatment, sometimes including expensive shock treatments? Is it because general physicians can use the technique successfully? I don't believe any of these is the answer. What is probably true is that megavitamin therapy is so opposed to what they have been taught that they refuse to consider seriously the possibility that it could work. This is mega-ignorance!

Since my studies have led me to chastise old-line, straight-Freudian psychiatrists, let me also chastise any readers who would recommend to someone in need of psychiatric care that he try megavitamin therapy without proper treatment by a scientific psychiatrist. The dangers are great. Dual treatment is required—learning to cope with the triggering problem and correcting the body chemistry. Delaying professional treatment could cause the disease to progress to the point that hospitalization is required or the patient commits suicide. Why gamble? Have the person contact a local schizophrenia society, the Huxley Institute for Biosocial Research (formerly the American Schizophrenia Association), 1114 First Avenue, New York, N.Y. 10021, or Schizophrenics Anonymous International, Box 913, Saskatoon, Saskatchewan, Canada, for the name of a local psychiatrist, physician, or institute practicing megavitamin therapy.

THE ADVANTAGES OF MEGAVITAMIN THERAPY

The vitamins used in megavitamin therapy are relatively inexpensive; furthermore, they reduce the need for expensive drugs. *Soon after megavitamin therapy is added to a drug regimen, the tranquilizer need is often cut in half. With continued megavitamin therapy over several months, tranquilizers can be reduced gradually until they can be eliminated.*

The drugs used to treat schizophrenia, chlorpromazine and haloperidol, are effective; but excesses produce symptoms similar to those of Parkinson's disease, including lack of coordination and uncontrollable tremors. Megavitamin therapy reduces the need for these drugs and protects against harmful side effects as well. An additional saving comes about because the psychiatrist or physician can treat more patients with megavitamin therapy added to his protocol than with drug therapy alone. The patient is spared much of the expense and trouble of visits to the office of the psychiatrist or physician. The reduced number of visits per patient allow a psychiatrist or physician to treat more patients. Dr. David R. Hawkins, Medical Director of

North Nassau Mental Health Center (New York), reported in a book he wrote with Linus Pauling, *Orthomolecular Psychiatry*, 1973, that the number of yearly visits required per patient dropped from 150 to 15 with the combined therapy. Hospitalization can be avoided, too. Dr. Hawkins cites a case reported in the *Philadelphia Inquirer* (December 10, 1972) in which a patient suffering from malnutrition resulting from a reducing diet was in and out of seven mental institutions over a period of five years before being cured, at a cost of $230,000.

Even when a patient is first treated in a hospital, the avoidance of rehospitalization is significant to the patient or taxpayers who support state hospitals. Megavitamin therapy in the North Nassau Mental Health Center in New York reduced the rehospitalization rate by 50 percent and saved the hospital $100,000 per year; rehospitalization stays were reduced to one or two weeks rather than months (*Orthomolecular Psychiatry*, 1973).

Cost is only a minor concern; the effect on human life is much greater. How well does it work? Generally speaking, when megavitamin therapy is combined with conventional drug treatment, it is twice as effective as drug treatment alone. The suicide rate, which in schizophrenics is 22 times the normal rate, drops to almost zero (*Orthomolecular Psychiatry*, 1973).

CLINICAL CONFIRMATION

Dr. [Abram] Hoffer, one of the original developers of megavitamin therapy, has reported a 93 percent cure rate for patients in combined therapy ill less than two years (thus not chronic).

Although psychiatrists and physicians treating emotional and mental problems with megavitamin therapy have files bulging with thousands of individual case histories, large-scale double-blind tests are not plentiful. Drs. George Watson and W. D. Currier reported a single-blind test (the patients didn't know what medicines they were getting, but the physicians did) in the *Journal of Psychology* (March 1960). Thirty patients given inert placebos were observed and rated according to a standard personality survey (MMPI). Of the 30 patients, 17 remained the same during the first phase of the survey, 7 improved, and 6 became worse. The personality survey score for the group improved on the average only an insignificant 4 units out of 220 units. When megavitamin therapy was substituted for the placebos over an equal period of time, 22 improved, 6 remained the same, and 2 became worse. (It is suspected that adding magnesium to the formula would have prevented the 2 from becoming worse.) The improvement in the personality test was a significant 17 points. When the megavitamin therapy was continued even longer, 24 improved, 5 remained unchanged, and only 1 was worse. The test score improved by an average of a highly significant 27 (out of 220) units.

Drs. [Abram] Hoffer and [Humphrey] Osmond compared two large groups of schizophrenics under long-term observation in institutions in Canada and New Jersey. The 350 patients who received standard treatment (drugs and counseling) combined with megavitamin therapy were contrasted with 450 patients receiving standard treatment alone. The 10-year cure rate of those receiving megavitamin therapy was over 75 percent, while the standard-treatment patients showed only a 30 percent cure rate without relapse after 10 years.

Dr. Hawkins reported a 70 percent recovery rate in 2,000 seriously ill schizophrenics at the North Nassau Mental Health Center with megavitamin therapy (*Orthomolecular Psychiatry*, 1973).

His study was published in 1971 by the American Schizophrenia Association. In his private practice he has treated over 4,000 schizophrenic patients (including 600 alcoholics); the vast majority have shown marked improvement or fully recovered. Dr. Hawkins reported in *Psychosomatics* (November 1970) that in a test situation, 80 schizophrenic patients receiving megavitamin therapy had only half the relapse rate of a control group of 80 schizophrenic patients receiving standard treatment.

Dr. Bernard Rimland of the Institute for Child Behavior Research, San Diego, enrolled 300 autistic children in nationwide volunteer megavitamin therapy in 1966. All enrolled children were under the medical care of their local physician throughout the study, and were placed on megavitamins for three months. After that time, they were asked to abstain from the vitamins for one month. Letters from parents to Dr. Rimland told of children returning to normal activity, talking and playing—instead of being withdrawn and virtually vegetables. Many parents refused to adhere to the abstinence portion of the experiment, as their children began to deteriorate again. During the course of the test 3 percent of the children (nine cases) became more irritable and difficult to manage. At Adelle Davis's suggestion, magnesium was added to the regimen, and the undesirable side effects disappeared overnight (from a paper delivered to the Canadian Schizophrenia Foundation, Toronto, 1973).

In 1963 Dr. G. Milner reported in the *British Journal of Psychiatry* a true double-blind study showing significant improvement on the part of 20 vitamin C-treated schizophrenic patients over a placebo group of the same number.

Dr. Hoffer reported in 1964 a ten-year follow-up of the treatment of schizophrenia with nicotinic acid in the *Acta Psychiatrica Scandinavia;* and, also in 1964, reported a controlled study on the effect of nicotinic acid on the frequency and duration of rehospitalization of schizophrenia patients in the *International Journal of Neuropsychiatry.* He commented in the first-quarter 1972 issue of *Orthomolecular Psychiatry* on the two studies just mentioned:

> It turned out that of the ten or so patients receiving nicotinic acid seven had remained well over that year. Of the ten or so nicotinamide patients, seven or eight had remained well, while of the ten placebo patients only three had remained well. Around 75 percent of the patients receiving vitamins had remained well, whereas only one-third of the patients receiving placebo had remained well. It is important to remember that about two-thirds of all the patients had also received shock treatments so that this was a study of the combination of shock treatments plus megavitamins.
>
> The results of the study were relatively clear cut, but it seemed very important to us not to report this until we repeated the study on a larger scale, to make sure there had been no hidden errors. We, therefore, started the second double-blind clinical experiment using the same design except that this time we did use nicotinic acid and placebo while informing the staff that we were going to follow the previous design. With our second study, we were able to treat 82 patients. The results were very similar.

MEGAVITAMIN TREATMENT FOR EMOTIONAL DISORDERS

In treating emotional and mental disorders, the following dosages of vitamins are generally given along with a low-sugar, high-protein, balanced diet.

Niacinamide (Vitamin B_3, or niacin) is given in high dosage as the keystone of megavitamin therapy. The dosage for adults ranges from 3 to 30 grams per day, although some use as little as 1 gram daily. Typical initial doses seem to be 6 to 8 grams daily. Children receive 1 gram of niacinamide for each 50 pounds of body weight.

Thiamine (Vitamin B_1) is given in 1- or 2-gram doses, although some prefer to use 1 gram (100 mgs) of thiamine for each gram of niacinamide (1:10 ratio).

Pyridoxine (Vitamin B_6) is included in the 100- to 500-mg level with 100 to 300 mg being typical.

Pantothenic acid used at the 200- to 300-mg level. Vitamin B_{12} (1 mg) is generally given by injection in addition to another 50 to 100 micrograms orally.

Vitamin C is used on almost an equal weight basis as niacinamide. Dosage ranges from 3 to 20 grams daily, with an average of 6 grams.

The alpha tocopherol (vitamin E) dosage is 400 to 800 mg.

A high-potency multiple vitamin and mineral formulation, liver tablets, and a B-complex formulation are generally included. Minerals, including zinc and magnesium, are important in megavitamin therapy. Lithium has been successfully used to treat manic-depressives.

Megavitamin therapy normally takes two to three months to produce dramatic results, although fatigue and depression are reduced very quickly. Some patients experience excellent results in a few days. Megavitamin therapy is typically given for a year; during this period, other medication is eliminated gradually. Most patients continue to take large maintenance amounts of the vitamins, but not at the initial treatment rate. When the deficiency has been extensive and prolonged, some irreparable damage occurs and complete cure cannot be obtained. . . .

Bibliography and suggested reading

Abrahamson, E. M., and Pezet, A. W. *Body, Mind and Sugar.* York: Pyramid, 1971.

Adams, Ruth, and Murray, Frank. *Megavitamin Therapy.* New York: Larchmont Books, 1973.

Blaine, Tom. R. *Mental Health through Nutrition.* New York: Citadel Press, 1969.

Cheraskin, E., Ringsdorf, W. M., and Brecher, A. *Psychodietetics.* New York: Stein and Day, 1975.

Fredericks, Carlton. *Low Blood Sugar and You.* New York: Constellation International, 1969.

Hoffer, Abram, and Osmond, Humphrey. *How to Live with Schizophrenia.* New York: University Books, 1966.

————. *New Hope for Alcoholics.* New York: University Books, 1968.

Kiernan, Thomas. *Shrinks, Etc.* New York: Dial, 1974.

Steincrohn, Peter J. *The Most Common Misdiagnosed Disease: Low Blood Sugar.* Chicago: Henry Regnery, 1972.

Weller, Charles, and Boylan, Brian Richard. *Hypoglycemia.* New York: Award Books, 1970.

|19| Diet and Hyperactivity: Any Connection?

THE INSTITUTE OF FOOD TECHNOLOGISTS' EXPERT PANEL ON FOOD SAFETY & NUTRITION and THE COMMITTEE ON PUBLIC INFORMATION

The Institute of Food Technologists is an international non-profit, scientific society founded in 1939. Its members are food technologists, food scientists, food engineers, and food-industry managers and executives, as well as government personnel and educators in the field of food science and technology and other individuals working in closely related fields.

From a Scientific Status Summary, by the Institute of Food Technologists, April 1976. Reprinted with permission.

The role of the diet in maintaining the well-being of the human body is fairly well understood, but questions are frequently raised about its effect on the psychological state as well. Recently, claims have been made that certain chemicals found in foods—some present naturally, others added in processing—may be responsible for much of the syndrome referred to as "hyperactivity." Those claiming to have demonstrated the relationship have prescribed diets which prohibit a large number of commonly accepted foodstuffs.

The most emphatic claims come from Benjamin F. Feingold, M.D., emeritus director of the Laboratory of Medical Entomology of the Kaiser Foundation Research Institute. He has attributed behavioral disturbances and learning disabilities to "salicylate-like" natural compounds in foods, to "low-molecular weight food additives" in general, and to artificial food flavors and colors in particular.

As therapy for hyperactivity, Dr. Feingold has prescribed a diet which eliminates a wide variety of natural and processed foods, and he claims dramatic improvements in patients so treated. On this basis, he has appealed to the U.S. Food and Drug Administration for complete label declaration of ingredients and the use of a special symbol to indicate the absence of synthetic colors or flavors.

WHAT IS HYPERACTIVITY?

Hyperactivity is essentially a symptom, which may be the result of a child's basic personality, a temporary state of anxiety, or subclinical seizure disorders; or it may reflect a true hyperkinetic state. It may also, according to the Council on Child Health of the American Academy of Pediatrics, be strictly "'in the eye of the beholder" (AAP Council on Child Health, 1975).

Descriptions of hyperactivity are generally given in behavioral terms, such as motor activity, attention span, frustration tolerance, excitability, impulse control, irritability, restlessness, and aggressiveness. Although these behaviors are measurable, they may not adequately reflect the kind of problems that different children have. Objective measures of attention span have been developed and have been used in some studies to help make the diagnosis, usually during tasks requiring continuous performance by the child. Standard questionnaires have also been designed, to be used by parents and teachers as they make observations at different times; such questionnaires provide useful evaluation information.

Researchers, however, acknowledge the difficulties of measuring these attributes and of interpreting the measurements. For example, in a study at the University of North Carolina designed to measure the motor activity and interest span of children diagnosed as hyperkinetic, Routh (1975) reported that of 78 referrals from physicians, teachers, and parents, only 47 percent of the children were judged to be overactive—despite the fact that all of the children were considered to be "problem children" by those referring them to the testing service. In a study of teacher ratings of hyperactivity conducted at the University of Iowa, older teachers rated more children hyperactive than did young teachers (Johnson, 1974).

Clinical experience also indicates that many factors alter the activity patterns of such children or the perception of the patterns by parents. Such factors range from the presence or absence of breakfast, weather conditions and resultant seasonal cycles that alter activities during cold seasons, to the interpersonal family relationships or existence of disruptive family problems.

Age of the child appears to be another determinant of detection of the syndrome of hyperactivity. The majority of cases are noted at about the age the child enters school, and there is usually a gradual diminution in the hyperactivity at puberty or slightly thereafter. While some observers cite isolated cases of identifiable hyperkinesis in older individuals, it is unusual. Also, in some areas of the world, the syndrome is not recognized as a problem by school authorities—again, an example of differences in perception or of occurrence.

HYPERACTIVITY OR HYPERKINESIS?

The terms "hyperactivity," "hyperkinesis," and "hyperkinetic syndrome" have been loosely employed in both lay and professional writings. Frequently, the term "hyperkinesis" is mistakenly used interchangeably with that of the syndrome of "minimal brain dysfunction," or MBD. MBD itself is poorly defined (Strother, 1973). There is no agreement—and little evidence—as to the extent to which several seemingly related syndromes overlap.

In an effort to clarify the terminology, Wender (1973) suggested that there is evidence for several subgroups depending on their origin. He further suggests that the "hyperkinetic behavior syndrome" includes a number of clinical features: hyperactivity; short attention span and poor powers of concentration; impulsiveness and the inability to delay gratification. There is diminished ability to experience pleasure and frequent rejection of disciplinary measures. Learning abilities are affected in variable ways, as are nervous functions and muscular coordination. Obviously, a child with the hyperkinetic behavior syndrome will exhibit significant underachievement and classroom disruption in school. The disorder will also disrupt family relations at home.

A variety of factors have been proposed as possible causes of hyperkinesis. They include low-level lead poisoning, carbon monoxide poisoning, oxygen deprivation at birth, fluorescent lights, and milk drinking, as well as food additives. Studies in experimental animals on lead and carbon monoxide poisoning (David, 1974; Silbergeld and Goldbert, 1974; Culver and Norton, 1974) and on oxygen deprivation at birth (Kalverboer et al., 1973) are convincing and well documented. Observations on man are not as well documented for any of the factors mentioned, and are largely based upon anecdotal evidence.

The origin and development of the disorder has thus not been definitely established. Indeed, it is not even certain whether this is a discrete illness or a syndrome of many causes. There is evidence to support the hypothesis that some minimal brain dysfunction is inherited, produced genetically by subtle central nervous dysfunction of a biochemical nature (Wender, 1973).

Estimates of the incidence of the syndrome in U.S. schools range widely, frequently being cited as from 3 to 10 percent. Feingold quotes estimates as high as 25 percent or more of all children in certain schools. Others estimate that a similar percentage of children are receiving drugs for the disorder (Sprague and Sleator, 1973). These variations in estimates reflect the inappropriate grouping of a variety of conditions under the general term "learning disabilities"—i.e., combining hyperkinesis and reading retardation (Minskoff, 1973).

The confusion pertaining to these conditions is emphasized by the statement of the AAP Council on Child Health (1975):

> One must be cognizant of the fact that there is probably more confusion in relation to diagnosis and appropriate criteria for the use of medication for the treatment of hyperkinetic children than there is regarding the actual medication. Many physicians, as well as the general public, do not truly appreciate the differential diagnosis of the overactive child. It may be the result of basic personality, anxiety, subclinical seizure disorders, strictly in the eyes of the beholder, or true hyperkinesis; the latter is the only condition in which stimulants might be expected to be beneficial.

The Council further notes:

> The hyperkinetic child is typically one of normal intelligence who fails to learn at a normal rate even though he is given the same educational opportunities as children with equal intelligence. He usually exhibits to some degree (1) short attention span, (2) easy distractibility, (3) impulsive behavior, and (4) overactivity. Although other behaviors ofttimes are seen in children with normal intelligence and academic lag, stimulant drugs seem to be most effective in the four behaviors just mentioned. Little is known about the effect of stimulant drugs on such things as poor motor integration, deficits in the perception of space, form, movement, and time, and disorders of language or symbol development.

THE FEINGOLD HYPOTHESIS

In June 1973, Dr. Feingold presented a preliminary oral report at the annual meeting of the American Medical Association (Feingold et al., 1973) in which he stated that hyperkinesis was associated primarily with the ingestion of "low-molecular weight chemicals." He included in this category salicylates, compounds which react in the body with salicylates, and common food additives. This presentation was followed by a signed editorial in the October 1973 issue of *Hospital Practice* magazine (Feingold, 1973). He also presented a paper in London in September of that year, which was later inserted in the *Congressional Record* by Senator Beall (1973) along with an account by a writer for the *Washington Post*. He later restated and expanded his position in a popular book entitled *Why Your Child Is Hyperactive* (Feingold, 1975).

In this book, Feingold states his hypothesis as follows:

• "The hyperactive disturbance is nonimmunologic." In contrast to allergic reactions, he says, "there is no natural body defense against it."

• "Those children who react to synthetic additives have genetic variations—not abnormalities—which predispose them to such adverse responses."

• An "innate releasing mechanism is involved in the disturbance."

The treatment he suggests is dietary, and is based on an "exclusion diet." Twenty-one fruits and vegetables reported by Feingold to "contain natural salicylates" must be omitted. In addition, all foods that contain artificial color and artificial flavor are prohibited; he lists fifty-four foods in his book as examples. According to Feingold, "an individual sensitive to artificial colors and flavors must avoid them throughout his life."

Dr. Feingold currently recommends the following public actions on the basis of work:

• *Full disclosure* on food labels of the use of flavors and colors in all food products.

• *A broad educational program* by the Food and Drug Administration to inform the public of what he terms the "inherent potentials" of these chemicals.

• *The use of a special symbol* on food packages to indicate the complete absence of synthetic colors and flavors. (By implication, of course, foods *not* bearing this special symbol would be assumed by the interested consumer to contain "synthetic" additives.)

It should also be noted that the Feingold regimen prohibits not only certain foods, but also a wide variety of *non-food* items which contain the compounds he lists. These items include many prescription drugs and over-the-counter medications, toothpastes and tooth powder, mouthwashes, cough drops, throat lozenges, antacid tablets, and perfumes.

EVALUATING THE HYPOTHESIS

In order to examine these claims from a variety of viewpoints, the Nutrition Foundation assembled a team of fourteen expert food, medical, and behavioral scientists, designated as the National Advisory Committee on Hyperkinesis and Food Additives, to conduct a thorough review of evidence on this subject.*

The committee was charged with the responsibility to: (a) review critically and objectively the nature of evidence relative to the hypothesized relationship; (b) recommend whether additional investigations were justified or desirable; and, if so, (c) provide guidelines for the experimental design of appropriate studies which would result in obtaining valid data upon which conclusions might be formulated. The members of the committee examined all the published materials available, as well as unpublished manuscripts of talks, research proposals, and other pertinent information obtainable from any of the participating sources, including Dr. Feingold's book.

The committee's conclusions on the basis of the current state of knowledge about hyperactivity and food additives in children were summarized in its report to the Nutrition Foundation (National Advisory Committee, 1975) as follows:

• No controlled studies have demonstrated that hyperkinesis is related to the ingestion of food additives.
• The claim that hyperactive children improve significantly on a diet that is free of salicylates and food additives has not been confirmed.
• The nutritional qualities of the Feingold diet have not been evaluated, and it may not meet the long-term nutrient needs of children.
• The diet should not be used without competent medical supervision.

HYPOTHESIS QUESTIONED

Dr. Feingold's use of case studies to support his thesis has come under criticism for various reasons:

More than diet changed

In Dr. Feingold's prescribed regimen, the entire family—not just the children—is placed on the diet and regimen, in order to ensure compliance.

---

*The scientists were selected by the offices of the following major scientific and medical organizations: American Medical Association's Council on Foods and Nutrition; American Psychiatric Association; American Association of Child Psychiatry; Society of Toxicology; Council for Exceptional Children; American Alliance for Health, Physical Education; Institute of Food Technologists; American Society for Clinical Nutrition; American Dietetic Association; The National Nutrition Consortium; Life Sciences Research Office of the Federation of American Societies for Experimental Biology; Committee on Nutrition of the American Academy of Pediatrics; and the Food and Nutrition Board of the National Academy of Sciences.

But diet is only one of several critical variables of the child's life which is changed. Parents are instructed to spend Saturday mornings making additive-free candy and cake with their children. Since hyperactive behavior in many children is often associated with family problems and lack of attention, it is quite possible that such alterations in the family dynamics may be related to the reported improvement in the child.

Suggestibility a factor

Hyperactive behavior and its rating on a severity score are both subject to suggestibility. Dr. Feingold has a charismatic personality, and is positive about the value of his program. It is possible that the confident expectations generated in the patient and the family affect the syndrome itself, or at least the parents' ratings of the altered severity of the behavioral pattern.

Observations not objective

Parents or teachers who rate the children know that they are on the diet, and this knowledge may influence their ratings. In addition, Dr. Feingold's improvement ratings tend to be highly general, rather than specific, and are not based on objective rating scales like that developed by Conners (1973).

Risk of nutritional inadequacy

The exact additive and nutrient content of the exclusion diet prescribed by Dr. Feingold is difficult to assess, since it manipulates a myriad of factors. A number of common sources of important nutrients are prohibited in the diet, making careful planning and food selection especially important to assure that nutrient requirements are met for any long-term period of restriction to the regimen. Also, carbohydrate intake is likely to be curtailed under the diet, and extreme care would be needed to incorporate sufficient quantities of some of the essential vitamins. Because of the potential risk of nutritional inadequacy, the National Advisory Committee (1975) recommended that this regimen should not be used without competent medical supervision.

Chemical basis undefined

The initial rationale of the elimination diet advocated by Dr. Feingold was to avoid salicylate and salicylate-like compounds which occur naturally or as a result of processing. Although data on the occurrence of salicylic acid (orthohydroxybenzoic acid) in foods is very limited, at least part of the molecular fragment represented in the salicylate radical occurs in a broad range of natural foodstuffs.

The nine artificial certified food colors which are given prominence in the Feingold hypothesis are composed of a variety of chemical structures. Only one of these, erythrosine, bears some resemblance to the salicylate radical. Tartrazine, which has been reported to induce reactions similar to salicylates, bears even less chemical resemblance.

Moreover, naturally occurring food pigments exhibit even greater variety in chemical structure than these synthetic colors do. The more-common ones include the chlorophylls, anthocyanins (120 types), flavonoids (600 types), purines, carotenoids (120 types), quinones (200 types), betalains (69 types), and myoglobin. These occur naturally in a variety of foods, particularly leafy green vegetables, most fruits, root crops, milk, butter, yellow vegetables, and meats.

In addition, there are hundreds of flavors, natural and manmade, and their chemical structures differ equally widely.

It is also worth noting that any distinction between "naturally occurring" and "synthetic" is vague and generally related only to origin, not chemical structure of the substance. The body cannot differentiate between chemically synthesized β-carotene, the precursor of vitamin A, and the chemically identical material naturally present in the carrot.

With these considerations in mind, the National Advisory Committee agreed that there was no identifiable single substance or group of substances which the Feingold diet specifically removes. More recently, Dr. Feingold himself has shifted emphasis from a suspected role of salicylates to other food ingredients.

Results similar to other approaches

Dr. Feingold has reported that his regimen and diet have effectively treated 48 percent of the children presented to him with hyperkinesis.

He reports that of the children who respond under his guidance, about two-thirds do so dramatically, the other third "favorably." It is important to note that Dr. Feingold claims a response in *only half* of the children treated and dramatic response in but two-thirds of these. This percentage of success is about the same as that which occurs following *cessation* of drug therapy (Sleator et al., 1974).

Response to drug therapy in cases of true hyperkinesis is unmistakable when it occurs; also, if the drug is omitted after the child responds satisfactorily to short-term treatment, the child will rapidly return to the base-line abnormal behavior (AAP Council on Child Health, 1975), which is immediately evident to those around him. In about 25 percent of patients, discontinuance of drug therapy after long periods of control is not followed by renewed symptoms. Because of this fact, many clinicians routinely discontinue the use of medication before each long school vacation. This allows the child to start a new year without medication. The medication is resumed only if the syndrome that initiated the original treatment returns and hinders satisfactory school progress.

For example, Sleator et al. (1974) published a study of 42 children known to be responsive to Ritalin; 13 had been followed for two years, and 29 for one year. The subjects were part of a double-blind placebo study on the effect of different dose levels of the drug Ritalin on behavior and school performance and were tested at one-month intervals. Twenty-six percent of those taken off medication exhibited no deterioration of performance; this is consistent with the results of other studies.

Preliminary studies of eight patients on the Feingold regimen, initiated by a Pittsburgh group (Goyette, 1975) soon after publication of Feingold's thesis, revealed that parents of the majority of those subjects felt that the patients exhibited improvement, sometimes continuously, regardless of which of two dietary regimens (the Feingold diet or a "control") they were following. However, there were discrepancies between the assessment of behavioral changes made by parents and the assessments made by teachers in a portion of the studies. Also, no teacher assessment was made in a considerable number of observational periods reported.

CONTROLLED STUDY CONDUCTED

The National Advisory Committee also developed a research design which the members felt could avoid the subjective aspects inherent in all earlier studies and obtain the definitive data needed for decisive interpretation.

Preliminary findings from a carefully designed study, incorporating many of the criteria developed by the committee, were reported in January 1976 (Harley et al., 1976). The study was organized and funded by the Food Research Institute of the University of Wisconsin, and was conducted in the university's Departments of Psychology and Neurology. It represented the first systematic investigation of Dr. Feingold's hypothesis to include objective psychological, psychophysiological, and classroom observations, in addition to parent/teacher ratings of behavioral changes associated with changes in diets.

Preliminary analysis of the data shows no significant overall effect from the Feingold diet, as measured either by classroom behavior or by parents.

The study was conducted on boys in two age groups—3 to 6 and 6 to

12—and extended over an 8-month period. It was designed to be "double blind," as far as possible, in the sense that neither the test subjects nor the observers knew which diet any individual was consuming at any given time. Some observers weren't even aware of the fact that diets per se were being investigated. Subjects in the test were typically observed for a two-week period on their normal diet to determine their base-line behavior. They were then switched either to a "control" diet containing the usual additives or to an "experimental" diet developed around the rules prescribed by Dr. Feingold. After three or four weeks, the diets were changed so that those on the control switched to the Feingold diet, and vice versa. A number of products in both diets looked alike, in an attempt to avoid subjective or placebo effects.

During the tests, fathers, mothers, and teachers were asked to rate each child's behavior on a specially designed questionnaire (Conners Parent-Teacher questionnaire) as *improved, no change,* or *worsened,* on a scale of +2 to −2. In addition, the children were observed during classroom activity, and data collected on various types of behavior (attentiveness, restlessness, and disruptive behavior). They were also observed under independent play conditions, and data collected on movement about a grid playroom.

In both age groups, there was a significant difference between the level of activity of the control subjects and the test subjects (tending to confirm their "hyperactivity"), but there was *no significant change* in either group's observed classroom behavior as they changed from one diet to the other. There were a number of cases in which the parents and teachers observed improvement, tending to support the hypothesis. But there were also a number of observations of *worsening* in behavior. In fact, in only 4 cases out of 36 did all observers agree on their observations.

Thus, their conclusion was that "with the possible exception of the youngest age sample, the preliminary analyses completed to date in the Wisconsin study do not appear to offer strong support for the efficacy of the experimental diet, at least with respect to group effect. . . . The frequency with which positive diet effects were judged to be present was highest in the parent ratings, declined sharply in the teacher rating data, and essentially disappeared in the objective classroom and grid room observational data. . . ."

The Wisconsin group, in releasing their findings, stressed the preliminary nature of their conclusions. They also stated that there were sufficient subjects who were rated by both parents and teachers as significantly improved on the experimental diet to warrant additional detailed future study.

ADDITIONAL CONTROLLED STUDIES UNDER WAY

The National Institute of Education funded a three-month study on 15 youngsters age 6 to 12 by a group at the University of Pittsburgh's Department of Psychiatry. These children were observed by their parents and teachers while on their normal diet for a one-month base-line period. They were then assigned either to an additive-free diet or to a control diet made up of non-overlapping foods containing synthetic flavors and colors. After one month, they "crossed over" to the opposite diet. At the end of each of these periods, teachers and parents were interviewed separately as to their impressions of the children's behavior.

The teachers rated the children as being significantly improved while on the exclusion (additive-free) diet compared with both the base-line and the control (additive-containing) diets. The parents noted a significant improvement while on the exclusion diet compared with the normal base-line diet, but no change compared with the additive-containing control diet.

Dr. C. Keith Conners, chief investigator in the Pittsburgh group, stated in conclusion, "Although the results favor the Feingold hypothesis, methodological limitations warrant caution as well as concern regarding possible long-term negative consequences of unmonitored diet fads among parents of hyperkinetic children looking for simple solutions to a complex group of disorders" (Conners and Goyette, 1976). He also has other tests under way, in which he is attempting to measure, in the laboratory and the body, changes in blood chemistry in patients whose behavior improves on the exclusion diet, when they are "challenged" with foods containing additives.

FURTHER STUDY MERITED

The human body represents a complex network of interacting systems. Many specific agents react negatively with specific parts of that network, and individual differences are the rule rather than the exception. That the complex mixture we call a "diet" can elicit certain negative reactions in specific individuals should arouse concern, but not surprise. Aspirin sensitivity, for example, has been recognized for a long time, and similar reactions have been found occasionally with specific food colors, particularly tartrazine.

In view of the proof of safety required by FDA for the approval of a food additive, the data presented against the use of synthetic colors and flavors as a class of compounds by Dr. Feingold does not justify additional limitations at this time. The FDA *has* agreed that a symbol denoting that no artificial colors and flavors are used may be employed. However, any implication that such additives are unsafe or unhealthy would be considered "misbranding" and would not be permitted.

The FDA has also formed an Interagency Collaborative Group on Hyperkinesis, composed of 29 specialists from a number of federal agencies and headed by Dr. Albert C. Kolbye, Associate Director for Sciences of the FDA's Bureau of Foods. The group released a preliminary report in early January 1976 (prior to release of the Wisconsin data) stating that studies to date "have neither proven nor disproven the hypothesis that a diet free of artificial food colors and flavors reduces the symptoms in a significant number of children with the hyperkinetic behavior syndrome" (ICGH, 1976).

The report added that "the evidence taken as a whole is sufficient to merit further investigation into the relationship of diet and the hyperkinetic syndrome."

AAP Council on Child Health, 1975. Medication for hyperactive children. Am. Acad. of Pediatrics. Pediatrics 55: 560, April.

Beall, J. G. 1973. Food additives and hyperactivity in children. Congressional Record. S 19736, Oct. 30.

Conners, C. K. 1973. Psychological assessment of children with minimal brain dysfunction. Ann. N.Y. Acad. Sci. 205: 283, Feb. 28.

Conners, C. K. and Goyette, C. 1976. Progress report of studies on hyperkinesis and food additives. Paper presented at Ann. Meet., Food and Nutrition Liaison Committee, Nutrition Foundation, Naples, Fla., Jan. 30.

Culver, B. W. and Norton, S. 1974. Reversible hyperactivity in young rats after single exposure to carbon monoxide. Pharmacologist 16: 208.

David, O. J. 1974. Association between lower level lead concentrations and hyperactivity in children. Environ. Health Perspectives 7: 17, May.

ICGH. 1976. First report of the preliminary findings and recommendations of the Interagency Collaborative Group on Hyperkinesis submitted to the Assistant Secretary for Health, U.S. Dept. of Health, Education and Welfare, Washington, D.C., January.

Feingold, B. F. 1973. Food additives and child development (signed editorial). Hospital Practice, October, p. 11.

Feingold, B. 1975. "Why Your Child Is Hyperactive," p. 212. Random House, New York.

Feingold, B. F., German, D. F., Braham, R. M., and Simmers, E. 1973. Adverse reaction to food additives. Paper presented at Annual Convention, Am. Med. Assn., New York.

Goyette, C. 1975. Personal communication to the National Advisory Committee on Hyperkinesis and Food Additives, January. Univ. of Pittsburgh, Pittsburgh, Pa.

Harley, J. P., Chun, R., Cleeland, C. S., Eichman, P., Matthews, C. G., Ray, R., and Tomasi, L. 1976. Hyperkinesis: Food additives and hyperactivity in children. Paper presented at Ann. Meet., Food and Nutrition Liaison Committee, Nutrition Foundation, Naples, Fla., Jan. 29.

Johnson, C. 1974. Personal communication. University of Iowa, Iowa City.

Kalverboer, A. F., Touwen, B. C. L., and Prechtl, H. F. R. 1973. Follow-up of infants at risk of minor brain dysfunction. Ann. N.Y. Acad. Sci. 205: 173, Feb. 28.

Minskoff, J. G. 1973. Differential approaches to prevalence estimates of learning disabilities. Ann. N.Y. Acad. Sci. 205: 139, Feb. 28.

National Advisory Committee on Hyperkinesis and Food Additives. 1975. Report to the Nutrition Foundation. Nutriton Foundation, New York, N.Y.

Routh, D. 1975. The clinical significance of open-field activity in children. Pediatric Psychology 3: 3.

Silbergeld, E. K. and Goldbert, A. M. 1974. Hyperactivity: A lead-induced behavior disorder. Environ. Health Perspectives 7: 17, May.

Sleator, E. K., Sprague, R. L., and von Neumann, A. 1974. Hyperactive children. A continuous long-term placebo-controlled follow-up. J. Am. Med. Assn. 229: 316, July 15.

Sprague, R. L. and Sleator, E. K. 1973. The effects of psychopharmacologic agents on learning disorders. Pediatric Clinics of North America 20: 719.

Strother, C. R. 1973. Minimal cerebral dysfunction; A historical overview. Ann. N.Y. Acad. Sci. 205: 6, Feb. 28.

Wender, P. H. 1973. Some speculations concerning a possible biochemical basis of minimal brain dysfunction. Ann. N.Y. Acad. Sci. 205: 18, Feb. 28.

ALCOHOL AND DRUGS

| 20 | ## Alcohol and Nutrition |

CHARLES S. LIEBER

Charles S. Lieber, M.D., is professor of medicine and pathology at the Mt. Sinai School of Medicine of the City University of New York. He is also chief of the Liver Disease and Nutrition Section and director of the Alcoholism Research Laboratory at Bronx Veterans Administration Hospital. He is the author or coauthor of 300 scientific publications. In recent years, he has served as president of the New York Gastroenterological Association, the American Medical Society on Alcoholism, and the American Society for Clinical Nutrition.

Reprinted from *Nutrition News* 39 (October 1976), pp. 9 and 12. © 1976, National Dairy Council. Courtesy of National Dairy Council.

Thirty years ago, researchers considered the possibility that malnutrition promotes alcoholism. More recently, this theory has been abandoned.

Malnutrition, as well as impaired digestion and absorption, is now considered a result of chronic alcohol consumption. Independent of nutritional factors, alcohol also directly affects the development of fatty liver, hepatitis, and cirrhosis.

MALNUTRITION

Malnutrition is common among alcoholics because alcohol, high in caloric value, displaces other foods in the diet. Each gram of ethanol provides 7.1

calories. Twenty ounces of an 86-proof beverage contain about 1,500 calories, or approximately one-half to two-thirds of the recommended daily dietary allowance (RDA) for calories.

However, the calories provided by alcohol do not fully "count," at least at relatively high levels of intake, especially among alcoholics.[1] One of the pathways of ethanol metabolism is wasteful. Ethanol does not effectively form high energy phosphate bonds, therefore heat is produced without conservation of chemical energy.

Although the alcoholic has a reduced demand for food to fulfill his caloric needs, alcoholic beverages contain few, if any, vitamins, minerals, protein, or other nutrients. The alcoholic's intake of foods containing these nutrients may readily become insufficient. Economic factors may also reduce consumption of nutrient-rich food.

Chronic alcohol consumption can also result in malnutrition by interfering with normal food digestion and absorption. Alcohol exerts a direct effect on the gut[2] and pancreas. At high concentrations, it causes erosions of the gastrointestinal mucosa. Even in the absence of these lesions, alcohol abuse reduces intestinal enzymes.

Alcohol may also impair absorption of a number of essential nutrients, including vitamins B_1 and B_{12}.[3] Combining malnutrition with alcoholism is obviously "adding insult to injury."

For all these reasons, deficiency diseases develop more readily in the alcoholic than in the nonalcoholic population. Pellagra, once common in the alcoholic, has now practically disappeared. Similarly, overt thiamin deficiency such as Wernicke's syndrome is uncommon. However, mild thiamin deficiency, as well as riboflavin and pyridoxine deficiencies, can be observed. One of the most common alcoholic vitamin deficiencies is of folate,[4] a major cause of macrocytic anemia.

Mineral deficiencies have also been reported in the alcoholic. Low serum magnesium has been described. Similarly, zinc deficiency occurs in alcoholics due, in part, to increased zinc excretion. While mineral deficiencies are relatively uncommon and rarely warrant specific preventive action, vitamin deficiencies are sufficiently prevalent to merit vitamin therapy in known alcoholics.

A number of alcoholics also have a history of poor protein intake which may result in protein depletion. However, it is somewhat difficult to differentiate protein deficiency from decreased protein production as a result of liver disease. Protein repletion must, therefore, be carried out cautiously in the alcoholic, since protein overload in those with severe liver disease may be harmful.

LIVER DISORDERS

While most vitamin deficiencies are now recognized as deficiencies due to inadequate intake rather than due to a direct toxic effect of alcohol, the reverse is true with liver disease. Traditionally, disorders affecting the liver were attributed exclusively to nutritional deficiencies accompanying alcoholism. Recent studies, however, show that alcohol itself is a direct cause of alcoholic liver disease. Experimental evidence and statistics gathered in France and Germany indicate that incidence of liver disease is correlated with amount of alcohol consumed rather than with deficiencies in the diet.

To determine if chronic alcohol ingestion leads to deposition of dietary fat in the liver, rats were fed large amounts of ethanol as part of a liquid diet.[5] Despite nutritionally adequate diets, the rats developed fatty liver. In addition, the rats displayed an ethanol dependence and had typical withdrawal seizures when their alcohol intake was terminated.

Human volunteers[6] were also tested to determine if alcohol ingestion in amounts comparable to those consumed by chronic alcoholics is capable of injuring the liver. Test subjects were fed a variety of normal[5] or high protein[7] diets under controlled conditions. Ethanol either supplemented the diet or replaced carbohydrate calories. All human subjects also developed fatty liver.

Fatty liver develops when alcohol replaces fat as the preferred energy source for the liver. Combustion of fat ceases and lipid accumulates in the liver.

Although alcoholics may display varying degrees of liver complication, ranging from reversible fatty liver to alcoholic hepatitis and finally irreversible cirrhosis, the relationship between these disorders has been the subject of much debate.

To test the progression of liver disorders, 16 baboons were fed a nutritionally adequate diet. However, 50 percent of their total calories consisted of ethanol. Their intake of alcohol was sufficient to result in periods of obvious inebriation. These animals all developed excessive fat accumulation in the liver. In addition, five showed alcoholic hepatitis and five others studied for two to four years developed cirrhosis of the liver.[7] The study demonstrated that fatty liver, alcoholic hepatitis, and cirrhosis can all be produced by prolonged alcohol ingestion, even with nutritionally adequate diets.

This is not to downgrade the importance of good nutrition in the alcoholic. Adequate nutrition is essential for the normal functioning of all organs, including the liver. In fact, the treatment of alcoholics includes restoration of vitamin, mineral, and protein levels reduced because of low intake, poor digestion, or malabsorption.

However, the alcoholic should not be led to believe that mere correction or prevention of nutritional inadequacies will fully protect against liver damage. To this end, control of alcohol intake is also needed.

References

1   Pirola, R. C., Lieber, C. S. 1972. The energy cost of the metabolism of drugs, including ethanol. *Pharmacology* 7:185–196.

2   Baraona, E., Pirola, R. C., Lieber, C. S. 1974. Small intestinal damage and changes in cell population produced by ethanol ingestion in the rat. *Gastroenterology* 66:226–234.

3   Lindenbaum, J., Lieber, C. S. 1969. Alcohol-induced malabsorption of vitamin B_{12} in man. *Nature* 224:806.

4   Herbert, V., Zalusky, R., Davidson, C. S. 1963. Correlation of folate deficiency with alcoholism and associated macrocytosis, anemia and liver disease. *Ann Intern Med* 38:977–988.

5   Lieber, C. S., Jones, D. P., DeCarli, L. M. 1965. Effects of prolonged ethanol intake: Production of fatty liver despite adequate diets. *J Clin Invest* 44:1009–1021.

6   Lieber, C. S., Rubin, E. 1968. Alcoholic fatty liver in man on a high protein and low fat diet. *Amer J Med* 44:200–206.

7   Lieber, C. S., DeCarli, L. M., Rubin, E. 1975. Sequential production of fatty liver, hepatitis and cirrhosis in sub-human primates fed ethanol with adequate diets. *Proc Natl Acad Sci USA* 72:437–441.

21 Liquor's Good Side: Wine and Cognac

JOHN F. HENAHAN

John F. Henahan is a biomedical writer who is particularly fond of Bacchus.

Reprinted from *Science Digest,* May 1976, pp. 36–41, by permission of the Hearst Corporation. Copyright © 1976 The Hearst Corporation.

Wonder drugs come and go, but one of the most useful and durable is still going strong more than 1,100 years after it was first distilled by an Arabian alchemist named Jabir ibn Hayyan. We're talking, of course, about ethyl alcohol.

In many respects that ancient drug is the kind of "magic molecule" that today's pharmaceutical companies often have to spend millions of dollars for, in hopes of developing a substance that will ameliorate one or more of the ills that afflict human kind. Yet, the ethyl alcohol molecule is extremely simple and cheap to make. Composed of only nine atoms, it can be produced at a cost of less than a dollar a gallon. Packed into that tiny combination of atoms, however, are many remarkable properties. It is an excellent solvent for many things, including other drugs; it is a rapid source of energy for ailing patients and it has been prescribed for heart disease, diabetes, arthritic aches and pains, psychological tension and several other afflictions.

Ethyl alcohol is produced in nature's laboratory by the fermentation of grain, grapes and other carbohydrate-containing substances. Although it is usually singled out as an evil, leading to alcoholism and all the personal, economic and social ills that go along with it, many physicians believe its beneficial effects are generally overlooked, scoffed at, or only poorly explored. But there is plenty of historical and up-to-date evidence that alcoholic beverages are indeed good for you, not the least of which is the Biblical passage in which St. Paul tells his friend Timothy:

"I charge thee before God and the Lord Jesus Christ; drink no longer only water, but use a little wine for thy stomach's sake and thine often infirmities."

In acknowledgment of its many beneficial qualities, alcohol is known in some cultures as *aqua vitae,* the water of life. In fact, the name whiskey is derived from *usquebaugh,* the Irish word meaning exactly the same thing. And in spite of the fact that the more troublesome facets of alcohol's personality are most frequently apparent in the lay media and even the scientific literature, it's worth remembering that until 25 years ago, brandy and whiskey were legitimate entries in the pharmaceutical industry's bible, the *United States Pharmacoepia.*

Happily enough, there now is a resurgence of scientific and medical interest in Jabir ibn Hayyan's concoction of more than a millennium ago and some of the beverages that contain it. Most of the new findings pertain to two types of liquor specifically: wine and cognac. Here's the good news on these two drinks:

WINE

In many hospitals and nursing homes throughout the country, wine is served regularly to lighten many of the psychological and physiological stresses which Plato summed up as "the sourness of old age." For instance, a study carried out at the Vallejo General Hospital in California showed that elderly patients who were given wine with their meals were much more cooperative and generally felt better than patients who were not given wine. The wine-sipping patients invariably gave higher marks to the care they were receiving from doctors and hospital staff than the other patients did, and appeared to suffer no adverse side effects from the dietary innovation. In addition, the elderly wine drinkers enjoyed their food more than the other group, slept better and were, in general, happier, more responsive, and better patients than the non-drinkers were.

As Dr. William Dock sees it: "Wine is the safest, most popular and highly recommended tranquilizer that's ever been stumbled on to."

Dr. Dock, who now runs a cardiac laboratory at Lutheran Medical Center in Brooklyn, has long felt that the medicinal advantages of wine and other alcoholic beverages have been slighted, and notes that he frequently prescribes wine to "nice little old ladies who never had a drink and don't like to take medicine, but who are perfectly willing to take a glass of port or sherry with their dinner because it makes them feel better. Like any tranquilizer, it is probably better for *people* than it is for any illness *per se.*"

Although the alcohol in wine is largely responsible for its pleasant tranquilizing properties, Dr. Maynard Amerine, professor of enology (the study of wine) at the University of California, thinks that some of its beneficial effects are probably due to one or more of the two hundred other substances it contains. Wine, he says, is a "chemical symphony," a veritable molecular grab-bag of sugars, aldehydes, ketones, enzymes, pigments, vitamins, useful minerals and more than 22 different organic acids.

Some researchers believe that the tannins, which give wine its characteristic astringency, also play a major role in regulating the rate at which alcohol is absorbed into the blood stream from the digestive tract. Other compounds, called polyphenols, seem to strengthen delicate blood vessels and may help to reduce blood cholesterol levels, according to reports from various laboratories. Also, because wine contains almost no sodium, it is frequently included in "low sodium diets" prescribed for certain patients with high blood pressure or heart disease.

Because so much energy is crammed into such a small molecule, the alcohol in wine or other beverages comes in handy as a quick pickup when patients for various reasons can't take in normal foods. For example, an ounce of muscatel wine supplies about 50 calories while the same amount of a red table wine provides a boost of 24 calories. Beer, in spite of its reputation as a fat promoter, only supplies about 15 calories per ounce.

Wine, in moderate amounts, is also prescribed to spur the appetites of people who must put on weight but, because of physiological or psychological reasons, just can't stand the sight of food. Again, physicians assume that it is chiefly the tranquilizing qualities that remove the patient's aversion to food, while others suspect that some of the organic acids it contains may be the real appetite-promoters.

Wine may also help get more nutritional benefit out of whatever kind of food you take in, according to research recently carried out by Dr. Janet McDonald and her colleagues at the University of California in Berkeley. Their 75-day-long study involved six adult males who were fed formula diets, which were supplemented either with regular California Zinfandel (a red wine) that contained alcohol or with a mock Zinfandel from which only the alcohol had been removed. At the conclusion of the study, says Dr. McDonald, the nonalcoholic wine appeared to have the greatest effect in enhancing the uptake of several important nutrients, including calcium, iron, zinc, magnesium and phosphrous.

"The differences were large enough to conclude that wine tends to have a beneficial effect on the absorption of these elements independent of an alcohol and is presumably due to the congeners [other chemical factors]," she said, noting that the chemicals which were responsible have yet to be identified.

On the other end of the scale, wine is often used to help people who eat too much but who find it difficult to stay with a reducing diet. Some physicians say that their obese patients feel a lot better about cutting down their food intake, if the diet is spiced up with several ounces of a dry red table wine. (Dr. Dock's tranquilizer strikes again.)

As for specific diseases, many physicians, particularly in Europe, routinely recommend moderate amounts of dry, sugar-free wine in the diet of diabetics. That recommendation is supported by a study carried out at the International Center for Psychodietetics in Rome, which found that from 0.4 to one liter of dry red wine per day helped maintain low blood sugar levels in diabetics who were on insulin, took oral diabetic drugs or were able to control their condition by diet alone. There are also some indications that wine and other alcoholic beverages may actually help counter hardening of the arteries (one of the major complications in diabetes) by widening the arteries and allowing better circulation throughout the body.

For the same reason, Dr. Dock and others suspect that wine is useful therapy for patients with heart disease, its main effect being to reduce the load on the overtaxed heart. Along those lines, an epidemiological study carried out in Europe 12 years ago found that in countries where wine is part of the national life style, the incidence of heart disease is significantly lower than it is in countries where the population shows less affection for the product of the fermented grape. Closer to home, Dr. Stewart Wolf and his colleagues found that wine-drinking Italian-Americans who live in Roseto, Pennsylvania, had a lower than average incidence of heart disease even though their diet contained large amounts of saturated fats (usually considered to be a contributing factor to hardening of the arteries and heart disease).

COGNAC

If more and more physicians seem to be singing the praises of wine these days, almost as many are intrigued with the healthful aspects of drinking cognac, a considerably more potent alcoholic beverage than the wines are.

A few months ago, for example, Dr. James A. Brussel sprang into print in a magazine called *Medical Dimensions* to announce that cognac—touted through history as the drink of the gods—is just what he and other doctors order for a number of heart ailments, including angina pectoris. The latter is a severe pain in the chest and shoulder which often is an indicator of impending heart attack.

There is no valid scientific evidence to explain why cognac should be useful in treating angina, Dr. Brussel admits, but he suspects that it may have something to do with the fact that cognac, like wine, dilates or widens the openings of the arteries which normally become constricted as heart disease progresses. By dilating the blood vessels, blood, with its life-giving cargo of oxygen, is better able to feed the undernourished heart. One good belt of cognac can usually produce an immediate dilatory effect which lasts for as long as two hours, says Dr. Brussel, former assistant commissioner of the New York State Department of Health.

Although wine also dilates blood vessels, Dr. Brussel says cognac does a better job because the arteries don't appear to "snap back" to the original constricted state as rapidly as they do when wine is given as the drug of choice.

At the same time, Dr. Brussel suggests, cognac's effects in a heart disease patient may be one part dilation and another part *elation*.

"With rare exceptions, when I give a person with heart trouble a drink of cognac, he shows an emotional uplift and grins as though his life had been saved," he says. Taking a leaf from his own prescription book, Dr. Brussel (who suffered his own heart attack 21 years ago) says that he now routinely sips three glasses of cognac a day to keep his blood vessels in good working order.

Echoing Dr. Brussel's sentiments in behalf of cognac, Dr. Paul Dudley White, who acted as the late President Eisenhower's heart physician, once said that in his opinion, alcohol, particularly in the form of cognac, was the most effective drug for heart disorders after the nitrates, the drugs that are traditionally used to prevent fatal heart attacks.

To move from life-threatening heart disease to the common cold, many physicians admit that distilled spirits, such as cognac, are by no means a cure, but that they can be beneficial in warding off the sniffles, snuffs and other symptoms of a cold after exposure to inclement weather and before the cold has had a chance to really take hold. Again, there is no strong scientific proof as to why that should be, but some scientists suggest that the alcohol apparently tends to restore the nasal mucosa to a normal physiological state by raising the temperature of the membranes inside the nose.

Like wine, cognac has many other desirable properties, including its effects as a pain killer and as a reducer of premenstrual tension. In addition, Dr. Fritz Fuchs of Cornell University Medical College says that cognac is also remarkably effective in postponing the premature birth of a baby.

A FINAL WARNING

As new data accumulates that alcohol in several of its drinkable forms is literally good for you, there is no getting away from the fact that the same simple molecule is a drug, and like other drugs should be used in reasonable amounts and with considerable caution. As with other tranquilizers, more alcohol does not mean that it will do a better job. It is also well known that alcohol, in combination with many other drugs, including the barbiturates, the tranquilizers, a few antibiotics and certain pain killers, can be a very troublesome mixture.

Aside from those hazards, physicians know that there are many individuals, including alcoholics of course, who should not be given wine, whiskey or any other alcoholic beverage for any reason. In some patients, even small amounts of Scotch, wine or cognac can produce pounding headaches, nausea and vomiting. Ordinarily, patients with stomach ulcers, sore throats or other types of inflammation are probably better off without the added irritation that alcohol can produce, although some doctors report that ulcer patients do very well when wine or diluted whiskey is part of their daily diet. Doctors also avoid prescribing alcohol in any form for patients who have gastrointestinal disorders, liver disease, viral hepatitis, kidney infections, gout, epilepsy or genitourinary disease. In these cases, liquor could possibly produce adverse reactions.

Not that all physicians are as enthusiastic as Dr. Dock is about wine as a tranquilizer or as certain as Drs. Brussel and White are that cognac is good for heart disease; in fact there are many who will disagree with both. Usually they object that the data supporting such views are inconclusive, inadequate or just plain wrong. Or they may be guided by the same natural suspicion of alcohol's adverse effects which spawned the prohibition movement and sentiments such as "lips that touch wine, shall never touch mine."

However, there is little doubt that the present interest in alcohol as a substance that can really be good for you has an eons-long basis in the history of medicine. Hippocrates swore by wine as a solution to many of the physical ills of his patients even before alcohol itself had been discovered. Galen, another ancient physician, wrote detailed analyses of different wines, the grapes and soils that produced them and the comparative medical advantages of various vintages. So, if longevity is any criterion of success, wine has proved its right to exist. On the same basis, it is very doubtful that any of the "wonder drugs" that have been developed even within the last 25 years will, with the passage of another 1,000 years, be able to claim the endurance record of wine, cognac and other beverages that contain Jabir ibn Hayyan's magic molecule.

| 22 | Drug-Vitamin Interrelationships

MYRON BRIN

Myron Brin is associate director for biochemical nutrition at the Roche Research Center, Nutley, N.J.

Reprinted from *Nutrition & the M.D.* 3 (November 1976), pp. 1–2, by permission of the publisher. Copyright © PM, Inc., 1976.

We live in a chemical world. Exposure to these chemicals may be inadvertent as with environmental chemicals (pollutants and others), or voluntary as with drugs. While in the past we considered the risk/benefit ratios of drug therapy only in terms of iatrogenic pathology, now we know there are also significant nutritional interrelationships.

Chemicals, including drugs, which are foreign to the body are metabolized by the "mixed function oxidases" of the microsomal particulate material in our tissue cells. These oxidases are often also referred to as the cytochrome P-450 enzymes. These enzymes, with vitamins acting as coenzymes, metabolize chemicals to facilitate their removal from the body. Furthermore, these mixed function oxidases are often induced by various drugs to increase their activity level.

VITAMIN EFFECTS ON DRUG METABOLISM

One may first ask: How do vitamin deficiencies influence the activity of mixed function oxidases? Deficiencies of vitamins A, B_2 (riboflavin), C, and E result in decreased metabolism of various drug and environmental chemical substrates. Vitamin B_1 (thiamin) deficiency, on the other hand, has been reported to cause increased metabolism. With vitamin E deficiency, there is about an 85 percent reduction in the ability to metabolize benzopyrene, a potent carcinogen. The same is true for the other vitamins, although the extent of decreased activity will vary with the specific chemical being studied.

Carbohydrate content of diets may also influence drug reactions. Increasing dietary carbohydrate, for instance, increases drug half-lifes and suggests reduced rates of metabolism and perhaps potentiation of drug action.

DRUG INFLUENCE ON VITAMIN NEEDS

Conversely, the administration of drugs and/or exposure to certain environmental chemicals (shown in Table 1) will have an influence on the vitamin needs of the individual. The consumption of alcohol results in reduced blood levels of thiamin (not in the table), vitamin B_6 (pyridoxine), and folacin. Alcohol interferes with the conversion of pyridoxine to pyridoxal

TABLE 1

Increased vitamin needs of man and animals as a consequence of drug and/or environmental chemical exposure.

Nutrient	Exposure resulting in increased vitamin needs or reduced blood levels
Vitamin A	Polychlorobiphenyls, benzopyrene, spironolactone, DDT
Folacin	Oral contraceptives, anticonvulsants, methotrexate, pyrimethamine, alcohol
Vitamin B_{12}	Biguanides, anticonvulsants, oral contraceptives
Vitamin B_6 (pyridoxine)	Isoniazid, thiosemicarbazide, pencillamine, L-dopa, hydralazine, oral contraceptives, alcohol
Niacin (vitamin B_3)	Polychlorobiphenyls, isoniazid, phenylbutazone
Riboflavin (vitamin B_2)	Boric acid
Vitamin D	Anticonvulsants
Vitamin K	Anticonvulsants, antibiotics
Vitamin C	Smoking, aspirin, oral contraceptives, nitrites
Vitamin E	Oxygen, ozone

phosphate, the co-enzyme (active) form of vitamin B_6, and with the absorption of both thiamin and folic acid.

Oral contraceptive steroids result in reduced blood levels of thiamin, riboflavin, vitamins B_6, B_{12}, C, and folacin. These estrogenic compounds also result in the excretion of abnormal tryptophan metabolites, an effect that can be corrected by large doses of vitamin B_6. Clinically, oral contraceptives may cause megaloblastosis of cervical mucosa and of erythrocytes and also may cause behavioral changes such as depression. These are sometimes correctable by folate and vitamin B_6 respectively.

INH, PENICILLAMINE, AND L-DOPA

Vitamin B_6 requirements are also increased by therapy with isoniazid (INH) and other hydrazines such as thiosemicarbazide and hydralazine and also with penicillamine. While vitamin B_6 levels may be decreased by the use of L-dopa, this vitamin may also interfere with the therapeutic effect of the drug.

Anticonvulsant therapy in children may produce rickets, which is correctable by vitamin D therapy. Anticonvulsants also may interfere with blood clotting and may reduce folacin and vitamin B_{12} levels in the blood.

POLLUTION AND NUTRITION

Environmental chemicals may also interfere with good nutrition. The pollutants polychlorobiphenyls (PCB) and DDT result in reduced blood levels of vitamin A and niacin. Vitamin C levels have been shown to be decreased in the blood of smokers, and in leukocytes after ingestion of aspirin and oral contraceptives. Administration of vitamin E to premature infants is reported to reduce the incidence and severity of retrolental fibroplasia resulting from exposure to high concentrations of oxygen.

If one were to generalize, one would say that vitamin insufficiency results in reduced capacity of the body to metabolize drugs, and that drug administration can cause vitamin insufficiency.

NEED FOR VITAMIN ADEQUACY

Ingestion of the daily Recommended Dietary Allowance of vitamins will usually correct the clinical effects of vitamin inadequacies resulting from drug therapy. When the individual is ingesting INH or other hydrazides, oral contraceptives, or alcohol, the doses of vitamin B_6 necessary to correct the metabolic problems may be 2 to 10 times the US RDA, varying with the drug given and the individual being treated. This also may be true for some of the other vitamins.

Physicians should obtain information concerning the nutritional status of their patients when prescribing drugs for specific indications. . . .

SUGAR

| 23 | Sweet and Sour

JOHN PEKKANEN and MATHEA FALCO

John Pekkanen is a free-lance writer and a Fellow of the Drug
Abuse Council, Inc., in Washington, D.C. Mathea Falco, an
attorney, is a special assistant to the president of the Drug
Abuse Council.

From *The Atlantic Monthly,* July 1975, pp. 50–53. Copyright ©
1975, by The Atlantic Monthly Company, Boston, Mass. Reprinted with permission.

It has come to be called "white gold." Some people
claim it is addictive, and many doctors and researchers believe it poses a
dire threat to our national health. It has created a black market. Many rock
music stations play songs which glorify it. On the average, each and every
one of us consumes nearly two pounds of it a week. Lest there be any
remaining mystery as to what it is, it is sugar.

Sugar comes under many names. Fructose is fruit sugar, lactose is milk
sugar, maltose is malt sugar, and glucose is blood sugar, which is what the
sugar we ingest becomes when it is metabolized. Our major source of sugar,
and the chief concern of nutritionists, however, is sucrose. This is the familiar
refined sugar—brown, white, and packaged "raw" sugar—which is commonly added to our food. Because it is so palatable, so highly concentrated,
and so freely available, we consume far more sucrose than any other type of
sugar.

Our individual consumption of refined sugar and other caloric sweeteners, such as molasses and corn syrup, now totals 130 pounds a year. Even for those who take their coffee black, avoid cake, ice cream, cookies, and assume somebody else must be eating enormous quantities of sugar because they are eating none, sugar is an inextricable, if unnoticed, part of their daily diet.

To gauge how much sugar is added to our food, read the labels listing the contents of the food you are eating. You will find that there is sugar in items as seemingly unsweet as canned soups, frozen vegetables, mayonnaise, mustard, peanut butter, baked beans, breads, bouillon cubes, dinner rolls, bologna, pastrami, chili—and for those of you who shop at the health food section, in flavored yogurts and natural cereals. In fact, it is almost impossible to avoid eating sugar unless one forgoes many processed foods and most restaurants.

Sugar consumption in this country accounts for nearly one-fifth of our total calorie intake. And because sugar provides "naked" calories, the burden on the remaining 80 percent of our diet to supply us with necessary vitamins and minerals is great. Yet even staggering price increases, coupled with the widespread antisugar campaigns waged by many grocery stores, have not inspired us to withdraw substantially from sugar.

"I don't think sugar is addictive in the sense that some drugs are," says Dr. Abraham Nizel professor of nutrition and dentistry at Tufts University, "but there is no question that many people experience a very strong craving for sugar when they try to give it up. I use the term 'sucroholics' to describe these people."

A recovered sucroholic, Mrs. Trudy Quick, a board member of Overeaters Anonymous, is convinced that refined sugar can be as addictive as alcohol. After years of sharing the experiences of other O.A. members, she has concluded that "many of us use sugar like a drug. It is our lover, friend, comforter, and when stress comes into our lives we reach for it automatically. Giving it up is terribly difficult; many people go through withdrawal and get the shakes. For some of us, complete abstinence is the only way out. We cannot be social sugar eaters just the way other people cannot be social drinkers."

Consider the entrapping world of sugar for the diabetic. Mrs. Edwin Ducat, president and founder of the Juvenile Diabetes Foundation, testifying before the U.S. Senate Select Committee on Nutrition and Human Needs in

February, 1974, said in part: "The diabetic in the United States lives in an alien, hostile environment. That is especially true of children. The diabetic child injects himself with insulin, then he goes to school where there are Coke and candy machines. He watches television and is bombarded with candy advertisements, sweet snacks, cereals, pies, cookies, cakes, ice cream, all of which are *verboten,* or 'poison' to him. A birthday party can become a painful experience if you are a diabetic child." So can Halloween, Christmas, Thanksgiving, and nearly every day of the year. Lollipops are doled out regularly by banks, barbers, and even some dentists.

A survey conducted in 1970 showed that almost two thirds of all food advertising specifically aimed at young television viewers emphasized heavily sugared foods or presweetened breakfast cereals, some, such as King Vitamin, Sugar Smacks, and Super Orange Crisp, ranging from 58 to 68 percent refined sugar. This compared to a total of only 6 percent of children's food commercials promoting milk and meat products. There was no advertising for fruits and vegetables. A later survey in 1972 revealed that during prime-time children's television, approximately ten commercials for candy, sugared drinks and snacks, and other heavily sweetened food products were aired every hour. Even the best intentioned parent finds it hard to battle an industry which spends hundreds of millions of dollars a year to push its sugared products to children.

The one widely accepted and advertised value of sugar—a supplier of quick energy—can in fact be obtained from many other foods which also supply minerals and vitamins. Refined sugar is an additive, a sweetener, a filler, a texturizer, and a preservative, but it not make us stronger or give us the sole source of quick energy. In fact, because of its effect on blood-sugar levels, some researchers believe it may do quite the reverse.

One disease for which sugar is unquestionably responsible is tooth decay. Often called the "arch-criminal of dental health," sucrose in effect creates a climate in which oral bacteria thrive and multiply. Candies like lollipops, which are held in the mouth for long periods of time, greatly enhance this bacteria growth. In view of the large amounts of candy children eat, it is not surprising that 98 percent of them suffer tooth decay.

High sugar intake might also be related to our number one killer, heart disease. Dr. John Yudkin, emeritus professor of nutrition at London University, believes that sugar's contribution to heart disease and other diseases is so clear-cut that sugar should be banned. Dr. Yudkin told the U.S. Senate

Select Committee on Nutrition and Human Needs in 1973: "Epidemiology supports the view that sugar is a cause of coronary disease at least as much as it supports the view that fat is a possible cause of coronary disease. . . . I think we have been in danger for a long time of assuming that coronary heart disease is simply a situation in which there is a raised level of blood cholesterol."

On the other hand, Dr. Ancel Keys, the American physiologist who performed studies linking heart disease to fat intake and its effect on elevated cholesterol levels, discounts the role of sugar in heart disease. He argues that the experiments and population data are misleading and do not support Yudkin's view. "It's really a matter of belief," says Dr. Richard A. Ahrens, associate professor of food and nutrition at the University of Maryland. "Either you believe the evidence implicating sugar or you don't. I, for one, do." Dr. Ahrens has conducted several experiments on sugar's effects on triglyceride levels. Elevated triglyceride levels may be a better indicator of heart attack risk for people under the age of fifty than elevated cholesterol levels. Triglycerides, fatty elements in the blood stream, are a form of storage for the excess carbohydrates we eat. Dr. Ahrens has found in recent animal studies that triglycerides caused by sugar intake are much more persistent than those caused by starch intake, and do not clear out of the blood stream very quickly after a radical dietary change.

Experiments now under way suggest another problem caused by sugar consumption. A recent study has found that animals previously fed sugar diets lose much less weight after an overnight fast than starch-fed animals. What this suggests to Dr. Ahrens, who conducted these experiments, is that sugar increases the body's fluid retention, which has a direct impact on elevated blood pressure. High blood pressure increases the risk of heart attack, stroke, kidney disease, diabetes, and other diseases. "I would speculate," Dr. Ahrens says, "that in twenty years, sugar in our diet will be shown to be a hypertensive agent. I don't think it will be possible for sugar's defenders to continue their claim that sugar is a harmless source of calories."

Diabetes—the one disease in which sugar often has been suggested as a causal factor—afflicts between five and twelve million Americans. Millions more are potential diabetics: 1000 new cases are reported every day. And the numbers are increasing geometrically—Mrs. Ducat of the Juvenile Diabetes Foundation predicts that by 1980, one in five people will have diabetes.

Some medical experts believe that diabetes, not cancer, is the second leading cause of death in this country. The actual death rate from diabetes may be even higher, since it accelerates other potentially fatal conditions, such as arteriosclerosis, stroke, heart attack, and kidney failure. Compared to the nondiabetic population, diabetics suffer heart attacks and strokes two or three times more frequently. Diabetes is the leading cause of new blindness in the United States and England, two of the world's leading sugar-consuming countries.

Diabetes is characterized by the failure of the pancreas to secrete sufficient insulin to break down blood sugar for storage in the body. Associated with inadequate removal of blood sugar is the accumulation of abnormal chemicals, particularly in the large and small blood vessels. Before the discovery of insulin in 1921, diabetes that could not be controlled through diet inevitably proved fatal. Even today the life expectancy of diabetes is only two thirds that of the general population.

No one argues that high sugar consumption alone causes diabetes; a genetic tendency must be present. Studies of isolated rural groups who have emigrated to countries high in the consumption of sugar show that while diabetes was virtually nonexistent in the land of origin, within twenty years in the new culture these groups developed a high incidence of diabetes. Dr. Aharon Cohen of the Jerusalem Hebrew University reported that immigrants from Yemen and Kurdistan, who had taken very little sugar in their diet, had virtually no detectable diabetes upon their arrival in Israel. However, veteran Yemenite and Kurdistan settlers who had adopted the dietary habits of the Israelis—which include a high sugar intake—later exhibited the same frequency of diabetes as the Israelis. This suggested that diet, and sugar intake in particular, was a factor that precipitated the onset of diabetic symptoms.

During times of sugar scarcity and limited caloric intake, diabetes drops dramatically. In England and Wales during World War I, diabetes mortality fell by 25 percent, and during World War II, when sugar was largely replaced by saccharin, or sweeteners were eliminated altogether, diabetes deaths dropped 40 percent. This and other evidence prompts Dr. Jean Mayer of Harvard to remark that despite the necessarily circumstantial nature of the evidence, sugar's implication in diabetes is "more than a mere allegation."

One study appeared to contradict the findings connecting high sugar intake with diabetes. It was done in 1966 and included several thousand sugarcane cutters in Natal, South Africa. It revealed that although they normally ate some 6000 calories a day, mostly derived from the sugarcane they constantly chewed, the cane cutters were entirely free of diabetes. However, some researchers believe the trace element chromium, which is present in sugarcane in exceptionally large amounts but almost absent from refined sugar, was the protective element for the cane cutters because trace chromium is vital in the maintenance of stable blood-sugar levels. If, in fact, the trace chromium in the natural sugarcane (and not merely the hard physical exercise of cutting cane, or genetic factors) was the critical protective factor, it suggests that the refinement process, rather than natural sugar, may be the culprit.

While some nutritionists and researchers regard the evidence linking sugar to heart disease and diabetes as too fragmentary to prove anything definitive, some refuse to accept even its possible implication. Dr. Fredrick Stare, chairman of the Department of Nutrition at Harvard University's School of Public Health and a frequent spokesman for sugar interests, says flatly: "There is not a shred of acceptable evidence to suggest sugar has a thing to do with heart disease," He says the evidence thus far collected is at best circumstantial. He dismisses as well the Israeli studies of the Yemenites and Kurdistanis. He argues that factors other than sugar intake probably accounted for the onset of diabetes. "If we didn't prefer foods with added sugar, it would not be added," he says. "Remember, eating is one of the real pleasures of life as well as a necessity . . . for most people, sugar helps other things taste better. . . . Sugar calories are not different from other calories, from calories obtained from protein, starch, fat, or alcohol." The calories may not be different; however, the nutritional value of the foods supplying those calories does vary widely, and refined sugar simply has no nutrients. Dr. Stare is among the minority of nutritionists who view our high sugar intake so benignly.

Some organizations are actively seeking ways in which changes can be made in our sugar consumption. One crusader group, called The Center for Science in the Public Interest, recently petitioned the Food and Drug Administration (FDA) to require a maximum sugar content for ready-to-eat cereals of 10 percent of total weight. For those cereals which do not meet this standard—and even some so-called natural cereals do not—the Center requested that the cereal boxes state the percentage of sugar content and carry a health warning saying "frequent use contributes to tooth decay and other health problems." The FDA rejected the petition. Says an FDA spokesman: "Ingredients are listed in order of predominance. The consumer can get the picture of the relative order of content by reading it." Relative order, however, is not the same as knowing specifically whether a food has 15 percent sugar content or 50 percent. To this the FDA simply says that the health hazards of sugar have "no solid scientific backup." The FDA historically has been slow to recognize the hazards of various substances, from drugs to food additives. However, even Dr. Stare believes the public has a right to know the sugar content of the food it buys.

Other governmental agencies seem equally willing to allow our sugar consumption to pass unnoticed. The U.S. Department of Agriculture (USDA), in its handbook *Composition of Foods,* does not differentiate the carbohydrate content of foods, which would allow a reader to know how much sugar versus how much starch he is getting in various products. However, the same book does differentiate between saturated and unsaturated fats in products. Although this omission may stem in part from our preoccupation with fats in our diet, the omission, some believe, is deliberate. Robert Choate, chairman of the Council on Children, Media and Merchandising— a consumer group watching out for the welfare of children in the marketplace—says: "I don't know of a single action by the Congress or the responsible federal agencies that has changed our national attitudes toward sugar use, or even to better inform us how much we are eating. The dental and health lobby is no match for the food and sugar lobby."

The sugar industry, as well as many segments of the food industry, would plainly prefer to see the sugar content of the American diet remain just about where it is. Most nutritionists, however, believe that our diet should contain not more than 10 percent sugar, and some believe that 5 percent should be the maximum. Even spokesmen for the industry concede that we should not consume more than 20 percent, a limit we have just about reached.

The inevitable question is: Where do we go from here?

An obvious first step is more research to verify or discount the possible links between high sugar consumption and disease.

Equally important is informing the American consumer of how much sugar he or she is actually consuming. All food products should carry labels which state *how much* sugar is contained therein.

The Federal Trade Commission should grant the supplemental petition submitted in April, 1973, by Action for Children's Television to ban all sugared-food advertising during children's prime-time viewing hours. "Sugar is a learned taste," says Dr. Nizel, "and it can with effort be unlearned." The FTC has not acted on the petition, saying only that it is awaiting the "advice" of the FDA on the health hazards of sugar. The FTC is also waiting for the FDA's advice before it decides whether or not to draw up special standards governing the advertising of sugared foods in general. Since the FDA has already rejected the cereal labeling petition on the grounds that sugar's hazards have "no solid scientific backup," it is unlikely that the American consumer will soon be better informed about his sugar consumption.

| 24 | Sugar Doctors Push Hypoglycemia

SYDNEY WALKER III

Sydney Walker III is a neuropsychiatrist with a private medical practice in La Jolla, Calif. He is director of the newly formed Southern California Neuropsychiatric Institute, which is devoted to the multidimensional evaluation of emotional and behavioral disorders in children and adults.

Reprinted from *Psychology Today* Magazine, July 1975.
Copyright © 1975 Ziff-Davis Publishing Company. Reprinted by permission.

A patient complains to his doctor that he feels weak, run-down, nervous, irritable. Sometimes his heart beats too fast, he breaks out in a sweat, and he is overcome by a vague sense of dread. The doctor does a routine physical exam, and everything checks out fine. This man's problem may be all in his head. But it could be in his bloodstream. He may be one of the thousands of people who suffer from hypoglycemia, a lower-than-normal level of sugar in the blood.

Sugar, or glucose, is not merely a source of energy; it is fuel for the brain. When there is too little of it in the blood, the brain and the rest of the nervous system cannot function properly. Sometimes behavior and mood are affected, and the patient becomes depressed, restless, or anxious. Friends and relatives begin to notice signs of emotional instability. On the surface, the person appears to be neurotic rather than physically ill. So if help is sought, it is often psychiatric or psychological, not medical.

Hypoglycemia has caught the popular imagination lately. Somehow it has managed to attract the public's interest and engage the passions of the medical community. Doctors who think the condition is being neglected have been making television appearances and writing popular books about it. Largely because of their efforts, hypoglycemia is now faintly fashionable, just as tuberculosis once was. Other doctors think the importance and prevalence of the problem have been grossly exaggerated; they accuse the "sugar doctors" of misleading a gullible public.

Whenever there is a medical controversy of this sort, the patient gets caught in the crossfire. If a person who suspects he has low blood sugar goes to an overly conservative doctor, he may soon find himself on the local psychiatrist's couch. Cases have been reported in which a real physical disorder has gone unrecognized and untreated for years. But if the person goes to an extremist on the other side, he may get roped into a long series of expensive treatments that are not really necessary. Clearly, the time has come for some straight thinking about hypoglycemia.

First, hypoglycemia is not a disease; it is a physiological state that can occur for various reasons. The process by which our bodies convert carbohydrates into glucose, and glucose into energy and fuel for the nervous system, is a very complicated one. It involves the liver, the adrenal glands, the pituitary and thyroid glands, the pancreas, and other organs. A dysfunction anywhere along the line can cause blood-sugar levels to be too high (diabetes) or too low (hypoglycemia).

Too much of a good thing

Sometimes there is an obvious physical reason for low blood sugar. For example, there may be a tumor of the pancreas. The pancreas is a large organ that produces a substance called insulin, which helps the body to utilize sugar. A tumor can cause the pancreas to produce too much of a good thing, and then the blood sugar plummets. In such cases, the symptoms may be severe. If the patient doesn't get glucose by eating, his blood sugar reaches a dangerously low level; he may even lose consciousness.

In other cases, there are symptoms that are much milder, and the causes are difficult or even impossible to discover. The patient's blood-sugar level may fall a few hours after eating, but fail to reach the extreme low level that doctors usually insist on before diagnosing hypoglycemia. Strictly speaking, the word "hypoglycemia" should not be used for this sort of carbohydrate abnormality, though it is often used loosely for the sake of convenience.

Subtle blood-sugar disorders may occur because of defects in metabolism that are congenital or the result of disease. Sometimes alcohol is the culprit; if you drink too much, you can damage the liver, an organ that plays an important role in carbohydrate metabolism. Sometimes low blood sugar is the precursor of diabetes, an illness characterized by a high level of blood sugar and a low level of insulin.

There are certain physical symptoms and signs that can alert a physician to the possible presence of hypoglycemia, if he or she has an open mind and does not automatically write off a patient's complaints as hypochondria. For instance, when a person has a carbohydrate problem, his body may produce too much urine and he may have to go to the bathroom at all hours of the day and night. He may also sweat profusely, especially after meals. Because he is losing fluid through urination and perspiration, he may feel thirsty much of the time and may appear to be losing weight. (In some carbohydrate disorders, though, people retain too much water and gain weight.)

Craving for sweets

Some patients complain of itching, skin rashes, or numbness in certain areas. These symptoms can be traced to the effect that low blood-sugar levels have on nerve endings. Sometimes hypoglycemic people complain of repeated urinary tract infections, and various skin infections, including boils and styes. If the patient is a woman, she may get frequent vaginal yeast infections that are hard to clear up. These symptoms stem from the fact that glucose problems can reduce the ability of certain body tissues to ward off infection.

Often, hypoglycemic patients report an excessive craving for sweets. In a sense, they try to treat themselves by ingesting large amounts of sugar. Unfortunately, that can overstimulate the pancreas and cause it to produce too much insulin. In turn, blood-sugar levels fall. So the self-treatment only makes the problem worse.

None of these symptoms is unique to hypoglycemia, and finding the right explanation for the patient's complaints can be very tricky. It's important for the doctor to listen carefully and respectfully to what the patient says. If you go to a physician because of chronic fatigue, anxiety, or emotional distress, you should expect him to take a complete history. He should find out if you have diabetes or liver disease in your family, and if you weighed more than 10 pounds at birth, because prediabetic and diabetic mothers often have babies who are heavy. He should ask if there have been any other endocrine disorders in the family, and if you've been exposed recently to any toxic substances.

The physician should do a multidimensional examination. He may notice such diverse signs as tremor, abnormal eye movements, changes in the retina of the eye, rapid heart beat, a generally dysrhythmic electroencephalogram (EEG), and delayed conduction times in the nerves. If several of these occur, the doctor may begin to suspect a carbohydrate problem. He should not draw any conclusions, though, until he does tests on the liver, thyroid, and adrenal glands, and studies the balance of various salts in the body, including sodium, potassium, and magnesium.

Finally, he must run a glucose-tolerance test. The patient fasts overnight and then gets a dose of glucose. For the next five or six hours, the doctor draws periodic blood samples, checks the level of sugar in the blood, and plots a glucose-tolerance curve that shows blood-sugar changes over time. He interprets this curve—or should interpret it—according to strict guidelines laid down by the American Diabetes Association. These guidelines allow him to detect abnormalities that are more subtle than the extreme forms of hypoglycemia or diabetes.

The case of an 18-year-old boy I treated illustrates the course of diagnosis. For some time the boy had been doing poorly in school because of an inability to concentrate. More recently he had begun to have emotional problems. He worried that he was worthless, he felt depressed, and he was unresponsive to friends. When I took a history, I learned that he wanted badly to be a lifeguard, but had recently been disqualified after failing an eye examination.

The patient reported frequent thirst, burning urination, and the need to go to the bathroom during the night. In addition, he said he had an excessive craving for sweets. The boy underwent a complete multidimensional examination. The physical exam revealed an acnelike rash over his shoulders and face that he said itched, but nothing else.

A test for emotional instability confirmed that the patient was morose and depressed. He had a serious vision problem, and his EEG was mildly abnormal.

We decided to do a glucose-tolerance test. Three hours into the test, the patient's blood sugar had fallen to 50 milligrams per 100 cc of blood (usually stated as "50 milligrams percent"). That is quite low. None of the other biochemical tests were positive.

Gratifying results

Taken together, the boy's symptoms and test results seemed to indicate hypoglycemia. The diagnostic process had been complicated, but fortunately the treatment was not. I recommended the standard treatment, advising him to avoid refined carbohydrates, to eat three sensible meals a day, and to snack between meals, though not on sweets. A hypoglycemic person's body usually produces too much insulin; if he avoids carbohydrates his body will produce less insulin and therefore the blood-sugar level will stay higher. Ironically, the less sugar ingested, the higher the blood-sugar level stays.

The results were gratifying. After a month the patient had new vigor, and his itching, thirst, and urination problems had disappeared. Though we hadn't predicted it, his sight also improved dramatically. Because foods that are high in refined sugar often contain artificial food additives, it is not possible to say for sure whether this patient's improvement resulted solely from the removal of carbohydrates from his diet; the removal of the additives might also have helped. In any event, a change in nutrition resulted in a return to normal health.

Another case shows what can happen when a hypoglycemic person is depressed and anxious. The patient was a 26-year-old woman. For a year before her first visit, she had been taking Valium, a tranquilizer, and had been undergoing psychotherapy. Twice she had admitted herself to a hospital because of her persistent thoughts about suicide. Nothing had helped.

A careful history turned up some of the symptoms I've discussed. The patient complained of episodes of leg and body numbness. She was always thirsty, craved sweets, and had skin problems. The general physical exam was normal, but other tests were not. Her potassium and calcium levels were low. She had a generally abnormal brain-wave pattern, and an eye-muscle weakness caused spasmodic vertical and horizontal movements of the eye. We did a glucose-tolerance test. After fasting, the patient's blood sugar level was 66 milligrams percent, and after four hours it fell to 57 milligrams percent. At this point she felt very weak.

No artificial boundaries

I recommended that the patient increase her calcium intake by consuming milk and other dairy products, that she increase her potassium intake by eating certain fruits, and that she avoid refined sugars. Within two weeks her physical symptoms cleared up. She was then in a position to reenter psychotherapy and benefit from it. After six months her emotional distress was relieved.

This patient's case illustrates that before you can get what you should from psychiatric treatment, you must have any existing metabolic problems corrected. There is no natural boundary between mind and body, and there should be no artificial boundary between physical and psychological methods of treatment.

But if doctors should be on the lookout for hypoglycemia in patients who come to them with behavioral problems, they should also be careful not to set their sights too narrowly—especially if their practice focuses on hypoglycemia. Most hypoglycemia doctors sincerely try to treat their patients in the best way possible, but in any practice that is limited to one condition, there is a danger of seeing that condition everywhere. Just as allergists look first for allergies and psychiatrists probe for neuroses, hypoglycemia doctors are often predisposed to find a carbohydrate abnormality and stop there.

Critics claim that some sugar doctors make up their minds before they do all the necessary biochemical tests on a patient. There are reports that a few do not always do a glucose-tolerance test, the pivotal test for diagnosing a blood-sugar problem. The usual prescription is a high-protein, low-carbohydrate diet, which is appropriate if the patient has hypoglycemia. Even if he does not, no harm is done by the diet, because it simply amounts to a sensible program of eating, something we could all use. But in addition, the doctor may require the patient to return again and again for special shots. The shots contain adrenocortical extract (ACH), which supposedly increases the level of glucose in the blood. In my opinion, and in the opinion of many other doctors, there is no good rationale for giving ACH. The dosage is usually too small to have any effect, and there is little reason to think that a larger dosage would help either. Although they probably are not dangerous, the shots can be quite expensive.

Never in haste

More important, once someone is labeled hypoglycemic and started on a program of treatment, both he and his physician tend to assume the problem has been solved. Therefore, if the real malady is not hypoglycemia but something else, it may go unnoticed. Since many neurological and endocrine diseases and infections produce the same symptoms as low blood sugar does, this is a real danger.

Recently I saw a young woman who had symptoms that could easily have been interpreted as indicating hypoglycemia. She reported a sudden weight loss, progressively increasing thirst, and frequent urination. She had double vision, balancing difficulties, and chronic weakness and pain in one leg. She also suffered from recurring urinary tract and vaginal infections.

But she did not have hypoglycemia—her glucose-tolerance test was normal. A complete examination, including biochemical, neurophysiological, neurological, and physical tests, revealed two important facts. First, she had no abdominal reflexes, and second, her cerebrospinal fluid was abnormal. These and other findings pointed to multiple sclerosis.

The moral is that a diagnosis of hypoglycemia should never be made in haste, and it should certainly never be made by the patient himself. The interaction between physical and neurological problems and emotional or behavioral ones is complex. I have sketched, in rough outline, some of the causes for hypoglycemia and some of the symptoms that can result from it, but having the symptoms does not necessarily mean you have hypoglycemia.

What you should do if you think you have a carbohydrate problem is seek a proper medical evaluation and ask lots of questions. After a thorough investigation of your history and a complete examination, your doctor may or may not feel a glucose-tolerance test is warranted. But you should not accept the verdict "It's all in your head" if your doctor has neglected to give you a thorough examination, especially if you have physical symptoms in addition to emotional ones. Too many people have been called emotionally disturbed when physical factors were contributing to their condition.

Because carbohydrate problems are so subtle, it makes little sense to take a position "pro" or "con" on hypoglycemia or to try to turn it into a social issue. Each case must be evaluated without bias. And that's the unsugar-coated truth.

CHOLESTEROL

|25| The Meaning of the Serum Cholesterol Level

DAVID KRITCHEVSKY

David Kritchevsky is associate director of the Wistar Institute in Philadelphia.

Reprinted from *Nutrition & the M.D.* 2 (December 1975), p. 1, by permission of the publisher. Coypright © PM, Inc., 1975.

The serum cholesterol level, or as it is commonly but erroneously referred to, the cholesterol count, has become a part of the household medical lexicon. If the average American were put through a word association test, when we said "cholesterol" he would say "heart disease" and vice versa. Is this commonly assessed serum value truly the harbinger of the impending coronary? Let us examine the present knowledge.

Cholesterol is a constituent of every cell, an integral component of the cell membrane. The many roles of cholesterol are not completely clear. In the brain and neural tissues it is believed to act as an insulator and in the skin as a lubricant. It is the parent compound of corticosteroids, sex hormones, and bile acids. The principal catabolic pathway of cholesterol is to bile acids.

The cholesterol in the blood (which can be regarded as another tissue) comes from two sources—the diet and endogenous synthesis.

Although a cholesterol-rich diet will tend to increase serum cholesterol levels, we know now that other dietary factors—protein (amount and type), carbohydrate (type), and fiber—also play important roles in determining cholesterol levels. Although almost every tissue can synthesize cholesterol, the two major sources of endogenous cholesterol are the liver and intestine. The cholesterol in the blood is generally of hepatic origin.

ALTERED CHOLESTEROL SYNTHESIS

The hepatic synthesis of cholesterol is under feedback control but the effect is not always total. The rat and dog will suspend cholesterol synthesis in the face of prolonged cholesterol feeding. In man, cholesterol ingestion reduces cholesterol synthesis by 30–70%. The liver cholesterol (and the absorbed dietary cholesterol as well) occurs in the blood as a component of a continuum of lipid-protein molecules called lipoproteins. Cholesterol, being an alcohol, can be esterified to fatty acids, and about 60–70% of the cholesterol in the blood is in the ester form.

The serum lipoproteins can be differentiated on the basis of their physical characteristics and are usually identified on the basis of their density. The beta-lipoprotein (based on electrophoretic mobility) comprises the very low density lipoproteins (VLDL), which contain about 50–80% triglyceride and 7–16% total cholesterol. The low density lipoprotein (LDL) contains 10% triglyceride and about 30% total cholesterol. The VLDL is also referred to as pre-beta-lipoprotein. The high density lipoproteins (HDL or alpha-lipoproteins) contain 45–55% protein (as against 20–25% in LDL and 2–13% in VLDL), 5–8% triglyceride, and about 12% total cholesterol.

SIGNIFICANCE OF BETA-LIPOPROTEIN

The susceptibility to heart disease is linked to high levels of beta-lipoproteins. Since this class of lipoproteins is cholesterol-rich, the connection with serum cholesterol is evident. In animal experiments it is virtually impossible to achieve atherosclerosis unless the beta-lipoprotein levels are elevated. There are some evidence suggesting that the triglyceride level may be a more important indicator of coronary disease. Here again, however, we are dealing with beta- and pre-beta-lipoproteins.

The serum cholesterol level is not constant. It has been shown to undergo diurnal as well as seasonal fluctuations. In addition, stress tends to raise cholesterol levels. All these factors vary from one individual to another, so that some patients may have consistent levels of serum cholesterol, while others may show considerable variation.

ASSOCIATION OF CHOLESTEROL AND CORONARIES

Solid data relate serum cholesterol levels to the probability of a coronary episode. As one example, the Framingham study* showed that persons whose cholesterol level was above 260 mg/dl were at three times the risk of those whose cholesterol level was below 200 mg/dl. The operative word is risk—this is a statistical rather than a medical diagnosis. Nevertheless, at present it is among the best diagnoses available and should be heeded. The converse of this theorem—that lowering cholesterol levels will reduce coronary disease—has not been proved conclusively. Some studies suggest that it may be true, others disagree. The duration of hypercholesteremia may be a determining factor.

The blood is in contact with all other tissues of the body and a significant part of the cholesterol accumulated in the aorta and coronary vessels is of criculatory origin. It follows then that with more cholesterol in the blood there is a better chance of some of it depositing in the vessels. But the vessels are also metabolizing tissues, so that the deposition of lipid is not passive filtration; some arterial trees can withstand the lipidic onslaught, others cannot.

OTHER RISK FACTORS

Furthermore, although high serum cholesterol represents a major risk factor, there are other important risks—elevated blood pressure, excessive cigarette smoking, stress, trace minerals. These factors interact to increase risk if several are present in one individual. So long as there is no unequivocal medical diagnosis, the search for other factors will continue and there will be controversy.

Current data indicate that elevations in serum cholesterol levels constitute an increased risk of coronary disease, but are not absolute predictors of the event. This would suggest that the normal person, in view of what we know, should be careful and concerned about his cholesterol level but, in view of what we do not know, should not become hysterical about it.

---

*EDITOR'S NOTE: In 1949 over 5,000 men and women in Framingham, Massachusetts, were enlisted by the U.S. Public Health Service to take part in a study of arterial diseases. The long study has been variously interpreted and criticized, but its highly influential findings built a strong case against cholesterol as one of the villains in heart disease.

| 26 | Normal vs. Pathological Variations in Serum Cholesterol Levels

RAYMOND REISER

Raymond Reiser is distinguished professor in the Department of Biochemistry and Biophysics at Texas A and M University.

Reprinted from *Nutrition & the M.D.* 2 (December 1975), p. 2, by permission of the publisher. Copyright © PM, Inc., 1975.

The advice to eat modified foods containing less saturated fat and cholesterol is based on the theory that the natural products increase the risk of coronary heart disease. This is an oversimplification and a distortion of the facts. Only under certain conditions can a limited number of people with pathological levels of serum cholesterol on a normal American diet reduce their chances (statistically but not necessarily individually) of a heart attack by reducing the amount of cholesterol they consume.

What are the normal and pathological levels of blood cholesterol? The National Cooperative Pooling Project collated data from most of the dependable studies relating concentration of serum cholesterol in various population groups to the number of episodes of heart attack in those groups. Their findings show that there were no more heart attacks among men with cholesterol levels between 225 and 250 mg/100 ml (6.7 attacks per 1000 men per year) than among those men with levels between 175 and 200 mg/100 ml (5.2 attacks per 1000). The difference is not statistically significant.

CORONARY RISK OVER 250 MG/100 ML

However, the data do show increasingly more heart attacks among persons whose levels were above 250 mg/100 ml. The incidence in the group with serum cholesterol between 250 to 275 mg was about 11 attacks per 1000 men per year, and about 16 per 1000 in the group with serum cholesterol levels above 300 mg. One must conclude, therefore, that serum cholesterol concentrations below 235 or 240 mg/100 ml are within the nonpathological range.

The next improtant question is, how many people have serum cholesterol levels in the pathological range? This varies with age and sex. In the third decade about 5% of both sexes are in the increased risk group, and this becomes greater with each additional decade. Of men between 50 and 70 years of age, about 20–30% have cholesterol levels in the pathological range; of women in that age group, 40% or more.

FEW BENEFIT FROM DIET

Thus, even if diet changes can lower serum cholesterol by a mathematically statistical amount, 70 to 95% of the population would gain no benefit by making the change. Of those with serum cholesterols above pathological level, some may benefit a little but many require drugs to reduce their serum cholesterol to nonpathological levels. People with serum cholesterol levels above 275/100 ml on the usual American diet have a genetic variable or even a genetic disease and should be under medical care.

But the 70–95% with levels below 240 mg/100 ml on conventional diets can eat all the eggs, butter, cheese, ice cream, and marbled beef they want without fear of increasing their risk of coronary heart attacks. It is an individual matter. Serum cholesterol assays should be routine so that the hypercholesterolemic patients may be screened and treated as individuals, similar to the screening and treatment of diabetic patients.

The failure to separate populations into normal and pathological groups could be responsible for the conflicting data and interpretations of many studies and experiments. Investigating committees of a number of important organizations have critically examined the data and report no relation between diet and coronary heart disease. Possibly, if the responses of people with pathological serum cholesterol levels were separated from those with normal levels, a relationship might be found. But it should be pointed out again that diet changes do not correct all hypercholesterolemic conditions.

ATHEROSCLEROSIS AND INFANTS

Some investigators and pediatricians fear that the fatty arterial streaks found in babies are the precursors of adult atherosclerosis. They recommend that infants be given low-fat milk and low-cholesterol diets. It is very unlikely that the fatty streaks found in the arteries of nursing infants are of any danger to the child. It is contrary to all that we know about animal development or evolution for nature to build into the milk of any mammal the seeds of its destruction (except for genetic aberrations such as familial Type II hyper-betalipoproteinemia).

The American Academy of Pediatrics, alarmed at the potential dangers of artificial manipulation of the natural food for babies, issued the following statement in 1974: "There is no scientific evidence that the incidence of atherosclerosis can be reduced by limiting cholesterol intake early in life. The Committee recommends against a radical reduction of saturated fats in the diets of all children until much more is known about the benefits versus possible adverse effects. Dietary restriction of saturated fats is indicated at present only for children with hereditary hypercholesterolemia . . . the indiscriminate consumption of low-fat milk by the general population might well deprive some children of needed calories" (Pediatrics, 53:576, 1974). Similar statements have been made by D. S. Frederickson, C. J. Glueck, and C. U. Lowe in a Symposium on Factors in Childhood That Influence the Development of Atherosclerosis and Hypertension (reported in Amer J Clin Nutr, 25:221–254, 1972).

| 27 | "Good" Cholesterol vs. "Bad"

MARK BRICKLIN

Mark Bricklin is executive editor of *Prevention* magazine.

Excerpted and reprinted by special permission from May 1977 issue of *Prevention*, Emmaus, Pennsylvania. Copyright 1977 by Rodale Press, Inc.

Several recent reports . . . give us an important new insight into the old problem of high cholesterol levels.

The first few reports present what scientists are calling "startling evidence" that cholesterol levels are currently being misinterpreted in many cases. The reason for that is that cholesterol has a good form and a bad form, depending on what type of blood fat it is bound up with. The two fractions of blood fat now receiving new attention are high-density lipoproteins (HDL) and low-density lipoproteins (LDL).

And what the new evidence tells us is that the LDL fraction of blood lipids or fats is the dangerous fraction. The HDL fraction, far from being dangerous, is actually *protective*. One major study has shown that the higher the level of HDL's in the blood fats, the less chance there is of the person suffering a heart attack. Even when the total cholesterol level is quite high, if the HDL fraction is large, that person is considered to be very fortunate.

Exactly why the HDL fraction is protective has not been determined. One theory is that it prevents the cholesterol in the LDL fraction from being deposited on the artery wall, while another theory has it that HDL simply removes cholesterol from the blood. In any event, as H. Bryan Brewer Jr., M.D., of the National Heart, Lung, and Blood Institute points out, a favorable blood-test result would show a low level of LDL and a high level of HDL.

WHAT LECITHIN DOES

Within days of the publication of this major discovery came a brief report from the Northwest Lipid Research Clinic at the University of Washington in Seattle (*Clinical Research,* vol. 25, no. 2, 1977). There, Marian T. Childs, Ph.D., and four colleagues decided to check out the claim that soybean lecithin is good for lowering cholesterol. Using 12 volunteers who did not have high cholesterol levels to begin with, they gave each 36 grams (a little over an ounce) of granular lecithin each day, which they gave in two divided doses along with water or juice. After three weeks they tested the blood of the volunteers to see what changes had occurred.

Not too surprisingly, they discovered that the overall cholesterol levels had not been lowered. (Past tests showing that lecithin lowers cholesterol have usually been done on patients who had abnormally high cholesterol levels which *needed* reducing.) But what they did find was that the lecithin lowered the LDL cholesterol—the harmful fraction—and, at least in women, raised the relative amount of HDL cholesterol, the fraction which helps protect against heart attacks.

Just to be sure that this wasn't simply an effect of all the polyunsaturated fat in lecithin, they also gave corn oil to the people and found that while it did reduce LDL somewhat, it did not boost the level of protective HDL.

Another food concentrate which seemingly does good things to cholesterol is pectin. Derived usually from the pulp of citrus fruits, pectin has been shown over and over again to reduce cholesterol levels in the blood, apparently by blocking the absorption of these fats. The latest report I've seen describes a study in which pectin reduced cholesterol levels by an average of 13 percent. The daily amount consumed was 15 grams, or a little more than half an ounce. A 13-percent reduction in plasma cholesterol would lower a cholesterol count of 275, for example, to 239 (*The American Journal of Clinical Nutrition,* February, 1977).

Calcium supplements have also been proven to be very useful in lowering too-high cholesterol levels. The usual amount taken ranges from about 800 to 1,200 milligrams, but since calcium is so concentrated, this amounts to no more than a few tablets—making calcium rather more convenient than lecithin or pectin. Or to look at it another way, a combination of the full amount of calcium and smaller amounts of lecithin and pectin seems to be a practical approach for whipping blood fat into line.

FIBER

28 | Fiber in Your Food: Assessment and Guidelines

LAWRENCE GALTON

Lawrence Galton is a medical editor, writer, and former visiting professor at Purdue University. He is a columnist for the *Washington Star Syndicate* and *Family Circle* and his articles frequently appear in the *New York Times Magazine, Reader's Digest,* and other national publications.

Taken from *The Truth about Fiber in Your Food* by Lawrence Galton. Copyright © 1976 by Lawrence Galton. Used by permission of Crown Publishers, Inc.

Many changes have occurred as man has become sophisticated. Certainly diet alterations have been many. Protein consumption has risen. Total carbohydrate intake has fallen. While carbohydrate supplied by sugar has increased manyfold, less bread and other cereal foods are eaten and what are eaten are almost wholly of refined white flour. Fat intake has increased. While fat supplies 10 percent of calories for rural Africans, the proportion is 35 to 45 percent in the United States, England, and other Western countries.

All these changes have come under study—all except, until very recently, one: the change in fiber content of the diet.

Fiber is undigested. It has no nutritional value. It seemed logical to pay it no attention as having any possible role in maintaining health. In fact, it was viewed largely as a contaminant, and its removal has even been believed to enhance the quality of food.

But if it is a contaminant—a totally unfortunate term—it is clearly an essential contaminant.

"Can I give you an illustration?" says Hugh Trowell.*

"The air is our environment. We breathe in air. And it has in it available air, which we call oxygen, 20 percent. And it has unavailable air, which is called nitrogen, 80 percent. And we and our ancestors have breathed this environment in those proportions for 400 million years, since life came out of the ocean.

"Now I am told by people who are experts that you could cut the nitrogen in air from 80 to 40 percent and increase the oxygen from 20 to 60 percent, and you could breathe such air as normal air and get away with it. But if you start cutting the nitrogen below half its normal figure, 40 percent, you run into trouble. In a premature baby you produce a serious eye disease. You mightily increase the hazard for ordinary people who, not adapted to such a proportion of the gases, develop new bacterial colonies, and many of them will be dead of pneumonia within a few weeks. An anesthetist who can juggle the mixture of oxygen and nitrogen is always careful not to give pure oxygen to anyone for very long.

"Now, similarly, we believe that we have eaten cell wall, which is dietary fiber, for 500 million years, since life started in the ocean. And we have always eaten it in a certain proportion because we were basically vegetarians, plant food gatherers.

"Only about a century or two ago did we say, 'Boys, let's really get the "goodness" out of the cell contents; we can forget about the cell walls.'

"And we believe that this is a very big change in terms of evolutionary adaptation. And that people who eat plant cell wall as my African patients did because they got the food out of the garden every day and other people who eat this in other parts of the world have a very different incidence, a tremendously lower incidence, of diseases than we 'goodness' eaters who have tossed away plant cell wall; and they have that lower incidence exactly because they haven't yet been exposed to our "goodness," our very civilized and highly refined 'goodies.' "

---

*EDITOR'S NOTE: Hugh Trowell is a British physician renowned for establishing the nature of the disease kwashiorkor and for his subsequent detective work on dietary fiber.

That, in a nutshell, is the fiber hypothesis. How well does it hold up?

An old tale—true—has it that Charles Darwin observed that only bumblebees with their long tongues could pollinate red clover effectively and that the prime enemies of bumblebees are field mice that devour both larvae and honeycombs. The better crops of clover near villages, Darwin remarked, had much to do with the control of mice by the village cats.

But another scientist went further, suggesting that since red clover was the staple diet of British cattle and bully beef the staple of the British sailor, a relationship might be shown between British naval victories and keeping cats.

Diseases, too, have relationships—much closer ones—and it has often been rewarding to ferret out these relationships.

Malaria and mosquitoes, cholera and contaminated water, lung cancer and tobacco smoke—these are examples of associations that have clarified causes and even made possible preventive measures.

Establishing relationships between symptoms also can be rewarding. Skin rashes, penile lesions, palate perforation, bone changes, and aortic aneurysms or balloonings out—observations that some or all of these conditions tended to occur together in the same patients led to the realization that they were manifestations of a single disease, syphilis, and a common cause.

The fiber hypothesis, of course, takes into account relationships—relationships, one with the other, of many common, troublesome, some of them deadly, diseases that at first blush would seem to be entirely unrelated; relationships of time and place, of increased prevalence; and relationships with concomitant environmental changes.

All are relatively new diseases. Coronary heart disease was considered a rarity by Sir William Osler in 1910 and was still newsworthy in 1925 when an English physician, Sir John McNee, described with some excitement two cases of this "rare condition" he had seen in the United States. Appendicitis was first described in 1812 and appeared to become common after 1880. Diverticular disease has become a major problem only in the last fifty years; hiatus hernia only in the last thirty years; hemorrhoids and tumors of the colon also appear to be recent developments; so, too, gallbladder disease, which has increased by 350 percent since 1940 in the records of the Bristol Royal Infirmary in England.

All these diseases, while common in all economically developed countries, are rare or unknown in rural Africa and all less-developed communities.

Moreover, not only are they geographically related; they are chronologically related. Where the incidence of one begins to rise, so does that of the others. Where, for example, diabetes surges upward, so later does appendicitis. Atherosclerosis and lesions of the colon then become common after another generation or so. With migration, too—from Africa to America, from Japan to America, and from country to city in Africa and Japan—these diseases become much more common.

And, beyond sharing geographical and chronological relationships, these diseases often occur in the same individuals. Most notable is the strong tendency for atherosclerosis, obesity, and diabetes to occur in individual patients.

The most compelling argument for relating these diseases to a fiber-depleted diet, of course, was the great rise in their prevalence after the removal, in the latter part of the last century, of most of the cereal fiber still remaining in Western diets.

Admittedly, this was only one dietary change. But rational explanations of how lack of fiber may cause the various diseases could be presented and . . . have been.

Is it an open and shut case, proved beyond all doubt, that lack of dietary fiber is the sole cause, or the major cause, of all these diseases?

Hardly.

Not one of the men who are studying fiber and its relationship to disease would say that.

"Nearly all disease," says Denis Burkitt,* "has more than one causative factor. Not in any of these diseases would I suggest that fiber deficiency is a sole causative factor, merely that it may be one important factor. What I would emphasize is that a fiber-depleted diet is a common factor, common to a number of characteristic Western diseases. It is a major factor, I believe, in some, a less important factor in others, but it is common to each of them and offers the only reasonable explanation put forward, I think, why these diseases are associated.

"I like to do everything with little pictures," Burkitt says. "I want to draw a picture—a little flask for each of these diseases. When the flask overflows,

---

*EDITOR'S NOTE: Denis Burkitt, an Irish surgeon who first gained fame for his discovery and cure of a cancer in children (now known as Burkitt's lymphoma), is a co-discoverer of the importance of fiber in the diet.

we can say, disease begins. The overflow would come from pipes leading into the flask.

"It may be that for some diseases—for example, coronary heart disease and diabetes—there are many, many pipes and for others, fewer. And the pipes may vary in size. But one pipe would be fiber-depleted diet. That pipe may be a very big one for diverticular disease. It may be very big for appendicitis. It may be a smaller pipe for coronary heart disease and diabetes. But that pipe would be there, common to all these characteristically Western diseases."

Because he has what he calls his "platform"—his renown in the medical profession for his lymphoma work—Burkitt is listened to when he talks at medical meetings. And all the more so because he emphasizes, as does Hugh Trowell and all the others who have been associated with him, that what he is presenting is a hypothesis about a dietary factor long overlooked but now certainly worthy of thorough investigation. He welcomes to the investigation any evidence in favor or against the hypothesis.

There are skeptics. In fact, to some, the very simplicity of the concept is offensive, as if only complicated explanations are likely to have any validity and simple ones none. Of them, Burkitt is likely to ask calmly, "But what alternative hypothesis do you have to explain the epidemiology and interrelationships of these diseases?" There isn't any as of now.

Burkitt has aroused interest. So have Trowell, [K. W.] Heaton, [Neil] Painter, and others with their journal papers and talks. And in the last three years or so there has been a mushrooming of research on fiber and its role in health—and on fiber itself: what it actually is and how many kinds of it there are. That research is going on now in many centers in England, the United States, and elsewhere in the world.

And that is exactly what Burkitt and his "fiber gang" want and are happy to have.

Many specific research projects could be valuable. They are not easy to do, and even as recently as a year or two ago would have had little chance of getting done. But with the rapidly growing interest, they could well be undertaken soon.

Alec Walker has suggested several projects. One would be to select from questionnaire surveys people who clearly are habituated to a higher-than-average intake of whole-grain products and lower-than-average intake of refined carbohydrate foods. Then it would be possible to determine what the prevalence was among them of the various diseases believed to be associated with low-fiber diets. If it were found to be much lower than for the population as a whole, that would count heavily in favor of the fiber hypothesis.

Another, suggests Walker, would be an experiment done with a random group of about 500 men, between 30 and 39 years old, who would be willing to include 15 grams of bran (about 2 heaping teaspoonfuls) in their daily diet for an indefinite period. Measurements, such as for bowel motility, constipation incidence, overweight, blood sugar and cholesterol and triglyceride levels, would have to be done at the start of the study, after six months, and after a year. In addition, studies on bile salt excretion and on bacterial colonies in the stools would be needed. Subsequently, investigations would be needed to learn if the beneficial effects achieved with bran could be further improved by reduction in the intake of refined carbohydrate foods, including sugar.

With these and other studies it would become possible to determine the minimum changes in diet needed to demonstrably lower the prevalence, or delay the onset, of the various diseases.

Fiber itself certainly needs study. It has long been surrounded by mystery, ignorance, and confusion.

It is a very complex substance. It consists of celluloses, of which there are thousands of different physical varieties. It also contains hemicelluloses, which got that name because they were once thought to be precursors of cellulose but now are known to have standing in their own right and are known also to consist of varied substances. And there are, as well, pectic substances and lignins. Some pectic substances are in apple pulp and the rind of oranges, for example, and are often used by food processors for jelling purposes. Lignins are "woody"-like materials.

No food table in the world even now contains a full analysis of all the fiber present in food. Food tables record only crude fiber. But crude fiber is not what we encounter. It is only the portion of total fiber that resists and is not dissolved out of food by acids and alkalis in laboratory determinations. But acids and alkalis dissolve out hemicelluloses which, in wheat, for example, are three to four times the weight of crude fiber.

There is confusion indeed. Recently Hugh Trowell suggested that a new term be adopted—and it largely has been—dietary fiber. It includes all the fiber, crude plus the rest. And roughly speaking, in many cereals dietary fiber is five times the figure for crude fiber.

It is all this dietary fiber not just the crude—the whole group of cell wall remnants—that remains intact in the small intestine and passes to the large bowel.

Only recently have there been any attempts to analyze what differences exist in the various dietary fiber components in various foods. Such analysis is far from simple, and until more work is done only a few broad generalizations can be made. Thus, plant cell walls eaten before maturity, such as occur in leafy cabbage and soft immature green peas, have little lignin, but much cellulose. Mature solid fruits, such as the apple, and fleshy tubers, such as the potato, have approximately equal proportions of hemicellulose, cellulose, and lignin. Cereals contain a large amount of hemicellulose and, when mature, also contain a fair amount of lignin.

Already, it has become evident that the components of dietary fiber have different properties. Cellulose, for example, acts as a moderate water absorbent in the bowel. Some of the other components such as hemicellulose are strong adsorbers. And water adsorption counts in making the stool moister and softer. Lignin, however, does not adsorb water to any significant extent, but there is some evidence that it does latch onto and bind bile salts to carry them out in the stool.

Undoubtedly, there are other differences in properties between the components of dietary fiber—and they could be significant differences. Many experimental studies have been done with bran to determine the influence of dietary fiber. But bran is a mixture of all the above components, and it is impossible to tell from the use of a mixture which particular component is responsible for any particular valuable effect. What are needed are intensive studies carried out with isolated components.

"As more work is done," says Denis Burkitt, "I think we may well find that the dietary fiber situation in the beginning—now—is much like the situation with B vitamins. At first, there were values attributed to the complex of B vitamins. Then came the studies that assigned specific values to the individual B vitamins—B_1, B_3, B_6, B_{12}, and the others. Similarly, I think, we may find specific values for the individual components of dietary fiber."

And that might mean that different plants, and even the same plants at different ages, could be analyzed for their specific arrays of fiber components, and diets might be based on overall optimal assortments of cereals, vegetables, and fruits, and perhaps even optimal assortments for individuals with specific problems or tendencies.

Actually, some of this work is being undertaken by David Southgate and

~~~~~~

FOOD FIBER

Food fiber, called "the latest dietary miracle," has been much in the news of late, with a rediscovery of the alleged virtues of bran and other roughage foods as means for lowering cholesterol levels, and as possible preventives of cancer. As to adding bran to the diet, we advise distinct caution. Many have jumped to the conclusion that, since bran is unquestionably a fibrous roughage food, a substantial daily intake of bran should be just what is needed. But bran does *not* provide all the benefits of a natural diet rich in fiber and it is not a proper substitute for the fiber present in most foods of the vegetable kingdom. . . .

Consumers' Research pointed out as long ago as 1936 that whole wheat bread consumed as a way of taking bran has its disadvantages, apart from the fact that whole grain flour is not in favor with the grocery trades because it has much poorer keeping qualities than white flour. The roughage of whole-grain wheat flour is not well tolerated by many people; it may be for this reason that the public demand has for many years been overwhelmingly for bread made from highly refined ("low extraction") wheat flour. The nature of bran in true whole wheat

bread is such that it presents digestive difficulties and may interfere seriously with the health of the digestive system.

A difficulty with brown flour, known as "high extraction" flour, is the presence of phytic acid, which interferes with the retention of calcium and phosphorus, essential in everyone's diet. The same applies to oatmeal.

Careful researchers found that calcium, magnesium, phosphorus, and potassium were less completely absorbed than the same minerals were in diets made up with a white 69% extraction flour.

As to brown bread, so often recommended as a good source of iron, this was found not actually to be a good source. In fact, absorption of iron (a dietary essential) was actually better in experiments with white flour than with 92% extraction (brown) flour.

There is no certainty at all that the sudden popular interest in fiber is justified. On balance, the evidence seems to favor some increase in the average person's intake of fiber in foods, but not as bran or other relatively harsh roughage.

~~~~~~

his group at the Dunn Nutritional Laboratory at Cambridge, and it is almost certain that more will be—and more, in fact, may already be—undertaken at other institutions.

PRACTICALITIES FOR THE READER

It is not, as you see, open and shut. There is going to be much more to come on dietary fiber. . . .

In determining whether it is a return [to a high-fiber diet] you wish to consider, you will, of course, use your own judgment in evaluating the existing evidence.

It seems to many informed physicians and scientists now that certainly more evidence is desirable but what is available justifies a return.

In the United States five scientists, four of them physicians, are calling for action by doctors, nutritionists, public health officials, and the federal government to increase the use of fiber in the American diet.

In a "white paper" on fiber and health, the five men—Dr. William O. Dobbins, director of the division of gastroenterology at George Washington University Medical Center in the District of Columbia, Dr. Franz Goldstein, chief of gastroenterology at Lankenau Hospital in Philadelphia, Dr. Daniel H. Connor, chief of the geographic pathology division of the Armed Forces Institute of Pathology, Dr. Stuart Danovitch, a Washington, D.C., gastroenterologist, and Michael Jacobson, PhD, co-director of the Center for Science in the Public Interest in Washington—review the evidence.

They conclude that increased consumption of dietary fiber would be a "prudent preventative measure," that "enough is known to justify informing people that a diet richer in unrefined plant products and thus higher in dietary fiber would increase the health of almost everyone."

They urge that the U.S. Department of Agriculture, which reaches millions through its extension service, school lunch, school breakfast, and food stamp programs, encourage consumption of fiber-rich foods through its TV spots, publications, press releases, and authority to approve foods used in its programs; that the Department of Defense, which buys and serves vast quantities of food, inform servicemen [and] civilian employees and their families of the health benefits of whole-grain products, bran, legumes, fruits, and vegetables; that the Department of Health, Education and Welfare encourage food editors, consumer writers, authors of cookbooks, schoolteachers, and medical school professors to inform their audiences of the value of fiber and whole-grain foods. . . .

Basic Guidelines

About carbohydrates—refined and unrefined. The most important energy source in the human diet, carbohydrate occurs in two forms. One, of course, is starch—composed of large, complex molecules—which is, in fact, a plant's energy store. The other is sugar—made up of small, relatively simple molecules. Among the well-known types of sugars are sucrose or cane sugar, fructose or fruit sugar, and glucose or dextrose, the latter being the form in which all sugar is absorbed into the blood. Starch—tasteless, incapable of dissolving in water—seems far removed from sugar; yet, in fact, it is converted to sugar in the intestinal tract before being absorbed into the body.

Unrefined carbohydrates are carbohydrates in their natural form; they may be cooked but they are not otherwise processed. In the natural state carbohydrates are never isolated and "pure." Instead, they are mingled with other materials. Without exception, starch is associated with protein, various vitamins and minerals, and with indigestible fiber, as in cereals such as wheat and rice and various vegetables. Sugars, too, in nature are always associated with fiber. Moreover, except in the case of honey, sugars in nature are in dilute form so that, for example, a fairly large sweet apple will contain only a teaspoonful of sugar.

Natural, unrefined carbohydrates provide vitamins and other nutrients, take chewing, tend to be filling, and are the only sources of dietary fiber.

On the other hand, refined carbohydrates—white flour, white rice, and sugar—are the products of the milling of flour that involves the use of steel rollers to pull out the starch-rich portion of the grain and of the extraction of sugar from sugar beet and cane.

For adequate restoration of fiber to the diet, it is necessary, as much as possible, to eat natural, unrefined carbohydrates and avoid the refined as much as possible.

Although it is possible to keep on consuming the usual large quantities of refined carbohydrates and restore some or even much or all of the refined-out fiber by using bran as a supplement, that, as we have seen earlier, is not the same thing as materially increasing the unrefined carbohydrate intake. One very important reason is that as the intake of unrefined carbohydrate is increased, the apparent digestibility of other constituents in the diet is decreased—a good thing in our overconsuming society.

About cereal fiber and vegetable fiber. Both are important. It appears from recent research that cereals contain fiber that is more resistant to digestion than that of many vegetables and fruits, and therefore more remains to function effectively throughout the gastrointestinal tract. Thus, there are grounds for considering cereal fiber as something special. But, again, other fiber as well is needed.

About wheat germ. The wheat grain is a tiny seed, which if left alone, will grow into a new plant. The grain has three main parts. The bran—somewhat like an eggshell—protects the softer inside. Unlike an eggshell, however, it has important roles in diet, providing dietary fiber and also vitamins and minerals. The endosperm of the grain, similar to the white of an egg, is largely protein and starch. Finally, there is wheat germ, the germ of the seed which, like the yolk of an egg, is rich not in fiber but in nutrients, including vitamins and minerals.

For use as a flour, wheat grain is crushed. Different kinds of flours can be produced, depending upon the extent to which various parts of the grain are removed or retained. These flours are differentiated by their extraction rates, indicating amounts of grain retained. Whole-meal flour, with 100 percent extraction rate, contains all the ground grain. White flour, now commonly of 70–72 percent extraction, retains only the endosperm, with both germ and bran removed.

With both germ and bran removed, there is a huge loss not only of fiber but of vitamins and minerals. According to a 1971 study* by Dr. H. Schroeder of Dartmouth Medical College, the losses are as shown on page 285.

No attempt is made to restore most of these nutrients to white flour. So-called enriched white flour has returned to it usually only vitamins B_1, B_2, niacin, and iron. While the use of bran as a supplement provides some unrestored nutrients, those from wheat germ would still be missing. And the use of wheat germ supplement along with bran supplement still would not provide the values of eating carbohydrates whole and unrefined. . . .

Knowing what to eat and what not to eat. The objective is to eat, as much as possible, natural, unrefined carbohydrates in place of the refined, that is, white flour and all things made with it, and refined sugar.

Any change of diet in that direction is helpful. The greater the change, the better. But the change can be made gradually, and you are likely to be motivated to make greater and greater change as you begin to experience what lesser changes provide.

---

*American Journal of Clinical Nutrition, May 1971, Vol. 24, pp. 467–69.

Nutrient	Loss in flour (in %)
Thiamine (vitamin B_1)	77.1
Riboflavin (vitamin B_2)	80.0
Niacin	80.8
Vitamin B_6	71.8
Pantothenic acid	50.0
Alpha-tocopherol (vitamin E)	86.3
Calcium	60.0
Phosphorus	70.9
Magnesium	84.7
Potassium	77.0
Sodium	78.3
Chromium	40.0
Manganese	85.8
Iron	75.6
Cobalt	88.5
Copper	67.9
Zinc	77.7
Selenium	15.9
Molybdenum	48.0

How much fiber? Exact requirements are not definitively established. Yet, there are useful guidelines. . . .

Excellent results in relieving common colon disorders—including constipation, spastic colon, and diverticular disease—have been achieved with the use of 10 to 15 grams ($\frac{1}{2}$ ounce; 15 grams are roughly 1 heaping tablespoon) of bran and 200 grams ($6\frac{2}{3}$ ounces) of appropriate fruit and vegetables such as carrots, apples, oranges, and brussels sprouts. . . . The 15 grams of bran contain the same amount of fiber to be found in about 75 grams (about $\frac{2}{3}$ cup) of whole-grain wheatmeal—and, for reasons we have noted, . . . greater reliance on the wheatmeal (and there are many ways to use it) than on bran is to be preferred.

That amount of fiber restoration, suggests Dr. Martin Eastwood of the University of Edinburgh, might well be universally adopted.

You are very likely to know when you are getting a suitable amount of fiber by the effects on the stools: they will become softer, well formed, and readily passed without straining.

Does that mean more calories? No. By replacing as much as possible refined carbohydrates with unrefined, you are not going to be adding calories to your diet. If anything, by such substitution, you are likely—even as you get the fiber you need—to be taking in less calories. . . .*

More about bran—a recent study by Dr. Eastwood and his associates at Edinburgh indicates that not all brans are equally efficacious. Coarse bran appeared to be much more effective than fine bran, they found, in reducing pressures within the large bowel and in reducing transit time. Bran with coarse particles held more water than did fine bran.

"The whole problem is not bran, it is dietary fiber," Eastwood wrote me. . . . "The evidence does not support any idea that bran is the sole panacea. The diet of Africans, against which comparisons are made, never has contained bran, and I think that it would be misleading to further this view."

Denis Burkitt, too, wrote: "I am increasingly convinced that Dr. Trowell is right in emphasizing the need for a diet from which the fiber has not been removed rather than merely adding lost fiber requirements."

If protection is to be gained from dietary fiber, not alone against constipation and diverticular disease but [also against] obesity, diabetes, and coronary heart disease, it will come not so much—in some conditions not at all—from the arrival once, twice, or several times a day of some separated-out bran in the colon. Instead it will come from intact dietary fiber still in place where it belongs in foods, intimately associated with those foods, helping to produce satiety, helping to prevent excessive absorption of starches and sugars and possibly cholesterol in the diet, helping to prevent excessively rapid absorption that may disturb the proper secretion of insulin by the pancreas, and helping in many other ways. . . .

---

*EDITOR'S NOTE: One theory behind this is that fiber-containing food requires more chewing than fiber-depleted food. Chewing slows down ingestion and stimulates the secretion of saliva and gastric juices, which, along with the food, help fill the stomach and promote satiety. In addition, of course, part of the fiber-rich food is nonnutritive, is not absorbed, and obviously cannot supply calories.

Part IV
The Health Food Controversy

*The traditionalist believes
that foolishness frozen into
custom is preferable to
foolishness fresh off the
vine.*

—D. SUTTEN

Introduction to

Part IV

Jimmy Durante once said that health foods don't actually make you live longer, they only make it seem longer. Nevertheless, an increasing number of people in America, convinced that the food in supermarkets is more atrocious than nutritious, have turned to the health food store for salvation. These supermarket dropouts, many of them young people, are frequently regarded as having been brushed by the wings of madness. "But in recent years," William Longgood states,

> a revolutionary theme has been preached by a hard core of researchers in nutrition. They hold that the *birthright of all living creatures is health,* and sickness and disease are perversions of the natural condition. Further, they contend, . . . if people eat the right foods they will enjoy good health.[1]

About 5 to 10 percent of any population today are earnestly looking for more nutrition information and for possible diet alternatives; perhaps another 5 percent are searching for a miracle to improve health.[2]

The suggestible, fearful miracle-seeker can become a fanatic—"one who," as Winston Churchill is supposed to have said, "can't change his mind and won't change the subject." Ruth Gay notes:

> Although we learned long ago to abandon magical thinking in connection with weather, crops, the care of animals, and other phenomena, it still has us in its grip when we think of diet. Our latest thinking about food, based on fear, is proportionately retrograde—willing to accept, indeed seeking out, the consolations of magic, the mute practice of peasants, and the quaint devices of folklore.[3]

But the health food "cult" is not restricted to a quasi-religious lunatic fringe. A large proportion of so-called food freaks, faddists, and fanatics are simply people who are determined to return to a dietary regime of foods validated by history. In their quest for nutritional nirvana they make some serious mistakes. But do they make as many mistakes as those who follow the standard American diet? While the health food store is stocked with some high-priced absurdities, it can hardly compete with that showplace of high-priced absurdities, the local supermarket. Simply because the dietary practices of natural-food adherents are so different from the norm, they are often attacked with almost pathological intensity. But as K. H. Pfeffer has pointed out, the different food habits of others do not necessarily represent faddism, cultism, or quackery.[4] Whatever the faults of this growing subculture, it has generated a more questioning attitude toward the standard American diet.

Those who express dismay over the cost and superfluity of food bought by natural-food advocates seldom direct their concern toward the staggering sums spent on fabricated foods that, in effect, are nutritional nullities. Although the public annually spends some $4 billion on carbonated beverages alone, health food stores, which take in about $1 billion, are continually being condemned for wasting the money and possibly undermining the health of their patrons. This is like trying to kill a gnat with a sledgehammer.

Health food stores, it must be said, are not necessarily bulging with nutritionally superior foods. Not a few items contain the very things that food faddists deplore, such as sugar and additives. Indeed, there exists such a marvel as junk-food health food. In a health food store, as in a supermarket, it pays to read labels and be selective. While a few items are actually cheaper than elsewhere, the markup on most is high; it is highest of all on vitamin and other supplements, which are the key to a store's financial success.

The food industry has become uneasily aware that there are some consumers who want neither their food nor themselves manipulated. To placate them, and to compete with the burgeoning health food enterprises, several companies are putting out some token natural products, free of chemical additives—and usually high in sugar and price.

The personnel in health food stores commonly accompany their sales with gratuitous and zealous nutrition information, much of it zany. Regular grocers are short on advice, believing that their primary function is to sell food; but many would prefer to sell nutritious food. Their disinclination to offer nutritional advice is well-founded: when a recent questionnaire was sent to selected grocers to test their nutrition knowledge and attitudes, their final combined score was a D.[5]

Health food hustlers are not a special breed, but merely an offshoot of the general hustler. As Sidney Margolius comments, "Revealingly, many recent entrants into the health food business are former insurance and car salesmen, and promoters of franchised computer schools and fast-food restaurant chains during the booms for those services in the late 1960's."[6]

A lot of hot air is expended in the charges and countercharges of tradition-alists and natural-food adherents. Traditionalists scoff that the claims of health foodists lack scientific proof, and health foodists reply either that they have scientific proof or that they don't need it. Each side resents the accusation that it doesn't know what it is doing or what it is talking about. And, as Margolius says, there is "nutritional exaggeration on both sides of the compost heap."[7]

In *Selection 29,* Margolius considers the pluses and minuses of the health food movement: the legitimate fears and concerns, the exaggerations, the sales pressure, and "organic chic." He examines with forbearance five major issues in the health food controversy and suggests that the movement's most salutary effects have been environmental and social. However, he concludes, the move-ment is inclined to be faddist and self-deluding and can at times even be self-endangering; moreover, some dedicated people are being exploited by the commercial health food industry in much the same way as the American public in general is exploited by manufacturers of all those other foods.

Dr. Victor Herbert, in *Selection 30,* is far less temperate as he writes about the distortions, exaggerations, and oversimplifications foisted on "brainwashed" health foodists. His opinions strongly reflect his belief that "most diseases have nothing to do with diet." Herbert emphasizes the simplicity of basing the diet on the "basic four" of good nutrition and warns about the dangers of excess vitamins. Contending that "health hustlers are usually charlatans and quacks," he offers 14 tips on how to recognize the food quack. In concluding, he exam-ines the weakness of the law in protecting the consumer against false or decep-tive health information.

Diametrically opposed to Herbert's views are those of medical maverick Alan Nittler in *Selection 31.* Dr. Nittler aims his words at the physician who knows little or nothing about nutrition, but his article is of equal interest to the layper-son. Conceding that there is some quackery and faddism in the field of nutrition, he argues that this is all the more reason why people who must now experiment on themselves need doctors who can separate nutritional untruths from truths. He explains how to gain nutritional know-how; and he suggests that the physi-cian rely less on drugs and more on nutritional therapy and that he or she not be wary of health food stores. Many of the periodicals and books recom-mended by Nittler at the end of his selection tend to be spurned by the physi-cian, who, he contends, has been "brainwashed"; the majority of the books appear on the "not recommended" lists in standard surveys.

Do you think the corner grocery, the produce stand, and the supermarket generally offer foods that are cheaper than and identical or superior to those found in the health food stores, or not? Do you put your faith in the supermarket or the health food store? Whatever your answer, these words of Wilson Mizener apply: "I respect faith but doubt is what gets you an education."

References

1   William Longgood, *The Poisons in Your Food,* new rev. ed. (New York: Pyramid Books, 1969), p. 171.

2   LaVell M. Henderson, "Programs to Combat Nutrition Quackery," *Journal of The American Dietetic Association* 64 (April 1974), p. 375. For an irreverent account of health food advocates past and present, see Ronald M. Deutsch, *The New Nuts among the Berries* (Palo Alto, Calif.: Bull Publishing Co., 1977).

3   Ruth Gay, "Fear of Food," *American Scholar,* Summer 1976, p. 438.

4   K. H. Pfeffer, "The Sociology of Nutrition, Malnutrition and Hunger in Developing Countries," in G. Blix, ed., *VIII Symposium of the Swedish Nutrition Foundation: Food Cultism and Nutrition Quackery* (Stockholm: Almquist and Wiksells, 1972), p. 30.

5   Johanna Dwyer and Jean Mayer, "Food for Thought: What Do Grocers Know?" *San Francisco Examiner,* August 3, 1977, p. 26.

6   Sidney Margolius, *Health Foods: Facts and Fakes* (New York: Walker and Co., 1973), p. 22.

7   Ibid., p. 197.

| 29 | Panic in Healthfoodland

SIDNEY MARGOLIUS

Sidney Margolius is one of the foremost U.S. experts on consumer problems and family money management. Included among his numerous books is *The Great American Food Hoax.*

From *Health Foods: Facts and Fakes* by Sidney Margolius. Copyright © 1973 by Sidney Margolius. Used with permission of the publisher, Walker and Company, Inc.

From young people on college campuses to Park Avenue socialites, many Americans have turned to "organic" and "natural" foods, and to the pursuit of health and even emotional stability through massive doses of vitamin pills.

They have become alarmed by a relentless stream of reports of misuses of chemical additives, pesticides, and fertilizers; by repeated charges of "poisons" in our food; by botulism incidents among some of the country's most trusted brand names; by revelations of fish contaminated by mercury, chicken by synthetic chemicals, powdered milk by salmonella organisms, and beef by growth hormones found potentially cancerous in lab tests; by the ban on cyclamates and the review of saccharin—in general, a constant bombardment of the public's nerves, let alone its intestinal tract.

Each new scare has given impetus to sales of organic foods, a leading New York supermarket operator reported in 1972.[1]

Many other people, even if not panicky about chemical additives, are finding that some nutritional beliefs they were raised on suddenly have crumbled. What can be "healthier" than an egg? Yet some eggs were found to be contaminated by PCB's, a chemical used in printing ink. Even the carrots which your own mother said would help you see at night now are under suspicion for concentrating in their innocent-looking bodies even more pesticides than other vegetables.

Eat your *spinach?* What was your mother trying to do to you? Now we learn that if spinach is left at room temperature for some time after cooking, or if a jar of baby-food spinach is left opened, nitrites may develop with potentially toxic effects for infants.[2]

The savory hot dog of your youth? That appetizing pink color comes from nitrites which are suspected of producing nitrosamines. These have been found to cause cancer and mutations in laboratory animals.

Milk? Butter? Sugar? You could get heart disease, according to various reports—or claims.

Even tap water is under suspicion in some areas for an excess of nitrates and other pollutants. In the nation's thoroughly impartial supermarkets, bottled water, although sometimes no purer, has become a best-seller along with nitrate-containing hot dogs and additive-preserved cereals.

Packages have turned hostile too. The dreaded PCB's can apparently be transmitted from packages to the foods inside them. Returnable plastic milk containers have come under suspicion in Oregon because strange tastes and odors have been reported, and children have become ill after drinking milk from such containers. The plastic, it seems, retains some foreign materials like a sponge.[3]

The healthiest habits, like brushing your teeth, suddenly seem fraught with danger, at least to the more anxious. Some toothpaste tubes were found by two Chicago medical researchers to contain "potentially hazardous" amounts of lead that contaminated the paste itself. While no instances of lead ingestion have been reported, the manufacturers involved scurried back to their drawing boards to develop new tubes without lead. Then another unsuspected lead hazard popped up. The FDA (Food and Drug Administration) revealed late in 1972 that it was working with manufacturers to reduce the amount of lead found in canned milk and infant formula by revising the soldering process used in canning.

Most of all, the threat of cancer now seems to lurk in every corner of your kitchen cupboard.

As well as the specter of a chemical assault on our bodies, many people fear that foods have been robbed of much of their nourishment by modern growing and processing methods. Rats have starved on white bread; breakfast cereals are said to have "no more nutrition than dirty fingernails"; our soils are said to be depleted of vital minerals. Other often-voiced concerns are that modern foods lose vitamins while being transported long distances; modern mass production of chickens has robbed them of both their flavor and nourishment; such staples of the American diet as cold cuts now are almost half fat and water; the blanching method used to can vegetables destroys much of the water-soluble vitamins, and if the canners don't, your own careless cooking habits will.

Even aluminum cooking utensils have been termed a health hazard because minute amounts of the metal dissolve during cooking. This attack, revealingly, is carried on by salesmen and manufacturers of stainless steelware.

Another factor underlying the unprecedented boom in the sale of health food is the American people's yearning for a return to a simpler time. The very real fear of the pollution of our environment and contamination of our food supplies is an outgrowth of the ten-year struggle between environmental groups and those advocating the use of chemical fertilizers, pesticides, and additives in food production.

The conflict, given impetus with the 1962 publication of the late Rachel Carson's book *Silent Spring,* has pitted scientific giants and powerful national organizations against each other. On the environmentalist side of this increasingly bitter fight over the future direction of our physical and social environment are the National Audubon Society, the Sierra Club, the Izaac Walton League, and the more recently organized Environmental Defense Fund. On the other side are influential farmer organizations, chemical and drug manufacturers, the U.S. Department of Agriculture, and leading agricultural scientists, including Norman E. Borlaug, winner of the 1970 Nobel Prize for the development of new wheat strains.

The crux of the issue is a compelling need to increase food production to satisfy the world's ever-growing population without endangering the earth's environment. The conservationists, in varying degrees, maintain that this need can be met through "organic" farming, which uses as fertilizer animal manures, decomposed vegetation and crop residues, and the treated sewage of the cities.

The appeal of these arguments lies mainly in the apparent motivations of their spokesmen: the preservation of the earth's natural beauties; the replacement of artificially flavored and chemically preserved foods with the home-grown, freshly picked produce of a bygone era; and the Don Quixote-like quality of their fight, that of small but indomitable groups pitted against the giant forces of government and agricultural and processing industries.

The influx of young people into the "food revolution" is especially noticeable. Some have joined communes in search of an alternative way of life that includes "natural foods," ecological care, and an effort to "try to save our sweet world," as a young California mother, although not in a commune, expressed it.[4]

But many older and usually well-to-do people too have become engrossed in organic gardening, "unadulterated" foods, and, even if belatedly, ecological concerns.*

There is a strong religious character, too, in the food movement, and especially in its booming vegetarian and raw-food wings. Many religions have made a ritual of certain foods and their preparation. Now the Loma Linda vegetarian foods of the Seventh Day Adventists have become popular with the new health foodists; the Zen macrobiotic dieters ascribe qualities of good and evil to different foods, and one of the current raw-food cults insists that if God wanted food to be cooked he would have provided a heat shield to cook it as it fell from the heavens. One woman, whose ten-year-old son

---

*While qualified psychoanalytic opinion holds that the current great interest in natural foods among young people to some extent represents a rejection of the customs of the older generation, at the same time their elders want to get into the swing too—not only with long hair and youthful fashions but with health foods. It is difficult to know where the youngsters can go next if their parents move into their communes and insist on eating and smoking the same commodities.

died from doses of LSD secretly fed to him in candy, blamed the drug traffic on the unavailability of "God's food," which has "nothing added."

But perhaps most significantly, many people no longer wholly trust the government, let alone the food industry, to properly police the wholesomeness and nutritional quality of food.

Unfortunately, there is some reason for this mistrust even if often exaggerated. Food worries no longer can be dismissed as faddism. When the Secretary of Agriculture, Earl F. Butz, derides what he calls "hysteria . . . to make everything safe," people are shocked.[5] But they are no less concerned when officials more thoughtful than Butz have reversed earlier reassurances and announced more stringent controls on additives, medicated livestock feeds, and pesticides, which they previously had reassured the public were safe enough under earlier regulations.

Thus, in the early 1970's, the government, among other actions, successively barred cyclamates; restricted the use of a number of pesticides; moved to curtail use of Red No. 2 dye, the most widely used and controversial color additive, and tried to reduce the use of diethylstilbestrol (DES), the bitterly contested livestock growth hormone.

It is revealing to see the change in the government's own attitudes in the past ten years. As one example, in 1963 the FDA announced that its "total diet" studies, based on foods collected from grocery stores, found that "pesticide residues detected were well within the amounts to be expected from compliance with sale limits established for individual crops." That was soon after Rachel Carson's *Silent Spring* came out. By 1972, of course, DDT, the major pesticide, was virtually banned for agricultural use, even for cotton crops, and use of a number of other pesticides was curtailed.

I do not question the sincerity of the FDA officials or the accuracy of their tests. But what they failed to realize, admit, or face up to were the ecological effects, the accumulation of pesticides in the soil, and the difficulties of controlling individual users. While undoubtedly Rachel Carson's book was one-sided and highly dramatic, its basic warning should not have been brushed aside.

One problem has been that at times when FDA officials acted decisively and courageously on behalf of public safety, they have had their hands held to the political fires. Thus in 1959, when the FDA just before Thanksgiving banned cranberries tainted by aminotriazole, a powerful weedkiller, the agency and the then-Secretary of Health, Education and Welfare, Arthur S.

Flemming, were thoroughly clobbered by farm organizations, many Congressmen, and the *Journal of the American Medical Association.* (Congress also paid off the growers for their misdeeds to the tune of $8.5 million.)

The result of all these both legitimate and exaggerated fears, sales pressure, faddism, and organic chic is that the number of health food stores has increased from 1,200 in 1968 to well over 3,000 in 1972; an estimated 1,300 in Los Angeles County alone, and some 150 in New York City where perhaps ten existed (the word of choice) a decade ago.

While health foods have been here for forty years, from 1970 to 1972 "growth has been almost straight up," a major wholesaler told its stockholders.[6]

As a sample of the recent proliferation, in 1971 there were twenty-one health food stores on Long Island. One year later there already were thirty-six.

Even this weedlike eruption of health food stores does not include the rush of supermarkets, department stores, drugstores, gift shops, and even karate and judo gyms to sell health foods and "natural" vitamins.

The boom also has produced a sharp increase in the number and size of health food restaurants. They are a far cry from the old-fashioned vegetarian eating places or health food bars with their small but devoted group of followers. Much of the clientele is youthful—almost completely so in the inexpensive East Village places in New York but largely so even in the chic health food restaurants uptown.

Health food dining rooms have been established at a number of universities. At San Francisco State University, where only a few years ago students put their bodies on the line in a bloody confrontation with the authorities, they now cultivate an organic garden in space provided by the university. At eight Eastern colleges the Barnes and Noble bookstores now sell Red Cheek apple juice, Tiger's Milk, soybeans, and vitamins along with the cram books.

Much publicity was given to the announcement that a majority of students, when offered a choice at the Santa Cruz campus of the University of California, preferred organically grown foods.[7]

Phyllis Hanes, food editor of *The Christian Science Monitor,* reports that the young people she encounters almost invariably ask her what they can make with yogurt, grains, and other "health" foods. "They would not be caught dead with meat and potatoes," Ms. Hanes comments.

There really are five main issues in what is known as the "health food movement" or "food revolution," depending on your age and temperament. In some of these issues, our investigation found, there is a grain, so to speak, of truth on the side of the health foodists. Some of their claims, however, are self-deluding and exaggerated.

The main issues are:

1. *The anxiety about foods "poisoned" by chemical additives and pesticides.* This is an exaggerated alarm, as shown by the unabashed use of the word "poisons" by organic food merchants, publishers, writers, and health foodists themselves. Even Rachel Carson used such scary imagery as comparing the American public to the "guests of the Borgias," while Odin R. Townly, a leading health food merchant, flatly told a public hearing that "known cancer-causing chemicals are used in many foods."[8]

These are only a handful of examples of scare language involved in the health food movement, especially its commerical wing. But even if exaggerated, this fear can no longer be dismissed merely as paranoid. Some incidents *have* occurred . . . and too many scientists have voiced misgivings, to disregard the warnings at least against careless or unnecessary use of chemical additives and pesticides.

It is not exaggerating the case to say that unnecessary chemical additives in processed foods, or even useful ones that have not been adequately tested, should be eliminated. Charles C. Johnson, Jr., a former U.S. Public Health Service official, has warned that the use of food additives increased 50 percent in ten years.[9] Each of us now consumes an average of five pounds of these chemicals yearly.

As impressive an authority as Dr. Orrea F. Pye, Professor of Nutrition at Columbia University and coauthor of *Foundations of Nutrition,* has said, even if in a notably understated way, ". . . consumers must be alert and keep well-informed to monitor the food industry, which may be motivated for profit."[10] (Note that Dr. Pye also said, " . . . it is naive to believe that the expensive products sold in health food stores are more reliable [than ordinary foods]," and that "many false claims are made by food quacks for . . . so-called natural foods. . . .")

2. *The belief that organic fertilizers produce nutritionally superior foods or, conversely, that chemical fertilizers "poison" foods.* These are the weakest of the health food movement's charges, with virtually no scientific evidence and only the most fragile speculation and "personal experience" to back these often self-serving claims.

While excessive or careless use of chemical fertilizers certainly has aggravated ecological problems, and some of the precepts of organic gardening are useful, by no means are they an answer to personal health problems, and they cannot possibly provide for the nation's food needs.

There is even a more likely danger of food contamination from some of the organic fertilizers than from chemical fertilizers.

3. *The belief that certain foods have such high nutrition that they are virtually miracle foods.* Some of the favored foods of the health food movement truly do provide high-quality nutrition, including whole grains ~ wheat germ, and blackstrap molasses. They do not, however, have special health-giving powers, let alone the curative powers sometimes ascribed to them. A few may be no more helpful than their "commerical" counterparts. Examples include the virtually cultist and even mystical use of honey by the health foodists, or the unfounded but no less unswerving belief in the greater nutrition of fertile eggs at twice the price, or even the revered granola cereals.

4. *The tendency to rely on special foods to cure personal health problems.* This is the dangerous aspect of health foodism, stemming, of course, from the belief that certain foods have remarkable curative powers. Many people, of course, would like to solve complicated personal problems in a simple way by swallowing something. These beliefs range from such risky ones as the unhesitating assurance that megadoses of niacin can cure schizophrenia, and that "happy people rarely get cancer," to such self deluding notions as that certain foods can cure arthritis or that eating meat clouds the mind, or the merely foolish notion, propounded by a Rodale editor, that you can achieve sexual vitality by eating halvah, or the claim that "natural cosmetics" can "calm" your skin.

The preoccupation of dedicated health foodists with their bodies is pervasive and constant. As one example, Adelle Davis has some worried people actually examining their tongues each day to see if they might have a deficiency of B vitamins, making sure, as she instructs, that the tongue is the right size and color and is evenly covered with taste buds.

5. *The belief that you regularly need to take vitamin or other food supplements because modern foods are nutritionally deficient, and also because various vitamins and minerals have special powers.* This is the fear that really powers the natural and organic food movement and is used to exploit its followers.

I am convinced by this investigation that without the large profits in "natural" vitamin pills, which often retail at actually three to four times their factory price, the health food industry and movement would be much smaller and much less aggressive in alarming the rest of the public about its claimed nutritional impoverishment.

The exploitation of anxieties about our food supply by the "natural vitamins" industry is not a conspiracy. It is simply that profits are to be found in scaring partially informed people about their health. The same manipulations have occurred before and go on today in other industries.

The most beneficent effects of the health food movement have been environmental and social; although in some cases, as in the highly emotional, ceaseless war against fluoridation of water, evidence indicates that the health foodists have caused harm. Despite their preoccupation with tongue-watching, pulse-counting, and vitamin-chewing, the organic or natural foodists have helped to focus attention on the environmental damage and some health risks of overuse of agricultural chemicals.

The most effective work in securing legislative remedies, however, has not been accomplished by the health food movement as much as by the national conservation associations and consumer federations.

But even in their concern for the environment, the health foodists overlook or oversimplify other pressing problems, such as the food and fiber needs of underdeveloped nations, including the underdeveloped nations in America's own ghettos. Bitter controversies are brewing over the greater concern for birds and animals than for human beings in slums. We even found "organic dog food" at a higher price than many people can afford to pay for their own canned hash.

The really committed health foodists usually harm only themselves, although sometimes others are affected. The harm is usually financial but sometimes can be physical as in the case of extreme diets, overuse of vitamins and of the most cherished health foods such as honey, or in pursuing food and vitamin nostrums instead of getting experienced, impartial medical or psychiatric advice. Often we, as have other investigators, found that health food clerks and vitamin sellers come dangerously close to prescribing health foods or vitamins as medicines.

This is not to say that there have not been some useful personal results. Several nutrition experts have commented that the concern over food adulteration has at least stimulated interest in nutrition among younger adherents. A vegetarian-oriented commune sought guidance from Mary Gullberg, a home economist for the Berkeley, California, co-ops. She found that their meals were balanced even without meat. They used eggs and milk products, and would prepare soybean and whole-grain casseroles with cheese and salads.

Similarly, Marian Burros, the *Washington Star's* food editor, reported that interest in health foods has stimulated home baking of whole-grain and sourdough breads and has turned attention to other relatively nutritious foods.

Another helpful fallout, John Darnton reported in the *New York Times,* is that the trend toward "natural living" and communalism, with its emphasis on organically grown foods, simplicity, and health, "is beginning to weigh against heavy drug use."[11]

Another unexpected benefit is that the high cost of health foods has brought together young people interested in vegetarian, whole-grain, and other diets in co-ops or "food conspiracies," as they are called in the Berkeley counter-culture. While their immediate objective, though partly self-deluding, is to save by buying organic foods wholesale, subsequently these groups often arrange for medical insurance and other needs on a cooperative basis.

The surprisingly strong vegetarian movement among young people also may spin off social and financial benefits by reducing the current high consumption of meat, which has added to cost-of-living problems.

But even with some truths on its side, and taken as a whole, the health food movement is still largely faddist, often self-deluding, and in a few instances even self-endangering. Many times the confused are leading the bewildered, as in the case of a health food clerk who advised researcher Steve Josenhans that to produce fertile eggs "you need a happy rooster in each flock, and such eggs contain equal amounts of lecithin and cholesterol, helping the body to assimilate the cholesterol in eggs."

But organic and natural foodists are convinced, dedicated, and angry. So are the standard nutritionists and medical authorities who at the least consider the organic movement's claims exaggerated, and at the most are likely to call their spokesmen quacks.

What *is* certain is that many sincere people concerned about their health and the environment are being exploited by the commercial health food industry itself—as arrogantly as the large commercial manufacturers often manipulate the public with their nutritional exaggerations and additive-bolstered concoctions.

References

1 "N.Y. Chain Climbs Aboard Organic Food Bandwagon," *Supermarket News,* September 29, 1971, p. 1.

2 I. A. Wolff and A. E. Wasserman, "Nitrates, Nitrites, and Nitrosamines," *Science,* July 7, 1972, p. 16.

3 *FDA Papers,* monthly magazine of the Food and Drug Administration, March, 1971, p. 30.

4 Judith Thomas, *Co-op News,* Berkeley, Calif., June 28, 1971, p. 11.

5 Jim Hightower, *Hard Tomatoes, Hard Times,* Task Force on the Land Grant College Complex, Agribusiness Accountability Project, Washington, D.C., 1972, p. 173.

6 Don Yeager, *Supermarket News,* interview with Richard D. Harrison, President of Fleming Co., May 1, 1972, p. 1.

7 Thomas H. Jukes, Division of Medical Physics, Donner Laboratory, University of California, Berkeley, "Fact and Fancy in Nutrition and Food Service," *Journal of the American Dietetic Association,* September, 1971, p. 203.

8 Odin R. Townley, President, Good Earth Natural Foods, Inc., testimony before New York City Consumer Affairs Department, December 9, 1971.

9 Charles C. Johnson, Jr., former Public Health Service official, at the Southern Regional Legislature Seminar on Current Public Health Problems, Atlanta, April 12, 1969.

10 Orrea F. Pye, *National Council of Women's Bulletin,* September, 1971, p. 7.

11 John Darnton, "Many on Campus Shifting to Softer Drugs and Alcohol," *New York Times,* January 17, 1971, p. 22.

30	# The Health Hustlers

VICTOR HERBERT

Victor Herbert, M.D., J.D., is clinical professor of medicine and clinical professor of pathology at Columbia College of Physicians and Surgeons.

We are being had. Most of what we read and hear about nutrition is wrong. Yet nutrition sells more magazines than sex!

We are in the midst of a vitamin craze. The health hustlers are cleaning up by stoking our fears and stroking our hopes. With their deceptive credentials, they dominate air waves and publications. The media hosts love them. Their false promises of super-health draw audiences of millions.

The situation now appears even worse than it was a decade ago, when the U.S. Food and Drug Administration Commission, George P. Larrick, stated:

> The most widespread and expensive type of quackery in the United States today is the promotion of vitamin products, special dietary foods, and food supplements. Millions of consumers are being misled concerning the need for such products. Complicating this problem is a vast and growing "folklore" or "mythology" of nutrition which is being built up by pseudo-scientific literature in books, pamphlets, and periodicals. As a result, millions of people are attempting self-medication for imaginary and real illnesses with a multitude of more or less irrational food items. Food quackery today can only be compared to the patent medicine craze which reached its height in the last century.

"Health food" rackets cost Americans over a billion dollars a year. The main victims of this waste are the elderly, the pregnant, the sick, and the poor.

THE "BASIC FOUR" OF GOOD NUTRITION

Have you been brainwashed by the hucksters? Do you supplement your diet with extra nutrients? Why? Do you believe that "if some is good, more may be better"? Do you believe, "It can't hurt"? Do you believe you are getting "nutritional insurance"? If you believe any of these things, you have been brainwashed.

The fundamentals of good nutrition are simple: To get the amounts and kinds of nutrients to maintain a positive state of health, all you need to eat is a moderate amount of food from each of the four basic categories (the "four basics"). Your daily average should be:

1   Fruits and/or vegetables and/or fresh fruit juices: four or more servings.
2   Grains and/or grain products (including cereals, breads, rice, macaroni, etc.): four or more servings.
3   Meats and/or meat products (including fish and/or poultry and/or eggs): two or more servings.
4   Milk and/or milk products: Two to four servings. (Except for infants, the requirement for this group is now recognized as more modest than previously believed.)

An easy way to remember the four basic categories is to think of a cheeseburger with lettuce and tomato—it has them all.

The health huckster doesn't tell you that the normal person needs no vitamin supplements if he gets the "four basics" each day. Why? Because his profits come from withholding that truth. Unlike your family doctor, he does not make his living by keeping you healthy, but rather by tempting you with rash, extravagant and false claims. Such claims raise his personal appearance fees and sell the products of companies in which (unknown to you) he may have a financial interest.

THE DANGERS OF EXCESS VITAMINS

When on the defensive, the quack is quick to demand, "How do you know it doesn't help?" The reply to this is "How do you know it doesn't *harm*?" Many substances which are harmless in small or moderate doses can be harmful either in large doses or by gradual build-up over many years. Just because a substance (such as a vitamin) is found naturally in food does not mean it is harmless in large doses. In fact, an entire book has been written on this subject (*Toxicants Occurring Naturally in Foods,* 2nd edition, published by a subcommittee of the National Research Council, National Academy of Sciences).

What do scientists mean by "excess" vitamins? They are referring to dosage in excess of the "Recommended Dietary Allowances (RDA)" set by the

Food and Nutrition Board of the National Research Council, National Academy of Sciences. The Recommended Dietary Allowances are the "levels of intake of essential nutrients considered, in the judgment of the Food and Nutrition Board on the basis of available scientific knowledge, to be adequate to meet the known nutritional needs of practically all healthy persons."

RDA's should not be confused with "requirements." They are actually more than most people require.

Quacks charge that the RDA's are set by a group which has a "conflict of interest to work to benefit the food industry." If you ever hear this, don't believe it. The RDA Committee of the Food and Nutrition Board consists of recognized nutrition experts from the Universities of California, Iowa, Wisconsin, New York State and Harvard as well as from the National Institutes of Health and the U.S. Department of Agriculture. There is not one representative of industry on the RDA Committee. Its work is supported by the National Institutes of Health, but members themselves serve without pay. Meeting at regular intervals, the RDA Committee sets its values after thorough study of the best evidence that scientists all over the world have developed. The only legitimate use of vitamins in excess of the RDA's is in treatment of medically diagnosed vitamin deficiency states—conditions which are rare except among the poor, especially among those who are pregnant or elderly.

Too much vitamin A can cause lack of appetite, retarded growth in children, drying and cracking of the skin, enlarged liver and spleen, increased intracranial pressure, loss of hair, migratory joint pains, menstrual difficulty, bone pain, irritability and headache.

Prolonged excessive intake of vitamin D can cause loss of appetite, nausea, weakness, weight loss, polyuria, constipation, vague aches, stiffness, kidney stones, calcifying of tissues, high blood pressure, acidosis and kidney failure which can lead to death.

Large doses of nicotinic acid or nicotinamide [niacin or niacinamide], recommended by purveyors of "orthomolecular psychiatry," can cause severe flushing, itching, liver damage, skin disorders, gout, ulcers and blood sugar disorders.

Excess vitamin E can cause headaches, nausea, tiredness, giddiness, inflammation of the mouth, chapped lips, GI [gastrointestinal] disturbances, muscle weakness, low blood sugar, increased bleeding tendency and degenerative changes. By antagonizing the action of vitamin A, large doses of vitamin E can also cause blurred vision. Vitamin E can also reduce sexual organ function—just the opposite of the false claim that the vitamin heightens sexual potency. (This claim is based on experiments with rats. . . . Quacks don't know that what may be true with rats may be just the opposite with man!)

Another way to look for health trouble is with large doses of ascorbic acid—vitamin C. Here the quacks take great pleasure in attempting to link themselves with one of the truly great men of our age, Dr. Linus Pauling, two-time Nobel Prize winner. Pauling's belief that vitamin C has value against the common cold has some validity, but its value is quite limited. Like an antihistamine tablet, in some cases it may reduce the symptomatology of a full-blown cold or completely eliminate the symptomatology of a mild cold (thereby creating the impression that no cold occurred). There is no reliable evidence that large doses of vitamin C *prevent* colds, and it is therefore not logical to take such doses in the absence of a cold.

Our laboratory has just published evidence that large doses of vitamin C can destroy substantial amounts of vitamin B_{12} in food.* If enough of your B_{12} is destroyed, you may develop a *very* dangerous deficiency. In addition, excess vitamin C may damage growing bone, produce diarrhea, produce "rebound scurvy" in newborn infants whose mothers took such dosage, produce adverse effects in pregnancy and cause kidney problems and false positive urine tests for sugar in diabetics. There may be other adverse effects. What should you do? Don't take more than 45 milligrams (mg) of ascorbic acid a day (the adult RDA) unless you have checked with your doctor, are pregnant (RDA 60 mg/day) or are breast-feeding (RDA 80 mg/day).

HEALTH HUSTLERS ARE USUALLY CHARLATANS AND QUACKS

The *Random House Unabridged Dictionary of the English Language* says that a charlatan is "one who pretends to more knowledge or skill than he possesses; quack." It then defines a quack as "1. a fraudulent or ignorant pretender to medical skill. 2. a person who pretends, professionally or publicly, to skill, knowledge, or qualification which he does not possess; a charlatan. 3 being a quack: a quack psychologist who complicates everyone's

---

*EDITOR'S NOTE: Although Dr. Herbert's conclusion has been in dispute, he has recently provided further evidence that it is correct. See the "Letters to the Editor" on "Destruction of Vitamin B₁₂ by Vitamin C," on pages 297–299 of the March 1977 issue of the *American Journal of Clinical Nutrition*, and the article by Herbert et al. on pages 253–258 of the February 1978 issue of the same journal.

problems. 4. presented falsely as having curative powers: quack medicine. 5. to advertise or sell with fraudulent claims."

The quack's pretense to greater knowledge or skill than he really has comes in various forms, some quite subtle. For example, the pretense often comes in the form of impressive-sounding credentials. It is typical for the talk show host to remark, when a quack and a genuine scientist are brought together as guests: "You both have such excellent credentials, and yet you make diametrically opposed statements. What is the layman to think?" What the layman should think is that one of the "experts" is very likely a quack.

Often the talk show quack will support his case by quoting the findings of a "great scientist" (another quack) who has "published over a hundred studies in scientific journals on vitamin E (or whatever)." Be cautious. He may be referring to publications which will publish anything submitted by almost anybody. Many journals do not have review systems to screen out garbage. The scientist knows which journals are scientific and which ones are not. The layman may not know this. But the quack does not care about the quality of his sources of information. He merely accepts any findings which appear to support him and rejects any evidence which contradicts his ideas.

Some quacks have a more modest-seeming approach, "I have published a few papers on this—maybe it takes more papers to convince some people." Don't let this fool you. It is not the number of papers which determines scientific truth, but the quality of the contents of each paper. One thousand poorly designed studies are one thousand pieces of junk. One well-designed study is worth its weight in gold. (The quack hates well-designed "controlled" studies.) Also keep in mind that when a quack refers to his own "research," what he really means is his unscientific combination of thoughts, plagiarized from two or more sources.

RECOGNIZING THE QUACK—FOURTEEN TIPS

How can you spot the health hustlers, the food quacks, the con men, the charlatans? The following should make you suspicious:

Tip #1: He advises that you go out and buy something which you would not otherwise have bought.

Ask yourself whether the friendly fellow with the benign smile who is recommending large doses of vitamin C or E, or some other vitamin or combination of vitamins, might have a financial interest in a vitamin company or two. Next time you hear someone on a talk show pushing a vitamin, call or write the station and ask whether he or the station has a financial interest, direct or indirect, in one or more companies selling vitamins. You might also ask whether Old Toothy Smile has ever been convicted of practicing medicine without a license. And whether any company in which he has or has had a financial interest has ever had its vitamin products seized by the FDA for mislabeling. The silence which greets your inquiry will astound you.

Tip #2: He is a Fake Specialist, with Imposing "Front" Titles. Credentials sell people. Because he knows this, and sometimes because he has grandiose character traits with messianic feelings, the quack often provides himself with impressive-sounding titles. Such include "Director" or "President" of the "X Nutrition Institute" or the "Y Nutrition Society," or "Nutrition Consultant" or "Nutrition Expert" or "World's Foremost (or Greatest or Leading) Nutritionist." Be suspicious of such titles. The "Institute" or "Society" will usually prove to be a "front" (created by the quack or his agents) with no standing among genuine nutrition scientists. The titles and institutes are rarely affiliated with legitimate scientific or academic institutions. When the quack is a "Nutrition Consultant," it will usually turn out to be to an organization which peddles misleading health information and/or vitamins and/or health foods. Often, the organization is controlled by him.

Information on who incorporated an institute or society is available from the State Attorney General where the institute is located. As for the title "World's Foremost (or Greatest or Leading) Nutritionist," there is no such title given by any reputable scientific organization. It is a "cover" anyone can use, no matter how ignorant he may be about nutrition. There is no law against it, just as there is no law against anyone calling himself "World's Foremost Lover."

Some reputable organizations which work for the advancement of science will accept any private citizen as a member. Quacks often join such groups in order to add "legitimate" credentials to their list. In order to protect the public, "open" membership organizations should forbid advertising of membership. The American Association for the Advancement of Science is one which does this. . . .

The largest private (non-government) group of genuine health research scientists in the world is probably the Federation of American Societies for Experimental Biology (FASEB). The American Institute of Nutrition (AIN) is the nutrition branch of FASEB, and the American Society for Clinical Nutrition (ASCN) is the clinical nutrition arm of AIN. These three organizations screen out quacks, so be suspicious if a "nutrition expert" does not list one of them among his credentials—especially if he includes some other group with "Nutrition" in its title. Some quacks try to seem more respectable by attacking other quacks.

Your doctor may be able to help you separate good nutrition information from nutrition nonsense. Unfortunately, a doctoral degree is not a guarantee of reliability. A few people with M.D., D.D.S., or Ph.D. after their names— who have received their training in reputable institutions—have strayed from scientific thought. Some of them have written books. The medical and dental degrees of Emanuel Cheraskin and the dental degree of W. M. Ringsdorf, Jr., did not prevent them from writing *New Hope for Incurable Diseases,* a book which stimulates false hopes that vitamins can cure various diseases which, at present, are incurable. An advertisement for this book deceptively states, "In an era of increasing faddism and misinformation about foods, the reader will benefit from the authoritative treatment of the subject contained herein." Unfortunately, the law does not protect you from this type of deception. When this ad was sent to the New York State Attorney General and the FDA, both replied that it was out of their jurisdiction. In the Fall 1972 issue of the *Journal of Nutrition Education,* Dr. C. E. Butterworth, Jr., Director of the Nutrition Program at the University of Alabama (where Cheraskin and Ringsdorf are on the dental faculty), wrote a devastating review of their book, closing with:

> There are a number of . . . statements throughout the book which are patently erroneous or misleading. . . . The main objection to this book is the tone and attitude of the presentation. There are subtleties and innuendoes readily apparent to an educated reader but which, alas, are likely to be missed by the lay public. One expects more from university professors who write interpretations of science for the general public. This book has apparently been written for the faddist fringe and "health" food store market and for readers who seemingly *want* to believe the miracles wrought by diet without regard for scientific evidence.
>
> Surely hope is an essential element of life. . . . But it is cruel to raise false hope under any pretense. In my opinion, this book raises nothing but false hopes, many of them not even new, in the mind of an uneducated reader. . . .

Tip #3: He says that most disease is due to a bad or faulty diet. This is not so. Inspect any medical school textbook of medicine or ask your doctor. They will tell you that most diseases have nothing to do with diet. Malaise (feeling poorly), tiredness, lack of pep, aches (including headaches) or pains, insomnia and similar complaints are usually the body's reaction to emotional stress, overwork, etc. The persistence of such complaints is a signal to see a doctor to be evaluated for possible underlying physical illness. It is not a signal to add vitamins.

Tip #4: He says that most people are poorly nourished (the old "Subclinical Deficiency" gambit). This is an appeal to fear which is not only untrue, but ignores the fact that the main forms of "poor" nourishment in the United States are undernourishment among the poverty-stricken and overnourishment among the economically well-to-do. The poverty-stricken can ill afford to waste money on unnecessary vitamins. Their food money should be spent on the "basic four," which contain not only all the vitamins in proper amounts, but also the other necessary nutrients.

It has been alleged that our advertising age has produced an addiction to snack foods, making a well-rounded diet exceptional rather than usual. This is an exaggeration, since the "basic four" need not be obtained in each meal, but rather over the course of an entire day. It is true that some snack foods are mainly "empty calories" (sugar without other nutrients). But it should be noted that acquiring the "basic four" is not all that difficult.

There is one form of poor nourishment which is particularly common in this country—fluoride deficiency. Fluoride is necessary to build strong teeth which resist decay. The best way for people to get an adequate amount of this essential nutrient is to adjust community water supplies so that the fluoride concentration is about one part fluoride for every million parts of water. Strangely, the quack is usually opposed to water fluoridation. It almost seems as if when he can't personally profit from the sale, he isn't interested in your health.

The quack tells you that everyone is in danger of "subclinical deficiency." Does the sound scary? It is meant to be. It is a typical sales tactic, like that of the door-to-door furnace huckster who tells you your perfectly good furnace is in danger of blowing up and you can only be saved by replacing it with his product. Scientists sometimes use the term subclinical deficiency to refer to the situation of a patient on the road to deficiency from an inadequate diet. But no normal person eating a wall-balanced diet each day is in any danger of "subclinical vitamin deficiency." As one well-controlled study reported, vitamin B complex and liver supplements "produced no improvement of . . . well-being and no decline in the incidence of minor illnesses among apparently healthy people on an adequate diet."

Tip #5: He tells you that soil depletion and the use of chemical fertilizers cause malnutrition. If a nutrient is missing from the soil, a plant just does not grow. Chemical fertilizers counteract the effects of soil depletion. The quack is dead wrong when he claims otherwise! He is also wrong when he claims that plants grown with natural (animal) fertilizers are nutritionally superior to those grown with synthetic fertilizers. The only "extra" you may get from an animal fertilizer is a good case of salmonella diarrhea or gastrointestinal parasites. Moreover, "natural" foods are more likely to have molds growing on them which produce aflatoxins which are among the most potent carcinogens (cancer-producers). Some food additives reduce the growth of these molds.

Don't make the mistake of thinking that the law forces people to tell the truth about nutrition. FDA regulations forbid only *labeling* claims that a deficient diet may be due to the soil in which a food is grown. But our laws do not protect you from the quack who states the same thing on TV or radio or in a publication.

Tip #6: He alleges that modern processing methods and storage remove all nutritive value from our food. This is a gross distortion of fact. It is true that food processing can change the nutrient content of foods. But the changes are not so drastic as the quack, who wants you to buy his supplements, wants you to believe. While some processing methods destroy nutrients, others add them. As long as you select your foods properly, you will get all the nourishment you need.

The quack distorts and oversimplifies. When he tells you that milling removes B vitamins and iron, he does not bother to tell you that enrichment puts them back. When he tells you that cooking destroys nutrients, he does not tell you that only a few nutrients are sensitive to heat. Nor does he tell you that these few nutrients are easily obtained by having fresh fruit, vegetables or fruit juice each day.

Tip #7: He says that you are in danger of being poisoned by food additives and preservatives. This is a scare tactic designed to undermine your confidence in food scientists and in government protection agencies. The quack wants you to think that he is out to protect you. He hopes that if you trust him, you will buy what he recommends. The fact is that the tiny amounts of preservatives used to protect our food pose no threat to human health.

. . . I would like to comment on how ridiculous quacks can get about food additives, especially those which are found naturally in food anyway. Calcium propionate, which is used to preserve bread, occurs naturally in Swiss cheese. The quack who would steer you toward (higher-priced) bread made without preservatives is careful not to tell you that one ounce of Swiss

cheese, which you may eat in a sandwich, contains enough calcium propionate to retard spoilage of two loaves of bread. Similarly, the organic food
quack who warns against monosodium glutamate (MSG) does not tell you
that wheat germ is a major natural source of this substance.

Tip #8: He tells you that if you eat badly, you'll be OK if you take a
vitamin or vitamin and mineral supplement. This is the "Nutrition Insurance
Gambit." It is dangerous nonsense. Not only is it untrue, but it encourages
careless eating habits. The cure for eating badly is a well-balanced diet.
Money spent for a vitamin or mineral supplement would be better spent for
a daily portion of fresh fruit or vegetable. With one exception, the "four
basics" diet contains all the nutrients, known and unknown, that normal
people need. (The exception involves the mineral iron. The average American diet contains barely enough iron to meet the needs of infants, women of
child-bearing age and, especially, pregnant women. This problem can be
solved simply by cooking in an iron pot or eating iron-rich foods such as soy
beans, . . . liver and veal muscle.)

Tip #9: He recommends that everybody take vitamins or health foods or
both. The nutrition quack belittles normal foods. He does not tell you that
he earns his living from such recommendations—via public appearance
fees, endorsements, sale of publications or financial interests in vitamin
companies, health food stores and/or "organic" farms. On the subject of
"health food" stores—the term itself is deceptive. Did you ever stop to think
that your corner grocery, fruit market, meat market and supermarket are
also health food stores? They are—and they charge less for food which is
identical or superior to that provided by "health food" stores!

The quack often makes nutritional claims for bioflavinoids, rutin, inositol
and other such food extracts. These "non-essential" ingredients have no
recognized nutritional value, and the FDA forbids nutritional claims for them
in labeling.

Tip #10: He claims that "natural" vitamins are better than "synthetic"
ones. This claim is a flat lie, and anyone who makes it should be immediately classified by you as a quack. Each vitamin is a chain of atoms
strung together as a molecule. Molecules made in the "factories" of nature
are identical to those made in the factories of chemical companies.

Tip #11: He promises quick, dramatic, miraculous cures. The promises
are usually implied or subtle—so he can deny making them when the Feds
close in. Such promises are the health hustler's most immoral practice. He
does not see, know or want to know the people who have been broken

financially or in spirit—by the elation over his claims of quick cure followed by the depression when the claims prove false. Nor does the health hustler keep count of how many people he lures away from proper medical care.

Quacks will tell you that "megavitamins" (huge doses of vitamins) can cure many different ailments, particularly emotional ones. But they won't tell you that the "evidence" supporting such claims is unreliable because it is based on inadequate investigations and other forms of sloppy research.

Tip #12: He uses testimonials and "case histories" to support his claims. We all tend to believe what others tell us about their personal experiences. When you hear someone claim that product X has cured his cancer, arthritis or whatever, be skeptical. He may not have actually had the condition he names. If he did have the condition he names, his recovery most likely would have occurred without the help of product X. (Most conditions recover with just the passage of time.) Establishing medical truths requires careful and repeated investigation—with well-designed experiments, not reports of what people *imagine* might have taken place. That is why testimonial evidence is forbidden in scientific articles.

Symptoms which are psychosomatic in origin are often relieved by any product which is taken with the suggestion that it will relieve the problem. Most headaches and minor aches and pains will respond to any enthusiastically recommended nostrum. For these problems, even physicians may prescribe a placebo. A placebo is a substance which has no pharmacological effect on a normal person, but is given merely to satisfy a patient who supposes it to be a medicine. Sugar tablets and vitamins (such as B_{12}) are commonly used in this way.

Placebos act by suggestion. Unfortunately, some physicians, like most laymen, really "believe in vitamins" beyond those supplied by a good diet. Those who share such false beliefs do so because they confuse placebo action with cause and effect.

Talk show hosts give quacks a tremendous boost when they ask them, "What do all the vitamins you take do for you personally?" Then, millions of viewers are treated to the quack's talk of improved health, vigor and vitality—with the implicit point: "It did this for me. It will do the same for you." A most revealing testimonial experience was described during a major network show recently which hosted several of the world's most prominent promoters of nutritional faddism. While the host was boasting about how his new eating program had cured his "hypoglycemia," he mentioned in passing that he no longer was drinking "20 to 30 cups of coffee a day." Neither the host nor any of his "experts" had the good sense to tell their audience how dangerous it can be to drink so much coffee. Nor did any of them suggest that some of the host's original symptoms might have been caused by caffeine intoxication.

Tip #13: He espouses the "Conspiracy Theory" and its twin, the "Controversy Claim." The quack claims he is being persecuted by orthodox medicine and that his work is being suppressed. He claims that orthodox medicine or the AMA [American Medical Association] is against him because his cures can cut into the incomes doctors make by keeping people sick. Don't fall for such nonsense. There is so much more medical business available than we doctors can handle that we import from other countries about as many doctors each year as we graduate from our own medical schools. Moreover, many doctors in health plans receive the same salary whether or not the patients in the plans are sick—so keeping their patients healthy reduces their workload but *not* their incomes.

The quack claims there is a "controversy" about facts between himself and "the bureaucrats," organized medicine and/or "the establishment." He clamors for medical investigation of "his" claims (ignoring the negative results of all past investigations). In reality, there is no fact controversy. The collision is between his misleading statements and the facts. The gambit "Do you believe in vitamins?" is one way in which he tries to increase confusion. Everyone "believes in vitamins." The real question should be: "Do you need additional vitamins beyond those in a well-balanced diet?" The answer is no.

Any physician who found a vitamin or other preparation which could cure sterility, heart disease, arthritis, cancer and the like could make an enormous fortune from such a discovery. Not only would patients flock to him, but his colleagues would shower him with prizes and awards—not the least of which would be the tax-free $100,000+ Nobel Prize!

Tip #14: He is legally belligerent. The majority of "nutrition experts" who appear on TV talk shows and whose publications dominate the "health" sections in bookstores and health food stores are quacks and charlatans. Why are they not labeled as such? Ralph Lee Smith, a former investigative reporter who became Associate Professor of Communications at Howard University, answered this question in the December 16, 1965 issue of *The National Reporter*. Writing in "The Vitamin Healers," a hard-hitting article which ripped the lid off Carlton Fredericks, Smith said it is the "question of libel":

A reputation for being legally belligerent can sometimes go far to insulate one from critical publicity. And if an attack does appear in print, a threat of libel action will sometimes bring a full retraction. Carlton Fredericks frequently threatens to take libel action against those who disagree with him. So assiduous has he been in this respect that he even writes threatening letters to physicians who have questioned his ideas in private correspondence.*

If a "nutritionist" travels with a lawyer and threatens libel actions against those who disagree with him, he is probably a quack.

As Smith noted, the threat of a libel action can be particularly effective when made against scientific and scholarly publications, especially those which are sponsored by publicly supported societies and universities.

Dena C. Cederquist is Chairman of the Department of Foods and Nutrition at Michigan State University. In March 1964, she testified at the hearings on health frauds and quackery held by a U.S. Senate subcommittee: "My salary is paid by the State of Michigan to teach, and yet on advice of our lawyer at the University, I did not write a criticism of the book *Calories Don't Count* [by Dr. Herman Taller, who was subsequently convicted of mail fraud, conspiracy and violating FDA regulations] for he said I would be liable and we simply could not afford this kind of thing." She further stated, about a paper relating to food faddism presented by Kenneth L. Milstead of the FDA to the American Dietetic Association in October 1962, "He submitted this paper first to the *Journal of the American Dietetic Association* and secondly to the *Journal of the American Medical Association,* and both organizations refused to publish it, a paper full of facts. They refused to publish it for fear of being hauled into court in one of those long, drawn-out law suits · . . , and so this very valuable bit of information which should have gone to all practicing dietitians in the United States—and could well have been read by all physicians—was not made available for publication.

The public feels that doctors should speak out against nutrition quacks because they have "nothing to fear" from a libel suit from a quack. Nothing to fear? Successful defense against a libel suit can take three years and cost the doctor $10,000 or more. We need "Good Samaritan" laws to cover the cost of defending libel actions brought by quacks! We also need vigorous enforcement of the laws against malicious prosecution. Any physician or genuine nutritionist who is sued by a quack should consider a counter-suit for malicious harassment.

---

*EDITOR'S NOTE: For some words in defense of Fredericks, see page 327.

This writer was threatened in connection with the 1974 David Susskind TV show "The Vitamin Craze." Just before the show was taped, I was handed a nutrition book written by a velvet-suited, silky-voiced co-panelist whom I had never heard of before—one Gary Null. After perusing it, I stated, "This book is garbage." Null immediately threatened me with a lawsuit if I repeated the statement. He told me he travels with two lawyers just to take care of people like me. Calling one of them over, he introduced us and asked his lawyer to watch me closely and hit me with a lawsuit if I said anything "out of line." Null told me he was "Director of the Nutrition Institute of America" and had 36 Nobel Prize winners on his board of directors. I replied that his Institute sounded like a quack "front" and that I did not believe it had 36 Nobel Prize winners on its board. (Subsequent investigation proved that I was correct on both counts.) With this warm-up, we went on the air. It was a lively program—one of the few in which the public heard immediate rebuttal of nutritional misinformation.

THE WEAKNESS OF THE LAW

Anybody can state, in any medium of his choice, any false, misleading or deceptive health information he chooses. The First Amendment (freedom of speech) protects him against the consequences of the harm he does, unless the false information is on the label of a product or the fraud occurs in the course of a provable doctor-patient relationship. Thus, the U.S. Food and Drug Administration, which can act against misleading labels, has no jurisdiction over misleading books.

Can the Federal Communications Commission (FCC) or the Federal Trade Commission (FTC) attack nutrition misinformation via laws which require broadcasters to operate in the public interest as well as laws which require "truth in advertising"? The FCC usually acts only after receiving complaints, and *a public that does not know it is being misinformed cannot complain.* The FTC appears to act only against very gross forms of advertising deception or deceptive trade practice. It does not appear to act against subtle forms of misleading information, and many complaints it receives are shelved for "lack of agency manpower." Purveying deceptive misinformation for profit appears on its face to be a deceptive trade practice. The FTC should be able to move against those who profit from public appearances in which they purvey false, deceptive or misleading nutrition information.

Why do the State Attorneys General not act? Isn't the presentation of misleading nutrition information perpetrating a fraud on the consuming public? If the First Amendment does not protect smut speech and writings which are alleged to injure mental health, why does it protect misleading nutrition speech and writings which can be proved to be harmful to both mental and physical health? When quack books were brought to the attention of the New York State Attorney General, however, he merely referred them to the FDA (which, of course, did not have jurisdiction over them).

The FDA has pointed out that excess vitamins can hurt you. How many Americans know this? How many preachers of nutrition gospel have ever mentioned this on a television talk show? This failure to mention should be prosecuted as negligence chargeable not only to the huckster, but also to his talk show host and sponsoring network. It also seems possible that the States and/or their courts can revise or interpret their "reckless endangerment" statutes to include reckless endangerment of public health by promotion of dangerous nutritional ideas. I also wonder whether the more dangerous of the quack's misrepresentations could be enjoined as a public nuisance. Perhaps a public-spirited prosecutor will try these approaches someday.

Under our civil laws, it may be possible for a private citizen to recover substantial damages if he relied on misinformation purveyed by the quack to the detriment of his health. He would need to establish that the quack had a duty not to mislead him. If a doctor recommends a remedy, he has a duty both to use care in selecting it and to warn of complications. If a patient is harmed because his doctor fails to do either one of these, he can sue for malpractice. Is it too much to expect that the unlicensed quack can be held responsible for the harm *he* does? . . .

. . . Many radio and television stations which broadcast nutrition quackery have been put on notice by scientists that they are creating an unreasonable risk of harm. Such stations might have serious difficulty defending themselves against suits by injured listeners.

When the charming quack does have an interest in a vitamin company, you can be sure that the labeling of his products makes none of the health benefit claims which he makes on the air or in his publications. This is because our laws forbid nutritional misinformation or outright lies only in connection with the sale of products. One way to find out whether someone on the air or in a book is telling the truth is to send him a label from a bottle of a vitamin preparation he sells. Attach the label to a sheet of paper stating the claims he makes for the product (in positive terms, such as, "This preparation will cure the following illnesses: —, —, —."). Ask him to sign the statement and return it to you with the label still attached. If he does not do so, you may assume that he is afraid that his signature on *labeling* can get him prosecuted for false statements.

Quacks project an aura of sincerity and public interest. They spout (un-provable) "case histories" and tales of personal experience. They cite sloppy research as "the great work of great men." Yet their deceptions dominate the media.

The food quack benefits only himself, collecting large fees for his public appearances, publications or "consultant" status to health food and vitamin companies which he often controls. The public is not only milked financially (for more than a billion dollars a year), but may also suffer damage from vitamin overdosage and from seduction away from proper medical care.

There is nutritional deficiency in this country, but it is found primarily among the poor, particularly among those who are elderly, are pregnant or are small children. These groups need to have their diets improved. Their problems will not be solved by the panaceas of the huckster, but by better nutritional practices. The best way to buy vitamins and minerals is in the rational combination packages provided by nature: the "basic four" of (1) fresh fruits and vegetables; (2) meats, fish and fowl; (3) whole grain or en-riched bread and cereal; and (4) milk products. . . .

Contrary to the health hustler's claim that "it may help," his advice not only does not help but may harm—both your health and your pocketbook. He will continue to "rip off" the American public, however, until the com-munications industries develop sufficient concern for the public interest to expose his quackery. And if the media cannot develop adequate social con-science on their own, they should be forced to do so by stronger laws and more vigorous law enforcement.

Recommended reading

The Great Vitamin Hoax, by Daniel Tatkon.
The Nuts Among the Berries, by Ron Deutsch (a history of food quackery).
Nutrition for Today, by R. Alfin-Slater and L. Aftergood.
The Bellybook, by James Trager.
Eating for Good Health, by Fredrick J. Stare, M.D.
The Family Guide to Better Food and Better Health, by Ron Deutsch.
Let's Talk About Food, by Philip L. White.

Megavitamin and Orthomolecular Therapy in Psychiatry, Task Force report of the American Psychiatric Association ($3.00 from Publications Services Division, APA, 1700 N. 18th Street, N.W., Washington, D.C. 20009).

Recommended Dietary Allowances, National Academy of Sciences ($2.50 from Publishing Office, National Academy of Sciences, 2101 Constitution Avenue, Washington, D.C. 20418).

List of Nutrition Books: Recommended, Recommended for Special Purposes, Not Recommended. Reliable guide to nutrition books. Compiled by Chicago Nutrition Association ($2.00 from Chicago Nutrition Association, 8158 South Kedzie Avenue, Chicago, Illinois 60652).

Nutrition Misinformation and Food Faddism. A collection of 17 papers published by the Nutrition Foundation ($2.50 from Nutrition Foundation, Office of Education, 888 17th Street, N.W., Washington, D.C. 20006).

| 31 |

How to Learn Nutritional Know-How

ALAN H. NITTLER

Alan Nittler, M.D., specializes in metabolic nutrition and is currently developing "ultrasonic-energy products," which are allied to homeopathic remedies. Dr. Nittler conducted a question-and-answer column for *Let's Live* magazine for five years and is also the author of *Health Questions and Answers* and *New Breed Digest of Metabolic Nutrition*.

From Alan H. Nittler, *A New Breed of Doctor* (New York: Pyramid House, 1972). Copyright © 1972 by Alan H. Nittler, M.D. Reprinted by permission of the author.

. . . There is no place to go for formal nutritional education. No approved medical institution looks favorably upon this subject. The usual medical curriculum includes some 4,000 total hours of medical education and only from zero to five credit hours of so-called nutrition, which is in reality dietetics, an entirely different subject. What *is* taught mainly includes such things as low-sodium diets for hypertension, bland diets for ulcers, low-cholesterol diets for arterial and heart problems, and calorie counting for obesity. All are sadly out of date by newer nutritional standards, and what's more, the public knows it! They are fed up with palliative measures and are losing confidence in the average medical practitioner and the drugs he uses to cover up symptoms. They are watching others, laymen and a *few* doctors, who are reversing illness. They (the public) are beginning to do the same things themselves through the newer concept of nutrition which teaches that the body is only as strong as what is put into it. Like a building, or a bridge, the body will endure stress and strain only if it is made of the best materials, of which the baby was created in the first place. These materials must be kept in constant supply in order to maintain good health. The public is reading, learning and using this approach with great success. There is no need for physicians to lose face during this revolution, which, believe me, is not temporary. My advice is, if you can't beat them, join them! Do as some doctors are already doing: educate yourself nutritionally. I will give you some tips on how to get started.

Many physicians recommend a good, nutritious diet for their patients when they themselves have neither been trained nor even have the faintest idea what a good, nutritious diet is! One young physician told me he believed that the body could get all the nutrients it needs from hot dogs, french fries and Cokes, so long as the person is kept free from hunger. Frankly, this man has a lot to learn. I could fill an entire page in this book with names of the chemicals and body-disturbing elements found in these items alone which may be stomach fillers but not body builders. Colorings, dyes, chemicals galore replace any nutrients which once may have existed in these foods but now add up only to a bunch of chemicals. Many of these very chemicals have been found to be cancer-causing in experimental situations.

I realize that the average doctor is beset by suspicions about nutrition. He has been warned it is quackery or faddism. A small percentage of it may be, but there is also a mass of growing research from laboratories the world over which is not quackery. Why do people fall for it indiscriminately? Because they have no doctor to guide them. They have to learn the hard way for themselves. Even at that, it may be safer for the patient in the long run than the doctor's use of experimental drugs. All too often these experimental drugs become demoted, one by one, because of their dangerous side effects. Let's face it, brainwashing takes place in the drug field as in any other. At least the nutritional fads won't kill people. People are clamoring for doctors who can separate the nutritional truths from the untruths so they won't have to experiment on themselves. At present, they are now learning by trial and error, by the hundreds of thousands. This army is increasing daily!

True science must develop demonstrable facts, not just opinions based on medical consensus. Testing can be tricky. To begin with, many tests are performed in subsidized laboratories which are trying to slant the results for ulterior reasons. Nutritional testing is especially difficult because there are so many variables. For instance, a test of a nutritional substance may fail because too small a dosage was used for too short a time. The false or incomplete verdict is then announced that the product is of no value. This has happened in the case of vitamins E and C. Both of these vitamins were rejected by the medical profession, but not the public, who used them with great success. In spite of attempts to slander or eliminate them, these vitamins have now become, when properly used, both accepted and successful. True science must be entirely objective and without bias.

~~~~~~

HOW MUCH DO AMERICAN PHYSICIANS KNOW ABOUT NUTRITION?

Excerpt from testimony given by Dr. Philip R. Lee (director of the Health Policy Program at the School of Medicine, University of California at San Francisco) in hearings held during summer 1976 before the Senate Select Committee on Nutrition and Human Needs:

SENATOR GEORGE MCGOVERN: "Are the graduates that are coming out of our medical schools now—that is, the doctors that are going to go out and practice and deal with patients—are they properly trained in your judgment on the importance of nutrition in overall human development?"

PHILIP R. LEE, M.D.: "Absolutely not. They know more about heart transplants than they do about basic nutrition. The technology has so taken hold of medicine, has sort of obsessed us all, and we instruct students in all kinds of technological advances. But in very basic things, like what is an adequate diet, we do not do an adequate job. . . . In the medical schools of the country, we are devoting tremendous resources to pediatric neonatal intensive care units to care for infants of mothers who were given inadequate nutrition counseling during their pregnancy. That is largely the fault of our own neglect of nutrition counseling in health care. . . . I would guess 90 percent of the graduates of our medical schools couldn't describe an adequate, nutritious diet that was appropriate for people at various stages of life."

~~~~~~

The public is now ahead of the doctors and is taking the bit in its teeth. The once respected, almost worshiped, medical profession is rapidly losing its public image. I repeat, the solution is: if you can't beat the opposition, in this case the unsatisfied public, join it! A joiner can become a leader. I realize that the average doctor is wary. He has spent years of his life learning the allopathic approach. He feels secure in his field. Unfortunately allopathy is meeting neither the needs of today nor the demands of an ever-increasing intelligent public. You would be amazed how much more the layman knows about this subject than the doctor. Even the press has discovered how important, as well as how popular, the subject of nutrition is to the general public, and is reporting laboratory findings as priority news. These reports are seized upon by a hungry public whose health is failing under the care of the busy, nutritionally unprepared and bewildered physician.

The only way I know to meet this challenge and survive professionally is to allow some time in your reading of medical literature for reading and studying nutritional literature. Read, study, learn. Attend any "health" conventions in your vicinity. Sure, you will find some crackpots, but you will also find other lecturers who have discovered nutritional truths which do work. You may shudder at the lack of education, as you know it, of some of these people who may not know the meaning of the word "documentation," and couldn't care less. They may just have rediscovered a natural remedy upon which some of our early pharmacology was based but is now banned in favor of more expensive drugs. Watch the people in the audience. Hear their testimonies. Pay attention to any of the outstanding well-educated experts in the field of nutrition who are devoting their lives to nutritional research and using it clinically with tremendous success. There may be only one or a few in this category at a convention because they are rare, overworked and hard to come by for public lecturing. They may have an M.A., a Ph.D., a D.D.S. or an M.D., so don't underrate their intelligence. They are merely educated in a field in which you are not but should be. The public is following them like Pied Pipers because they not only promise better health but they deliver it! Nutritional reporters often make reports on scientific studies and practical concepts many years before the ideas are actually accepted by contemporary medicine. Acceptance usually comes only after a battle with the status quo. In getting your postgraduate education, don't be afraid to listen to a lecture or read a book by a "crackpot." You might learn something, even only one point of importance. I have been called both "crackpot" and "beloved physician."

After you read and listen, and I implore you to do both with an open mind, then begin to experiment. A little now and a little later is enough at first. Try nutrition on yourself, as I did. You can expect some surprises. As you gain confidence, add more nutritional tools to your trade. If you are a specialist, try it in your specialty. I know of several physicians who have been amazed with the increased success of the nutritional vs. the drug approach in their particular fields. Don't give up if you have a failure. Try to learn why it did not work and keep trying. Believe me, you have no need to fear that your practice will fall off. The nutritional M.D.'s I know are so swamped with delighted patients that they are establishing more confidence than ever. The word-of-mouth publicity is bringing a never-ending line up to their doors.

Where can you find such information? I list the sources I know of at the end of this chapter.

As you add to your nutritional knowledge, you will wonder what products are the best to use. I have tried many. I have definitely rejected the synthetics, except in a few situations for temporary control only. I have found that whole, truly natural supplements, not just those products which pretend to be natural, bring the best results in the long run. I have finally settled down to a few sources, though I am not absolutely rigid about clinging to these alone. New and good products, as well as questionable ones, are coming out all the time. I try to keep alert for the good ones. If they measure up, I add them to my armamentarium. . . .

Before I list some suggested reading to help you in your postgraduate nutritional education, let us here and now dispel some myths. As you scan the names of the authors, you may react against some of them because you have been led to believe they are "quacks," "faddists" or "health nuts." I assure you they are not or I would not have listed their publications. . . . I urge you, as a doctor, to use common sense in making judgments about something or someone about whom you have *heard* or read derogatory remarks. Let's face it, there is usually a reason for continuous attacks, often unwarranted, on new methods, procedures or remedies. This is the history of medicine! When you have been warned again and again that a person or a remedy is useless or dangerous, put on your own thinking cap. Why did the government insist for so long that insecticides were perfectly safe, when they are now forced to admit that they are killing off wild life and upsetting our ecology and also poisonous, even carcinogenic, for people? Did it ever occur to you that the chemical insecticide industry may have been playing

STAMP OUT FOOD FADDISM

Food faddism is indeed a serious problem. But we have to recognize that the guru of food faddism is not Adelle Davis, but Betty Crocker. The true food faddists are not those who eat raw broccoli, wheat germ, and yogurt, but those who start the day on Breakfast Squares, gulp down bottle after bottle of soda pop, and snack on candy and Twinkies.

Food faddism is promoted from birth. Sugar is a major ingredient in baby food desserts. Then come the artificially flavored and colored breakfast cereals loaded with sugar, followed by soda pop and hot dogs. Meat marbled with fat and alcoholic beverages dominate the diets of many middle-aged people. And, of course, white bread is standard fare throughout life.

This diet—high in fat, sugar, cholesterol, and refined grains—is the prescription for illness; it can contribute to obesity, tooth decay, heart disease, intestinal cancer, and diabetes. And these diseases are, in fact, America's major health problems. So if any diet should be considered faddist, it is the standard one. Our far-out diet—almost 20 percent refined sugar and 45 percent fat—is new to human experience and foreign to all other animal life. . . .

It is incredible that people who eat a junk-food diet constitute the norm, while individuals whose diets resemble those of our great-grandparents are labeled deviants. . . .

From an editorial in *Nutrition Action* (a newsletter of the Center for Science in the Public Interest, Washington, D.C.), March-April 1975. Reprinted by permission.

footsies with certain members of government agencies to prevent the publication of such information, which would be a large burden financially?

Why has the government insisted for so long that this country does not suffer from malnutrition, as preached by some governmental spokesmen, while others in the same bureau have conducted respected research with contrary conclusions? The government finally was forced to admit this discrepancy. Could it be that the food processors—who claim that our food is the best in the world and that natural foods, vitamins, minerals, etc., found in health foods are useless—are robbing the public of millions of dollars for worthless foods? Could it be that these health stores, which more and more people are patronizing while searching for unsprayed foods or whole foods untampered by man, are a financial threat to the food processing industry?

Don't cringe at the thought of health food stores. True, they are not perfect and everything they carry is not a "health food." They were sold a bill of goods, for instance, on the cyclamates by the manufacturers who supplied other stores, too. These stores *try* to live up to their stated purpose. To my knowledge they are the only sources of natural grains, other organic foods and natural supplements. The personnel, it is true, are often not educated according to our standards. In their defense, however, they still may know more about the natural health field than doctors. They operate these stores, or did at least until recently, because they themselves have experienced improvement in health through nutritional methods. They are trying to spread the message to others. The propaganda that they are rolling in money is ridiculous. Except for the few large stores, most—and this also includes some mail-order businesses—are operating on a shoestring. The products they sell, particularly the fragile natural produce and grains, are hand-processed, making them more expensive than machinery and mass-produced and man-tampered foods. In order to make a profit at all, they have to add a 30 percent buffer to cover overhead costs. Yet, in spite of competition from supermarket prices, they manage to stay alive because people are searching for quality.

It is true that a change is taking place. The revolution I spoke of earlier, in which the public is becoming fighting mad because they have been hood-winked by pesticide-doused and chemically laden processed foods, is in full sway. They are taking matters into their own hands and surging into the health stores and organic food markets in self-defense. It is about time. Other retailers, who previously spurned such foods, now see that they are in the minority and have decided to get on the bandwagon to make a fast buck. Some are labeling foods "natural" which are not natural, and produce "organic" which is not organic. Real discrimination, label reading and protective standards are now necessary to offset this food prostitution.

Did you ever wonder why information about the healing effects of natural herbs were belittled? The true claims made for the use of these simple, harmless herbs, fresh from the garden or forest, are causing many herbs to be banned. . . . Did you know that those who have made claims have been put behind bars even though many drugs include derivatives from these same herbs? Did it ever occur to you that—following the announcement by Linus Pauling, a scientist and Nobel Prize winner, concerning his findings with vitamin C for colds—the rash of counter-claims, name-calling and pooh-poohs against vitamin C might have resulted because Mr. Pauling stated that cold drug-remedies were useless? Did it ever occur to you that the drug industry will stop at nothing to remove competition which threatens its financial structure? Now that the highly touted Pill, on which the drug companies made billions and fought tooth and nail any attempts to discredit it, is falling into disrepute, they are announcing, almost daily, hopeful substitutions in an attempt to recover their high profit status.

We doctors live in glass houses. I am reminded of the science editor of a highly respected literary publication who, on seeing several doctors' names used as endorsement for some new "wonder drug" in an ad in a professional magazine, became suspicious. He wrote to these physicians at the addresses given. The letters were returned with the notation "No such address." For physicians who need to have office addresses and phone numbers so that their patients can reach them, this was somewhat mysterious. The science editor then tried to reach these men by phone and telegram. Same answer. It turned out that *there were no such doctors!* Their endorsement had been faked merely to convince other doctors that they should buy and use these drugs on their patients.

I will no doubt be taken to task for telling you the truth and there will be attempts to discredit this book. However, I have already had it. One more blow will not stop me. Other forms of persecution, including unsavory articles in medical magazines and the loss of membership in the AMA [American Medical Association], have not stopped me. The public is now aware. They are beginning to catch on to what is happening and to fight our battles for us who dare to rebel against such domination.

Again, I assure you, if you have been "brainwashed" that the following authors are quacks because they dare to tell the truth about the natural health movement, nutrition, and what both can accomplish, brush away the cobwebs of prejudice and reevaluate your thinking. For example, Adelle Davis, a leader in this field, is NOT an uneducated quack.* She studied at Purdue University, Columbia University and the University of California, and has a master's of science degree from the University of Southern California Medical School. She served as a dietitian at Bellevue Hospital in New York City, and as supervisor of health education in the public school system of Yonkers, New York. Her successful nutritional clinical practice, which she . . . abandoned in favor of writing, was gratefully received by thousands.

Linda Clark, nutrition reporter, has attended three universities and has a master's degree. With a few added hours of study she could be eligible for a

---

*EDITOR'S NOTE: Adelle Davis died in 1974.

Ph.D. She has rejected this higher degree because the prerequisities do not offer the research in nutrition she trusts and respects. So she has obtained the information on her own, without benefit of the Ph.D. In her first book, *Stay Young Longer,* she researched information for its contents for ten years in New York City's Academy of Medicine Library. She documented every finding stated in the book. This documented research was either conducted by a scientist, a physician or a laboratory in good standing. As a result this book is used as a textbook in several schools and universities. She will no longer reveal their names, because when she has, pressure is brought to bear on the schools (by guess who?) and the books have to go! Many public libraries have been asked to have a book-burning party for both Adelle Davis' and Linda Clark's books (again, by guess who?).

You may have heard denunciation of Carlton Fredericks, Ph.D. His only crime was to announce nutritional truths for fifteen years on his radio program, which originated in New York City and was dedicated to educating people about nutrition. He is an expert on the subject. He denounced on the air such worthless foods as white bread and white sugar. He was called a liar and a crackpot (by guess who?) as he impressed his avid listeners. Yet, when Roger J. Williams, Ph.D., professor of chemistry at the University of Texas ·found recently that rats fed an exclusive diet of white bread died in approximately forty-five days, Carlton Fredericks' detractors ran for cover. Meanwhile he had already been thrown off some fifty radio stations in this country (by guess who?) for telling the truth.

I hope, by this time, you get the idea. You will get it still better if you will read these books, which represent years of respected nutritional research. They have been ignored by organized medical circles because they are controversial. This need not be. Nutrition could be a tremendous breakthrough to success for all doctors and patients.

Herewith, a list of some of the available periodicals which can be read to obtain nutritional knowledge.

1 *American Journal of Clinical Nutrition:* Scientific nutritional investigation. 9650 Rockville Pike, Bethesda, Maryland 20014.

2 *Science:* Scientific papers on nutrition on occasion. American Association for the Advancement of Science, 1515 Massachusetts Avenue, N.W., Washington, D.C. 20005.

3 *Nutrition Abstracts & Reviews:* Review of world's literature on nutrition. Commonwealth Bureau of Animal Nutrition, Bucksburn, Aberdeen, AB2 9SB, Scotland.

4 *Journal International Academy of Applied Nutrition:* Nutritional research publication International College of Applied Nutrition, Box 286, La Habra, California 90631.

5 *Nutrition Today:* Practical application of nutrition in medicine. Enloe, Stalvey & Associates, Inc., 1140 Connecticut Ave., N.W., Washington, D.C. 20036.

6 *Journal American Medical Association:* Occasional articles of nutritional importance. American Medical Association, 536 North Dearborn, Chicago, Ill. 60610.

7 *Biodynamics:* Devoted to better farming for better health. Biodynamics, Farming & Gardening Association, Inc., R.R. 1, Stroudsburg, Pennsylvania 18360.

8 *Let's Live:* A "prestige" magazine devoted to better health for the layman. Oxford Industries, Inc., 444 North Larchmont Blvd., Los Angeles, California 90004.

9 *The Miller Message:* Very comprehensive technical review of aspects of nutritional literature. Miller Pharmacal Co., P.O. Box 229, West Chicago, Illinois 60185.

10 *Natural Food and Farming:* Better farming for better health. Natural Food Associates, P.O. Box 210, Atlanta, Texas 75551.

11 *Organicville Newsletter:* Bi-monthly informal chat on nutritional information. Organic-Ville, 4177 W. 34th St., Los Angeles, California 90005.

12 *Rodale's Health Bulletin:* Current nutritional events. Rodale Press, Inc., Emmaus, Pennsylvania 18049.

13 *Prevention:* Health and better health by prevention. Rodale Press, Inc., Emmaus, Pennsylvania 18049.

14 *The Summary:* Shute Foundation for Medical Research, London, Ontario, Canada.

15 *Applied Trophology:* Standard Process Labs., 2023 West Wisconsin Avenue, Milwaukee, Wisconsin 53201.

The following books may be ordered through book stores or found in health stores. For a few I will list special sources, but don't be surprised to find them "out of print," which is a polite way of saying they have been banned because they were too hot for the competition. The following authors are not the only reliable ones, but they will get you started and will refer you to other sources you will wish to follow up. I have listed them alphabetically, not in order of importance nor by subject. I have omitted publishers too, since many are now in paperback.

E. M. Abrahamson, M.D., and A. W. Pezet, *Body, Mind and Sugar.* One of the earliest texts on hypoglycemia.

Franklin Bicknell, M.D., and Frederick Prescott, M.D., *The Vitamins in Medicine.* An invaluable textbook and reference.

Herbert Bailey, *Vitamin E: Your Key to a Healthy Heart,* with a foreword by Miles H. Robinson, M.D. The suppressed record of vitamin E.

Emanuel Cheraskin, M.D., D.M.D.; W. M. Ringsdorf Jr., D.M.D., M.S.; and J. W. Clark, D.D.S., *Diet and Disease;* also *New Hope for Incurable Diseases.*

Linda A. Clark, M.A., *Stay Young Longer;* also *Get Well Naturally;* and *Secrets of Health and Beauty* (contains some recent important nutritional research).

Adelle Davis, M.S., *Let's Eat Right to Keep Fit;* also *Let's Have Healthy Children;* and *Let's Get Well* (a superb reference book on nutritional research findings on specific diseases); and *Let's Cook It Right* (a nutritional cookbook).

John M. Ellis, M.D., *The Doctor Who Looked at Hands* (a fascinating story of vitamin B_6).

Catharyn Elwood, *Feel Like a Million!* (contains excellent laboratory nutritional research findings).

Dr. Carlton Fredericks and Herbert Bailey, *Food Facts and Fallacies.*

Dr. Carlton Fredericks and Herman Goodman, *Low Blood Sugar and You.*

Walter B. Guy, M.D., *Chemistry in Therapeutics* (out of print—the chemistry of acid-base balance).

Beatrice Trum Hunter, *Consumer Beware!* and *The Natural Foods Cook Book.*

W. Jennings Isobel, M.R.C.U.S. (University College, Cambridge University, England), *Vitamins in Endocrine Metabolism* (Charles R. Thomas, Springfield, Illinois).

D. C. Jarvis, M.D., *Arthritis and Folk Medicine.*

Royal Lee, D.D.S., and William A. Hanson, *Protomorphology** (a textbook on protomorphogens).

W. Coda Martin, M.D., *A Matter of Life* (a blueprint for a healthy family).

Sir Robert McCarrison, M.D., *Studies in Deficiency Disease** (with photographs—invaluable and informative); *Nutrition and Health,* with H. M. Sinclair, M.D. (available from Faber and Faber, Ltd., 24 Russell Square, London).

Lester M. Morrison, M.D., *The Low Fat Way to Health and Longer Life* (a deceiving title for an excellent overall book on nutrition).

Weston A. Price, M.S., D.D.S., F.A.C.D., *Nutrition and Physical Degeneration* (a survey of worldwide tribes correlating diet and health with photographs). A MUST! Available through the International College of Applied Nutrition.

Sam E. Roberts, M.D., *Ear, Nose and Throat Dysfunctions Due to Deficiencies and Imbalances;* and *Exhaustion: Causes and Treatment.*

Wilfrid E. Shute, B.A., M.D., with Harold J. Taub, *Vitamin E for Ailing and Healthy Hearts.*

G. M. Thienell, *My Battle with Low Blood Sugar* (Exposition-Banner Books).

"Three Years on HCl Therapy"* as recorded in *Medical World* (a must for understanding acid-base problems).

Roger J. Williams, *You Are Extraordinary* (an approach to nutrition through anatomy). Excellent.

H. Curtis Wood, Jr., M.D., *Overfed but Undernourished. . . .*

---

*Try to procure these books from Lee Foundation for Nutritional Research, Milwaukee, Wisconsin 53201. This foundation has been so mercilessly persecuted they are almost afraid to answer letters, but try.

Part V
The Politics and Economics of Food

The liberty of man consists
solely in this: that he obeys
natural laws because he has
himself recognized them as
such, and not because they
have been externally imposed
upon him by any extrinsic will
whatever, divine or human,
collective or individual.

—MIKHAIL BAKUNIN

Introduction to

Part V

"Why," you may ask, "should I worry about the politics and economics of food, when what I'm really interested in is gaining information that I can apply directly to my life?" One of the best answers is given by Ross Hume Hall:

> Psychologists tell us that man has an innate need to continually explore his environment, whether natural or artificial, and to exercise his personal judgment. However, the judgment of the individual and that of the mother—the member of the family unit most responsible for food safety and wholesomeness—has been replaced by the corporate wisdom of technical organizations. . . .
>
> Corporate wisdom expresses itself through government agencies, special committees, food company scientists, and university departments concerned with food and its production. These groups have assumed the responsibility to exercise what was formally a personal judgment.[1]

The American public is not totally blind to the forces that are undermining personal judgment. A Harris poll in May 1977 revealed the extent of disenchantment with food manufacturers: they ranked highest on the list of industries that Americans would like to see investigated or changed. During the same month Esther Peterson, special assistant to the President for consumer affairs, stated that the Grocery Manufacturers of America and other big-business representatives "have attacked the consumer protection agency bill with forces that Gen. Patton would have envied."[2] Unfortunately, some of the consumer protection now being offered by the Food and Drug Administration and other government regulatory agencies is not too stalwart, and their interplay with the very food manufacturers whose operations they are supposed to regulate tends to make their pronouncements and decisions suspect. This does not mean that "government decision-makers are corrupt, but that their sense of public duty is constantly eroded by industry contacts and the consideration of short-term effects on industry instead of long-term effects on consumers."[3]

333

Food processors market almost 9,000 new fabricated items a year (or about two dozen a day), of which roughly 500 survive. There is a widely held notion that it is consumer tastes that influence industry, that the food industry gives the people what they prefer. This overlooks the possibility that those preferences might have been conditioned by the industry. John Kenneth Galbraith, in an analysis of other sectors of the industrial economy, has made some remarks that can be applied to the food industry:

> The initiative in deciding what is to be produced comes not from the sovereign consumer who, through the market, issues the instructions that bend the productive mechanism to his ultimate will. Rather it comes from the great producing organization which reaches forward to control the markets that it is presumed to serve and, beyond, to bend the customer to its needs. And, in so doing, it deeply influences his values and beliefs. . . .
> . . . The subordination of belief to industrial necessity and convenience is not in accordance with the greatest vision of man. Nor is it an entirely safe thing to do.[4]

Advertising—that ubiquitous instrument of social control—ceaselessly encourages self-indulgence when what we need is self-restraint. Three cereal companies (General Mills, Kellogg's, and General Foods) together spend about $42 million annually for television advertising. In a typical year between 8,500 and 13,350 commercials for edibles—mostly sugar-laden cereals, candy, cookies, and soft drinks—appear at times when children, especially young children, are exposed to them. "With television," a Kellogg spokesman remarked about 15 years ago, "we can almost sell children our product before they can talk."[5] Cola-drink companies spend some $100 million every year on advertising. On the other hand, the U.S. government disburses about $70 million annually for nutrition education, or only some $5 million more than the yearly advertising budget of Coca-Cola. Although the government's expenditure is considerable, the quality of its nutrition programs and publications has been strongly questioned.[6]

Vending machines contribute to narrowing our choices: coffee and soda pop make up 60 percent of all vended food, and candy, gum, and the like another 20 percent. Recently the Los Angeles School Board and almost all the principals of the schools involved voted to continue the sale of junk food in school vending machines in order to provide funds for athletic and other programs. In 1975 alone the machines brought in $2 million.

The shopper who agonizes over the high cost of meat and produce frequently buys high-priced processed food under the illusion that it is convenient and economical. In many cases, the package rather than the contents influences judgment. Luxury foods—or, in trade parlance, "self-gratifying" products—can run as high as 90 percent of total purchases. And what is more, "supermarkets steal no less than $2600 million from us every year—through overcharges alone. By this the [Federal Trade Commission] refers to false weights and measures and other deceitful business practices, and not to whatever mistakes cash register operators may make by hitting the wrong keys."[7]

According to Joan Dye Gussow, chairman of the Nutrition Program at Columbia University's Teachers College: "It is our view that the policies of the last 20 years—policies which have resulted in an increasing centralization of food production and processing in the name of economic efficiency—will succumb to increasing recognition that such a system is energetically, ecologically and socially insane." She asks rhetorically, "Should health be left to the 'free-workings' of the marketplace?"[8]

In *Selection 32,* Jennifer Cross elaborates on many of the policies of both government and business that have helped promote unwise eating habits and enormous wastefulness. She also considers the economic and political changes needed to revolutionize America's food habits.

Johanna T. Dwyer and Jean Mayer in *Selection 33* examine the factors that stymie the development of practical and acceptable policies regarding food and nutrition. Their focus is the disciplinary limitations that have prevented physicians, nutritionists, and economists from collaborating with government to forge an integrated, broad-based nutrition policy. The authors show why policy-planning must take into account a wide spectrum of human values, involving not only a fusion of disciplines but greater elasticity within each one.

As the Manufacturing Chemists' Association has pointed out: "Most Americans like to try something different, a trait that makes the job of creative food technology doubly exciting!"[9] The result, as Ross Hume Hall shows in *Selection 34,* is that the farmer's crops are no longer merely whole foods to be eaten as part of a meal, but rich sources of raw materials to be manipulated and manufactured into diverse products. Hall discusses how basic food elements are processed, how the chemical industry has diversified into food, how technologists deal with the problems of texture and taste,[10] why nutrition science contributes little to food technology, and why totally synthetic food may be part of our future.

Increasingly often, professors of nutrition and food science are being called upon by government agencies for aid in formulating policies and by reporters for information. The question has been raised as to how unbiased and objective some of these professors are and whether financial ties to big food corporations are shading their views and their expert testimony. To air the problem, *Selection 35* is presented to demonstrate why criticism has arisen and *Selection 36* to show why it may be unwarranted. Perusing the first selection, by Benjamin Rosenthal, Michael Jacobson, and Marcy Bohm, you might bear in mind that only a handful of nutrition educators out of the hundreds in this country have been singled out for criticism. However controversial their report, in concluding it the authors offer sound recommendations for discouraging conflicts of interest.

In *Selection 36,* Ronald M. Deutsch reiterates some of the charges made in the preceding article, briefly refutes them, and questions whether consumer organizations, however well-intentioned, are "sources of truth without prejudice."

If personal judgment is as quiescent as the selections in Part Five imply, what can be done to revive it and broaden our choices? Part Six provides some clues, and so does Ross Hume Hall when he writes that

> everyone contributes in some way to the industrialization process. Everyone to a greater or lesser degree adapts his personal lifestyle to the demands of a technical world. There are those who wish to modify that world in some way, to bring the technical system into rapport with the realities of nature and the spirit of man. Such deliberate change will not be easily accomplished without understanding the major forces flowing through society. Not to change is to risk the continued impoverishment of natural processes. Man is an integral part of these processes and his lot in a rapidly evolving technologic system will be no better than that accorded any other living organism.[11]

References

1 Ross Hume Hall, *Food for Nought: The Decline in Nutrition* (New York: Vintage Books, 1976), pp. 57, 58.

2 Esther Peterson, quoted in "Consumer Plan Attacked," *San Francisco Examiner,* May 12, 1977, p. 14.

3 Jacqueline Verrett and Jean Carper, *Eating May Be Hazardous to Your Health* (New York: Simon and Schuster, 1974), p. 96.

4 John Kenneth Galbraith, *The New Industrial State,* 2d ed., rev. (Boston: Houghton Mifflin Co., 1971), pp. 6, 7.

5 Judith Van Allen, "Eating It! From Here to 2001," *Ramparts,* May 1972, p. 27.

6 Michael Jacobson, "Nutrition Education and National Policy," *Nutrition Action,* October 1977, pp. 9–11.

7 John Keats, *What Ever Happened to Mom's Apple Pie? The American Food Industry and How to Cope with It* (Boston: Houghton Mifflin Co., 1976), p. 107.

8   Joan Dye Gussow, quoted in Paul McKenney, "The Politics of Food," *Pomona*, February 1977, pp. 6, 7.

9   Van Allen, "Eating It!" p. 27.

10 For an amusing and informative account of the efforts to create crispness and crunchiness and provide the consumer with "aural thrills," see Ron Rosenbaum, "Crunch!" *Esquire*, July 1976, pp. 57–60, 114.

11 Hall, *Food for Nought*, p. x.

| 32 | The Politics of Food

JENNIFER CROSS

Jennifer Cross, a British free-lance journalist, is director of the San Francisco Consumer Action Group and author of *The Supermarket Trap*.

Reprinted from *The Nation*, August 17, 1974, pp. 114–116, by permission of the publisher. Copyright © by the Nation Associates, Inc.

How do you get people to understand that millions of Americans have adopted diets that will make them at best fat, or worst dead? That the $139 billion food industry has not only encouraged such unwise eating habits in the interest of profit but is so wasteful in many of its operations that we are inadvertently depriving hungry nations of food? That our agricultural policy is chauvinistic and short-sighted, primarily because the Agriculture Department, like most regulatory agencies, has been captured by business? That unless we can control inflation, stop playing politics with food and invest our money in people instead of corporations (especially those making unproductive weaponry), the world is probably headed for disaster?

These were the harsh issues underlying the mountain of testimony at the recent National Nutrition Policy Study in Washington, D.C. Few of them were met head-on, because they are a perfect example of a prevailing social dilemma. Well-motivated people suggest humane and necessary reforms, but these will not be carried out because they run counter to the interests of the power structure. However, changing the power structure is such a monumental job that people of good will bury themselves in displacement activities. Since they nevertheless still care deeply about social problems, they keep suggesting reforms, most of which end up gathering dust in the Library of Congress.

The National Nutrition Policy Study was a collection of several hundred doctors, dieticians, educators, food manufacturers, consumerists and fad-dists, who testified for three days before the Senate Select Committee on Nutrition and Human Needs. They were organized into six panels to deal with different aspects of the subject—consumer involvement, special (i.e., poor) groups, health, government, availability of food and the international situation. Together, these panels drew up a blueprint suggesting how America might best produce and distribute food in a world where people either do not have enough to eat or are eating the wrong things.

One of the most disheartening conclusions was the extent to which infla-tion has brought the war against poverty-related hunger to a standstill. Since the 1969 White House Conference on Food, Nutrition and Health . . . again brought poverty into the limelight, national spending for food programs has gone up about three and a half times, until they now reach 15 million people. Yet the special groups panel stated: "The 1970 Census listed nearly 26 million persons as living below the poverty line. Estimates of the number of persons eligible for family food programs ranged around 30 million until the beginning of 1974, and now range from 37 million to 50 million as the result of recent major increases in eligibility limits." Meanwhile, food prices have gone up 30 per cent in the last two years, forcing millions below the poverty line and millions more of the marginally poor to tighten their belts.

Overseas, the situation is still more bleak. World population continues to outstrip the food supply—each year the human race grows by 2 per cent, but eats 3.1 per cent more grain. We are increasingly at the mercy of droughts and poor harvests (as happened in 1972) and the kind of climatic changes now being experienced in the Sahara. The world is running short of fertilizer, argicultural land and water. We have scoured the seas, and the anchovies have fled.

Problems of scarcity are being compounded by the rising demand for food in fat-cat nations. And inflation, which hurts everyone, is pricing food beyond the reach of the world's poor. In addition to periodic local famines, we are now seeing what economist Lester Brown calls "a silent crisis of malnutrition," which "may be denying 1 billion human beings their basic right to realize the physical and mental potential of their genes." The differences in food intake between rich and poor nations is striking. The average American consumes nearly a ton of grain a year (mostly in the form of meat, milk and eggs); the average Indian gets only 400 pounds of grain a year, mostly consumed as cereals.

At the Indian level, tightening your belt means starvation. Even in America, where "poor folks' food" like beans and rice have gone up in price disproportionately, many families are being reduced to such fare as pet food, stale coffee and chocolate bars; or they face a bare cupboard at the end of each month, when the food stamps run out. Not surprisingly, the health problems of underfed Americans are exacerbated by inadequate or nonexistent medical care.

Not that prosperous Americans are in any great shape. Many of them overeat, and at least 40 percent of them are overweight. They also eat the wrong foods—too much meat, eggs, fat (especially saturated fat), salt, sugar, coffee, and alcohol. Add to this mixture stress and lack of exercise, and the result is an epidemic of diet-related diseases, not only here but in many other fat-cat countries. As the (predominantly medical) panel on nutrition and health services pointed out, 25 million Americans have high blood pressure, which can lead to coronary heart disease, our number-one killer (38 per cent). Diabetes mellitus and gallstones, both associated with obesity, are on the rampage; so are dental problems. And 15 million Americans have a drinking problem bad enough either to endanger their livers (if they don't eat properly) or to make them fat (if they do).

One reason for unwise eating is that people increasingly prefer snacking to three square meals, and fewer women prepare food from scratch—hence they buy more processed, snack and "fast" foods. It does not take a dietician to realize how many of these are fatty, salty, clog the arteries and embellish the waistline. Unfortunately, they are also found to be delicious to the point of being addictive; coffee, sugar and alcohol are quite literally so.

Last year the food, beverage and grocery products industries spent $2.9 billion on media advertising (nearly half of it on TV, where one out of every five commercials is for food or drink), plus another $3 billion on coupons and other promotions. As usual, about half of this was for inedible items, or for foods empty of nourishment—beer, liquor, coffee, soft drinks, snacks, candy and cold breakfast cereals. A good deal of the money was invested in advertising foods seductive to children.

As the consumer panel pointed out, "The economic interests of advertisers put advertising support behind high-profit, highly processed foods which are not necessarily nutritious, instead of the unprocessed, healthful foods." The result is a vicious but tasty cycle. We like seductive foods, they are more profitable to market, so that's what we eat, and what we see on TV. And since it's impossible to embody a nutritional message in ads for soft drinks, chips, beer or candy bars without raising a laugh or an FTC [Federal Trade Commission] lawsuit, and nutrition education provided by TV is practically nil.

It hasn't been much better elsewhere, because nutrition education is still considered Mommy's business, and chances are that she teaches about nutrition no better than she teaches about sex. Few children learn much in school home economics courses, and what little they do is quickly countered by TV and the omnipresent vending machine. Students rarely learn more at college, or medical school for that matter, unless they specialize in home economics or dietetics. Small wonder we have been called "a nation of nutritional illiterates."

Despite many pleas at the 1969 White House conference for improved nutrition education, there has been real progress in only two directions: the Expanded Food and Nutrition Education Program of the Agricultural Education Service, which caters to poor families; and the nutrition labeling of food products that make health claims, . . . required by the Food and Drug Administration on packaged foods after January 1975.

A third change, too new to be confidently called "progress," is the tremendous resurgence of interest in health foods. Thousands of Americans, many of them young, claim to have seen God in Crunchy Granola, yoghurt and mu tea—but pay inflated prices for produce which may or may not be "organic," and for vitamin and mineral supplements which may or may not be needed. Perhaps half the gospel of food is misinformed; the other half is ahead of its time. No one quite knows which is which.

What would it take to revolutionize the country's food habits? The Nutrition Study made the usual sensible suggestions: a special federal department of nutrition (modeled perhaps on the Council of Intergovernmental Relations), linked to a national network of community nutrition centers; plus much more research on how much of what food is eaten by whom. We need better, more appealing nutrition education at all levels, beginning with pre-school. Similarly, education should be included in all government food programs and health care services. We also need to be sure of what we are

eating: the consumer panel made a strong case for more nutrition information on food packages, open dating, unit pricing and a better system of
grading for quality. Finally, *all* Americans need the guarantee of a good diet,
which would ideally follow from more job opportunities or a guaranteed
annual income but at least from an improved and expanded food-stamp
program.

Unfortunately, most of these recommendations have been kicked
around, in some form, since the 1930's. Meanwhile, business as usual keeps
rolling along. On the same day that doctors on the Nutrition Study emphasized that we should eat less meat, U.S. Department of Agriculture-Sec-
retary Earl Butz instructed American housewives that buying more meat was
their patriotic duty. While the study produced figures showing that meat
production was a costly and inefficient way to use world grain resources,
Congress hastily debated a bill which would bail out the overstocked cattlemen once again with government loans, and Butz—though school was just
out—announced bulk-meat purchases for the school lunch program. As the
consumer panel bravely recommended that food advertising on children's
TV be banned, or at least restricted, Marian Burros, a panel member, reported on NBC-TV that the Federal Trade Commission, which had been
working for months on a children's TV advertising code, had been so intimi-
dated by the food industry's objections that it hadn't even dared to publish
its preliminary proposals.

Well-intentioned as the Nutrition Study is, it does not come to terms with
the politics of its concern. How do you get a top-level nutrition department
when the present Administration is not interested either in nutrition or in
tacking another layer onto government bureaucracy? And even if you got
one, what assurance would there be that it would not go the way of the U.S.
Department of Agriculture, the FTC and the Food and Drug Administration—which is to say, either captured by big business or cowed into varying
degrees of inactivity? How can the poor hope for more than token help,
when the Administration spends $100 billion a year on defense and openly
subsidizes big business, yet would veto expensive anti-poverty programs on
the ground that they fan the inflation? How can people be persuaded to eat
less meat, when the cattlemen's lobby has enough political clout to defy the
laws of supply and demand?

What can improved nutrition education accomplish without correspond-
ing changes in food marketing practice and industry structure? For one
thing, education is terribly slow, and the world is running out of time. Fur-

thermore, education may not work. As a Nutrition Study witness said, you can spend $1,000 and devote a whole year to educating a low-income mother on how to feed an obese, anemic baby, and the odds are 1 to 10 that the lesson will stick. . . .

It is easier to go on publishing more nutrition studies than to grapple with basic political force. But consumers do themselves an injustice if they fail to use what money and power they do have, while recognizing that they are not yet a match for the political and economic establishment. For a start, they could adjust the balance of power somewhat in their favor by pressing for the Consumer Protection Act of 1974, which would set up a Cabinet-level department of consumer affairs. They could encourage (or kick) the FTC into issuing a *strong* code on TV food advertising, starting with children's programs.

Citizens should also recognize the connection between big business, big advertising, monopoly and waste. It has been amply documented that the food and agricultural industries have been taken over by large, monopolistic or oligopolistic corporations. They are politically powerful, but they are not necessarily efficient, since they indulge in wasteful nonprice competition and price-fixing. They are also slaves to the ideas of growth and profit.

Putting more teeth into existing federal agencies and laws already on the books could turn the tide in favor of the medium-small corporation and farm. The use of farming and cattle feeding for tax-loss purposes should be discouraged, and price-fixing arrangements (starting with milk) should be eliminated.

Meanwhile, civic-minded groups could work out with the food industry ways of putting more profit into marketing nutritious foods without pricing them out of consumers' reach. A degraded transportation system is slowing down the movement of perishable produce. Grocery store margins might be altered to promote the sale of more nutritious foods. What would happen if stores devoted better display space, say, to milk rather than to soda pop, to fresh produce instead of potato chips? If the good foods still didn't sell, we could at least (judiciously) enrich the junk.

Sooner or later, the politics and economics of scarcity will force changes in our eating habits. Food is becoming scarcer worldwide, and as we learned from the Russian wheat deal, America is in competition with fat-cat countries, and will have to expect rising agricultural prices. Against this setting, the American way of eating is an irresponsible luxury. And the agricultural revolution is running out of steam in this country. As Dr. Jean Mayer, the

Nutrition Study coordinator, said: "We are on the diminishing returns part of the curve in the relationship of production to fertilizer. The same million tons of fertilizer which would produce 22 million tons of grain in India will only produce 11 million tons here. It is going to cost $750 million, according to the best estimates, to produce the same amount of grain and ship it to India . . . three times the $250 million it would cost to produce the fertilizer and send it to India."

The food industry consumes *huge* amounts of energy, all the way from heavily mechanized farms to elaborate processing and packaging and ending with the customer, who *drives* to and from the local supermarket several times a week. We spend $20 billion a year on packaging materials, and these are also getting scarce and expensive. Sooner or later we may have to give up many processed foods—and eat less meat—because they have been priced out of reach.

Despite rising costs, America (and other developed countries) have a responsibility to provide more aid than casual handouts under PL 480. Senator George McGovern outlined a "Ploughshares for Peace" policy— including larger world grain reserves, more agricultural research, and more aid to help developing countries grow more food for themselves. . . .

Right there one runs into the politics of population control, which is so horrendously difficult to accomplish that diplomats prefer to exchange money, missiles and trade agreements rather than take a hard line with obstinately fertile nations. We shall have to change or even reverse [the] policy of "produce, produce, produce, sell, sell, sell," since developing countries can less afford to buy, and American food reserves have hit a twenty-year low. Yet discussion of reserves is unpopular in the Corn Belt, which fears the effect on domestic prices if these are suddenly dumped on the market. The country must do a better job of regulating its international trade—which has produced not only the infamous grain deal but recent horrendous swings in grain and meat supplies and prices—all brought about by lack of planning. Planning, too, is a dirty word down on the farm, and among food manufacturers and exporters. Yet "business as usual" allows farmers to boil baby chicks and slaughter pregnant cows to keep prices up. It allows exporters to make (reputedly) outsize profits, and even to "corner" the soybean market, as in 1973. It also permits big governments to wheel and deal in scarce commodities, and . . . threaten and blackmail one another to protect their own producers.

The road is not going to be easy. Very profound changes must occur in the basic political and economic systems, not to mention the eating habits of whole nations. Are we going to *plan* these changes, and for the dislocation that will follow, or will we let time and accident decide?

At least the Nutrition Study has opened up the country's whole agricultural policy for public comment, and focused renewed attention on nutrition. It may influence some pending legislation, for example, Senator Hubert Humphrey's S.R.329, which calls for more aid to developing countries (and correspondingly bigger agricultural reserves); Senator Richard Schweiker's bill for medical education; the Kennedy-Mills health insurance proposals; and Senator Charles Percy's food and nutrition bills—all of which could usefully embody some provisions for nutrition education. To do much more would probably take a revolution. Instead, we will very likely continue to spend more on government food programs for the disadvantaged.

As I bade farewell to Dr. Jean Mayer on the steps of the Senate Office Building, I said, as cheerfully as I could, "See you in five years, Doctor!" He gave me a Gallic smile.

| 33 |

Beyond Economics and Nutrition: The Complex Basis of Food Policy

JOHANNA T. DWYER and JEAN MAYER

Johanna T. Dwyer is director of the Frances Stern Nutrition Center, New England Medical Center Hospital; associate professor, Tufts University School of Medicine; and lecturer in maternal and child nutrition, Harvard School of Public Health. Jean Mayer, professor of nutrition at Harvard University from 1950 to 1976, is now president of Tufts University. An expert on the problem of human obesity, he has published some 650 papers and several books, the latest *A Diet for Living* (1975). Dr. Mayer has served as a consultant to several United Nations agencies. As chairman of the National Council on Hunger and Malnutrition in the U.S., he was instrumental in calling the nation's attention to the nutrition problems of its poor.

Reprinted from *Science* 188 (May 9, 1975), pp. 566–570, by permission of the authors and the American Association for the Advancement of Science. Copyright © 1975 by the American Association for the Advancement of Science.

Governmental nutrition policy, given appropriate conditions for the feasibility of its development, is determined by the body politic. Inasmuch as nutrition is usually recognized to be, at least in part, a technical area, scientists (health specialists, nutritionists, and economists) are generally called upon to advise legislators, cabinet ministers, and planners in the formulation and implementation of policy.

Let us at the outset recognize that scientists have had a considerable favorable influence in the past 50 years, not only in their purely technical roles (for example, quantitative definition of nutritional requirements) but also in an ethical framework (such as implicit recognition that all human beings must be fed a similarly adequate diet). This article, however, is not concerned with past achievements but with trying to examine the factors that are hampering the development of practical and acceptable policies in the fields of foods and nutrition. In particular, we shall analyze the disciplinary limitations that prevent physicians, nutritionists, and economists from working together with governments to present coherent, broad-based plans in these fields.

OBJECT OF A NUTRITION POLICY

We shall assume in this article that the government has decided that adequate nutrition for all the people is an appropriate national goal, as an alternative to the traditional practice of letting nutrition status be secondary to agricultural policy, foreign trade, health policy, social policy, and economic conditions (1). This being accepted, there are a great many different possible means, some direct and some indirect, for bringing about positive nutritional effects. A number of such means are listed in Table 1 (2).

Consideration of this table shows that means of influencing the state of nutrition are extremely varied. This observation, evident to the nonspecialist, is often lost sight of by nutritionists, physicians, and economists, each of whom tend to consider only those means which can be activated exclusively within the confines of their own disciplines. Thus, physicians will usually be concerned solely with medical intervention—whether preventive, curative, or rehabilitative—dealing with deficiency diseases, nutrition-related infections, and degenerative diseases. Nutritionists will be concerned with supplementary feeding, nutrition education, food advertising, and labeling. Economists, if they are at all concerned with levels of food consumption, will consider measures having to do with production, imports, and income policies. The consumer is perforce broader in his interest and will be aware, however inchoately, of a multiplicity of factors impinging on his nutritional well-being.

INADEQUACIES OF PRESENT MODELS: RATIONING MODEL

While nutrition scientists may be uniquely qualified to define nutritional targets and goals, they sometimes are strangely unsophisticated in discussing the means to be used in reaching these objectives. Their models seem almost uniformly to be based on considerations that are applicable only under conditions of total war and are carried out by a well-informed government, a large and well-organized bureaucracy, and a highly disciplined population (such as in Britain in World War II). Under such conditions, food supplies are tailored to physiological requirements for nutrients by strict rationing systems. The social conditions are adjusted so that everyone can obtain the foods covering the requirements ascribed to his or her classification (sex, age, reproductive status, and intensity of physical labor). In turn, the national procurement policy is conducted so as to cover the collective national nutrient requirements. At most, adjustments are made from time to time to replace certain sources of calories and nutrients by equivalent amounts of appropriate alternative foodstuffs. That such systems, based on the calculations of nutritionists, worked as well as they did in the United Kingdom and in Switzerland during World War II is a tribute to the scientists, the governments, and the populations of these two countries (3). A less elaborate system worked reasonably well in the United States at the same period. However great these achievements, similar rationing schemes do not represent satisfactory models for peacetime food and nutrition policies in countries, whether wealthy or poor, that do not have simultaneously the scientific resources, the organized bureaucracy, and the coercive governments necessary to carry out nationwide, prolonged rationing schemes. Total control of production, distribution, and information is needed for such programs to be successful, and there is a question as to whether, even under such conditions, rationing can go on indefinitely. Awareness of the inevitable inequalities and inefficiencies eventually destroys the best-planned directive measures for food control. While consumers may be willing to undergo inconvenience and deprivation during wars and revolutionary periods, they are usually loath to do so indefinitely. . . .

The prerequisites for highly centralized direction of all aspects of the food supply do not exist at present in most countries. Thus, models for intervention other than adjusting supplies and distribution directly to requirements must be sought.

CONTROLLED DEMAND, NONINCOME MODELS

While most nutritionists are resigned to the idea that they cannot, under normal conditions, control supplies, they often strive for a utopia in which they control demand. Their ideal is a development of popular nutritional awareness so total that price, income, and taste can be eliminated as factors of practical importance in determining demand. They often forget the primacy of economics in influencing patterns of consumption and concentrate almost exclusively on the duel (indeed, the crusade) of education against advertising, which, in their view, represents the decisive factor in determining what people will eat. For many nutritionists, this viewpoint leads directly to a yearning for a directive banning all food advertising. In their view, the elimination of this enemy would lead in due time to the provision of a balanced diet for all consumers. Unfortunately, while there is abundant evidence that demand can be modified to a degree by limiting or eliminating unjustified claims or misinformation in food advertising, as well as by consumer information and health and nutrition education, there is also overwhelming evidence that such economic factors as price and income have at least equal importance, if not much greater influence. To focus exclusively on the cognitive aspects of food choices to the exclusion of economic means of intervention is to limit drastically the possibilities of implementing a nutrition policy.

Ignoring actions that modify supply as well as demand is to be equally myopic and self-limiting. Whether the middleman, fast food service institutions, food processing, "factory farming," agribusiness, and the entire food distribution system are in any way villains, which some groups declare them to be, is of little significance. The fact is that every component of the food system can be acted upon to bring about improvements of the nutritional status of large numbers of people. Similarly, income policies are crucial to raising the nutritional levels of large numbers of people. The most successful nutrition education system and the total elimination of noxious advertising, however desirable, will not substitute for an income adequate to bring an inexpensive but nutritionally satisfactory diet conforming to national preferences. Unless all these factors are taken into account in the elaboration of a planning model, the development of a sound nutrition policy is seriously hampered.

ECONOMIC MODELS THAT ARE NOT HEALTH-DIRECTED

Economists suffer from their own limitations. They are unwilling to pay much attention to those commodities that do not travel through channels of trade (in fact, most of the foodstuffs produced in subsistence farming areas) or to those commodities—fruits, vegetables, and small amounts of home-grown animal products, human milk, eggs, rabbits, and the like—that make a considerable contribution to good nutrition but are difficult to quantify. They thus arrive at such statistics as calculating average incomes for entire populations as equivalent to, say, less than $50 a year, a conclusion that does not lend itself to any international nutrition comparisons. Another bias of economists is their preference for theoretically cost-efficient measures such as fortification with added nutrients, however impractical and inadequate these measures usually are in the developing countries that are supposed to benefit most from them. It sometimes seems that the economists' models, consisting as they do of quantifiable food tonnages that move or can move through channels of trade and of the products of industrialization, suggest an ideal diet made of a homogeneous mixture of the

TABLE 1 ACTIONS AND INTERVENTIONS THAT MAY ALTER NUTRITIONAL STATUS

Category	Action
Need	Actions affecting health and biological utilization of food
	Supplying missing nutrients on either a prophylactic or curative basis
	Alterations of environmental sanitation that have indirect impact on health and biological utilization of foods
	Altering physiological requirements of persons by environmental manipulation
	Surveillance and treatment activities to assess special nutrient needs of the ill or otherwise handicapped
	Actions or events decreasing the numbers of persons at risk of malnutrition by various means
Supply	Altering production factors (land, labor, capital, technology) or inputs needed to raise food
	Changing type of foods produced or how they are used
	Altering processing and manufacturing of food products
	Altering marketing efficiency
	Foreign trade regulations modifying the food balance of a country
	Provision of food aid to the poor within the country or from abroad via food distribution programs which, in effect, transfer food or purchasing power specifically for food from more affluent to more needy groups
	Enrichment or conservation of food in the home or at the point of consumption
Demand	Increasing income by raising gross national product, or distributing income to poverty groups so as to increase their purchasing power
	Government interventions to affect price structures and hence demand
	Government programs to influence consumption
	Education
	Altering food habits and mores
	Favoring or promoting conservation of breast-feeding and increasing its prevalence and duration

dominant regional cereal (preferably one variety) and one variety of soybean, this mixture to be fed to humans or farm animals, to travel, or to be distilled depending on available systems and local incomes. If health problems are taken into consideration at all, they are often dealt with through suggestion of appropriate fortification with vitamins and amino acids. However convenient the oversimplified diet of economists may be for the purposes of international negotiations (the Rome World Food Conference dealt almost exclusively with cereals, with few mentions, at most, of soybeans and sugar), it bears little resemblance to the diets that are examined by health and nutrition workers for nutritional adequacy. The two groups must come closer in their definition of "food" if adequate food and nutrition planning is to evolve.

PREREQUISITES FOR JOINT PLANNING

We must emphasize that economists and planners appear unreceptive to qualitative statements, however well established. The statement that problems of malnutrition are severe and must be eradicated is unlikely to bring about changes in their economic plans. Their tools involve quantifiable variables, and unless the problems are presented to them in quantitative terms, they are unable to grapple seriously with them. Specifically, the information they require is the following: (i) the size and nature of the malnutrition problem, expressed in terms of the demographic and socioeconomic characteristics and number of persons who are malnourished or at risk of malnutrition; (ii) short-term and long-term targets, again in quantitative terms; and (iii) yardsticks for measuring progress.

Before these data are furnished, little is likely to be done. At the same time (except for extreme emergencies, when cases of starvation, edema, severe weight loss, or acute deficiencies can be counted with little margin for disagreement between experts), the data that economists want are in the very areas where clinicians and nutritionists are most loath to come out with flat, numerical statements. Health professionals will agree that the definition of malnutrition—entailing, as it may, choices between clinical, anthropometric, biochemical, or dietary criteria—is uncertain and subjective; that the standards for all of these criteria are arbitrary; and that small variations in cutoff points will yield widely different prevalences of malnutrition. Faced with this confusion and lack of agreement on the part of health and nutrition experts, economists and planners are likely to ignore the problem of malnutrition or to go ahead on the basis of indirect but quantitative estimates, such as a "poverty line" based on income, or budget study data compared with the food purchases of "representative" families. In the United States, it was only in the 1970's that partial baseline data on malnutrition were obtained in the course of the Ten State Nutrition Survey (4). Even then, nutritionists were hard put to summarize clearly the results of this (partial) survey or to recommend targets for action and yardsticks for measurement of progress.

Nutrition scientists must be encouraged to formulate serviceable definitions of malnutrition that can serve as necessary bases for action. Definitions worked out by nutritionists, although not infallible, should come closer to the realities of health than do those worked out by economists, managers and politicians. That the politicians have been willing in the past to attempt such definitions, unaided as they were by specialists, has been in many cases the prime impetus to development of socioeconomic conditions leading to better nutrition.

WHO ARE THE NUTRITION EXPERTS?

Nutritionists have another complaint about economists and planners for which lack of communication between the two groups must again be blamed. They understandably object to the unfortunate tendency of economists to check with the wrong people when matters nutritional arise. In the absence of a permanent, constructive dialogue with nutritionists, the economist · when faced with claims that economic and agricultural conditions are leading to many people being ill, logically enough calls in a physician as adviser. Unless the economist is particularly well counseled or lucky, he or she may, however, have the wrong adviser. The reasons for this are several.

First, deficiency diseases and diseases exacerbated by malnutrition are overwhelmingly diseases of the very poor, the class least likely to be seen routinely by physicians. When the poor finally receive medical treatment, usually very late in the natural history of the disease process, the nutritional factors in the etiology and pathogenesis of their health problems may be camouflaged by other, more dramatic medical conditions that have also gone untreated, and the underlying malnutrition may be disregarded.

Second, in developing countries and even in rich countries, the poor are least likely to be seen by the influential private physicians or senior academics among whom advisers to planners are likely to be recruited.

Third, throughout the world, and particularly in the United States, senior physicians are more likely to be enthused about dramatic methods of curative medicine than about the drabber, although ultimately more useful, preventive aspects of medicine, of which nutrition is the most important example.

Finally, even when physicians are conscious of the importance of nutrition as a discipline, they are almost invariably unable to translate "nutrition" into foods and their relation to habits and patterns of various socioeconomic and ethnic groups, or, for that matter, into the nuances of microeconomics and food distribution within the family. Thus, their opinion in feeding programs, food assistance interventions (whether in the form of money, food stamps, or other distributive measures), nutrition education, consumer education, and so forth, are generally far less factually based and authoritative than their views on, say, the etiology and treatment of acute diseases. Unless the physician who is asked to serve as adviser on nutritional problems is well versed in epidemiology and public health nutrition and has some knowledge of food science and the sociology of nutrition, his advice may be useless or misdirected.

NUTRITION, SOCIOECONOMIC ANALYSIS, AND ADVOCACY

All too often, nutrition scientists seem unable to correlate their findings about the state of nutrition of individuals with socioeconomic variables. This inability, coupled with overcaution in analysis of economic determinants of consumption, means that advocacy is all too often left to consumer spokesmen with no real understanding of health priorities in human nutrition. The often exaggerated or inaccurate statements of such spokesmen, instead of prompting nutrition scientists to take over the advocacy role and put it on a firm factual and scientific basis, seems, on the contrary, to frighten them even farther away from such a role. As a result of this attitude (probably due to overdefensiveness about their colleagues' opinion), interventions necessary to correct nutritional inadequacies are not undertaken, and no systematic trials and evaluations are conducted to assess what the best method for attacking nutritional problems may be or what progress is being made. As an example, since the 1969 White House Conference on Food, Nutrition, and Health (5), federal expenditures on food programs (food stamps, school lunch and breakfast programs, summer food programs, community meals and meals-on-wheels for the elderly and shut-ins, and special programs for pregnant and nursing women and infants) have risen from $600 million to over $6 billion without adequate monitoring of their relative effectiveness.

The surveillance of the state of nutrition of the nation, recommended by the conference, has not been organized, and the American people have gone through a massive change in the nature of the food supply, massive increases in the price of various foods, profound changes in welfare and social security legislation, a deep economic recession, and an explosive increase in the size of government food programs without any serious effort being made to follow the consumption levels of the various groups in our population. Indeed, the decennial consumption survey conducted by the U.S. Department of Agriculture has been postponed by at least one year. The moribund state of nutrition as a tool in social engineering encourages its neglect by economists and the filling of the gaps by amateurs and extremists.

NUTRITION AND PUBLIC EDUCATION

A recent essay on science literacy distinguishes three distinct but related forms: practical, cultural, and civic (6). This framework can also be used to determine the objectives of nutrition science orientation needed by various members of society.

The most obvious need of laymen is for practical nutrition advice given in ordinary language. Such knowledge can be coordinated with that given in formal educational settings. The bulk of the informational effort should be coordinated through the nonformal mass media. Nutrition scientists should be involved in the preparation of this message, but are they always qualified? Who are those nutritionists? Those falling under this umbrella term may include those having doctoral degrees in the biochemistry of nutrition, food science, or public health nutrition; physicians specializing in clinical nutrition; dietitians; home economists; food technologists; and educators with special expertise in food and nutrition. Unfortunately, the top of the pecking order belongs to the biochemists and clinicians, who, however deep their knowledge of intermediary metabolism or the treatment of acute conditions, are rarely prepared to dispense the necessary advice on menu planning, food buying, and food preparation. Their social concerns incline heavily toward support of research and academic institutions, and most of them have not bothered to inform themselves seriously about consumer problems. The situation is complicated by the fact that specialists are usually extremely timid at dispensing information about fields other than their own. Thus, a biochemical nutritionist will not be willing to publicly hazard an opinion on additives or food prices. For the general public, these are part of nutrition, and our expert is immediately classified as useless. The home economists are usually better prepared to give advice on a broader range of public concerns, but even they are usually afraid to venture in some fields, such as food toxicology or food assistance programs, and their prestige is low as compared with physicians and scientists.

Cultural nutritional literacy must be instilled in as large a part of our population as possible if nutrition considerations are going to be incorporated into the culture and broad academic programs. Nutritionists all too often fail there as well. Instead of making a serious effort at teaching the science of nutrition to the intelligent public, they often insult it by presenting it with quasi-scientific utterances about "good food habits," "balanced diets," or the "basic four," which tend to be vague, uninteresting, and, in the case of the last example, misleading. Fortunately, we are beginning to see some interesting and scholarly and at the same time readable approaches to nutrition as a cultural topic.

Our major concern here being with nutrition policy, it is the element of civic nutrition education that is crucial for our purpose. The aim of imparting civic nutritional literacy is to enable professionals, both those specialized in nutrition and those whose actions affect nutrition, to become more aware of the nutrition-related issues and to interpret those issues in policy-making. Such civic literacy involves some acquaintance with a broad range of issues, from agricultural policy to health to related social and economic issues. Civic literacy implies an interest in numerical, nationwide data on nutritional problems, an ability to evaluate advocacy, and to follow public actions likely to affect the nutritional well-being of large sections of the nation's population. In an increasingly interdependent world, civic literacy involves seeking information, forming quantitative opinions, and endorsing action on the international plane as well.

MISCLASSIFICATION OF NUTRITION INTERVENTION

In the absence of qualitative baselines, yardsticks, and targets pegged to nutritional health, it is understandable that economists all too often neglect health as a major aim in considering policies affecting food and nutrition. However, they often also fail to realize that certain "nutrition" programs may have objectives that far exceed the narrow nutritional goal that dominates their classification. For example, the nutritional benefits derived from such popular programs as the community meals for the elderly or school lunches could be hard to justify on a cost-effectiveness basis: they both, at best, supply a fraction of the total number of meals consumed during a year;

the same amount of money put, for example, into food stamps should guarantee more nutrition. On the other hand, if they are regarded as distributive measures with social welfare spin-off benefits—such as decreased isolation and increased opportunity for health surveillance and education of the elderly, socialization and nutrition education of children, and employment of neighborhood mothers as school lunch aides—the yardsticks applicable become quite different. Even though both the lay public and most nutritionists look at them as food and nutrition programs, the fact is that nutrition is not the only or even the main aim of these activities.

On the other hand, programs that are not thought of as nutrition programs by either nutritionists or economists may have a great deal to do with nutrition. These include actions that affect income and prices (particularly food prices). For example, the levels of family assistance allowances, social security, the coverage of minimum wage legislation, the broadening of the vesting of pension rights, unemployment insurance, and the price of the main staples are all of major significance to the nutritional status of much of the citizenry.

NUTRITION AND PLANNING OF ECONOMIC DEVELOPMENT

Economists are inclined to view nutrition as one of the unproductive personal and social expenditures that compete with reinvestment. Improvement in nutrition is thus seen as inimical to economic development. The case can be made, however, regarding nutritional expenditures as being, at least in part, an investment: it is becoming clearer that malnutrition during pregnancy, infancy, and early childhood may produce serious consequences for physical and mental development (7). Large expenditures in health and education later may be necessary to partly reverse these defects, whereas good nutrition during the growth period may contribute positively to productivity. Moreover, nutrition may also be thought of as an organizing principle for development of a sound, stable food industry and its ancillary activities such as packaging and for cutting down food waste, a major factor in all countries.

Neglect of nutrition considerations tends to lend economists to neglect small agricultural enterprises and subsistence agriculture, and thus to ignore the major part of the population in developing countries (8). The neglect of the importance of fruits, vegetables, small domestic animals, and small-scale production of animal products, which are the major sources of many nutrients in the diet, has led even rapidly developing countries to nutritional disasters at the same time as their gross national product was shooting upward. Ironically, lack of understanding of the role of foodstuffs other than those that are less perishable (cereals, legumes) or easily counted (large farm animals) leads to production figures which are usually underestimates and, hence, to costly mistakes in planning, particularly in import policies. In developing countries, this systematic bias, together with that voluntarily introduced by tax-shy farmers with regard to their production figures, means that consumption studies conducted by home economists often offer a better basis for the evaluation of production figures than do surveys directly attempting to obtain such figures.

FORTIFICATION AND OTHER "INSTANT" SOLUTIONS

Economists are constantly on the lookout for cheap and relatively straightforward solutions to nutritional problems. This occasionally degenerates into unwarranted enthusiasm for unproven solutions, such as fortification of staple foods with imported synthetic amino acids. Certainly, there are some well-established examples of the benefits of certain types of fortification. The elimination of goiter through iodization of salt, of rickets and osteomalacia through the fortification of milk with vitamin D (or periodic administration of large doses of vitamin D), the decrease in dental caries through fluoridation of water supply, and the prevention of blindness related to vitamin A deficiency through periodic administration of large doses are well documented. The benefits of other types of enrichment are often more doubtful. Recent data suggesting the importance of fiber and the deleterious effects of high levels of saturated fat, cholesterol, and sugar in the diet add to the complexity of nutrition policy and make us wary of instant solutions. Nonetheless, nutritionists may sometimes be too leery about the possibilities of enrichment and fortification, and prefer instead to advocate foods rich in the missing micronutrients as supplements to the diet; generally, these foods are so expensive that their cost far exceeds that of the enrichment-fortification approach and thus limits the number of persons that can be reached.

NUTRITION AND THE LIMITATIONS OF MACROECONOMICS

Understandably, perhaps, in view of their training, economists take as gospel the dictum that the primary way to change demand is by income and price alteration. While they are willing to give lip service to education, they are unlikely to take it seriously as an effective intervention technique. Elasticity coefficients derived from income and price relationships in the past are taken as being predictive of what will obtain in the future. Unfortunately, as we have seen in the recent past, in both meat glut and meat scarcity situations, these coefficients do not tell the whole story, however useful they may be.

Furthermore, focusing on aggregate supply and demand may lead to overlooking the importance of certain intervention tactics on groups with low effective demand, such as the poor. Similarly, focusing on society as a whole may lead to ignoring the effects of interventions on young children and other nutritionally vulnerable groups, who are unable to vote with their purchasing power. Children's diets may be exposed to nutritional risk by the interplays of supply and demand at the macroeconomic level, but also at the microeconomic level of the family. Greater attention must be devoted to microeconomics, especially as it applied to individual family members, in the analytical studies of economists.

Essential as income is to nutrition, the problems of malnutrition cannot automatically be solved by income increments. Food beliefs, other health practices deleterious to nutritional status, and maldistribution of food within the family may still be a problem. Also overlooked are the pressures of other felt needs, such as the buying of consumer goods, which may take precedence over nutritional needs as preceived by the family purchasing unit. Income is spent in a variety of ways, only one of which is food. What is seen by the family as discretionary income may vary greatly from one household to the next. Also, even if discretionary income is spent on food, it may be spent on foods that in fact do little to improve nutritional status.

BEYOND FOOD AND ECONOMICS TO NUTRITION POLICY

Physicians, nutritionists, and economists are not likely to solve the problems they must address within the realm of food policy simply by trading disciplines. Their disciplines are too narrow for this to accomplish much. What is necessary is beyond all of these disciplines, and involves policy-planning objectives based on broader considerations than dollars or health considerations alone. Other humane considerations based on other human values and views must be taken into account. Such policy-planning involves a fusion of disciplines, with different (for instance, health) objectives than would be usual for the discipline of economics and broader intervention strategies than the other professionals would normally employ.

References and notes

1. J. Perisse, F. Sizaret, P. Francois, *FAO (Food Agric. Organ. U.N.) Nutr. Newsl.* 7 (No. 3), 1 (1969); T. Cooke and J. Pines, *Planning Nutrition Programmes: A Suggested Approach* (Office of Nutrition, Agency for International Development, Washington D.C., 1973); J. Toro, *Final Report: Interagency Consultative Meeting on National Food and Nutrition Policies in the Americas* (SIAC/PNAN-1, United Nations, New York, 1973); F. J. Levinson and D. L. Call, in *Nutrition, National Development, and Planning.* A. Berg, N. S. Scrimshaw, D. L. Call, eds. (MIT Press, Cambridge, Mass., 1973), pp. 165–197; J. Mayer, ed., *U.S. Nutrition Policies in the Seventies* (Freeman, San Francisco, 1973); J. B. Orr, *Food, Health and Income* (Macmillan, London, 1936).

2. J. T. Dwyer, in *Priorities in Child Nutrition,* J. Mayer and J. D. Dwyer, eds. (UNICEF, New York, in press), vol. 2, Chap. 7.

3. A. H. J. Baines, D. F. Hollingsworth, I. Leitch, *Nutr. Abstr. Rev.* 33, 653 (1953); R. J. Hammond, *Food: The Growth of Policy* (Her Majesty's Stationery Office and Longmans, Green, London, 1951), vol. 1.

4. Center for Disease Control, Public Health Service, Department of Health, Education, and Welfare, *Ten State Nutrition Survey* (Government Printing Office, Washington, D.C., 1974), vols. 1–5.

5. *White House Conference on Food, Nutrition, and Health* (Government Printing Office, Washington, D.C., 1970).

6. B. P. Shen, *Sciences (N.Y. Acad. Sci.)* 15, 27 (1975).

7. A. Berg and R. Muscat, *The Nutrition Factor: Its Role in National Development* (Brookings Institution, Washington, D.C., 1973).

8. H. G. Farnsworth, *Food Res. Inst. Stud. Agric. Econ. Trade Dev. (Stanford)* 2, 179 (1961).

(We thank A. Ratner for editorial assistance and typing of the manuscript.)

34 | Crops as Raw Materials

ROSS HUME HALL

Ross Hume Hall is professor of biochemistry at McMaster University, Hamilton, Ontario. He is the author of *The Modified Nucleosides in Nucleic Acids* (1971) and editor of two journals: *Plant Physiology* and *Nucleic Acid Research*.

From Ross Hume Hall, *Food for Nought: The Decline in Nutrition* (Hagerstown, Pa.: Harper and Row, Medical Dept., 1974; New York: Vintage Books, 1976). Copyright © 1974 by Ross Hume Hall. Reprinted by permission.

The technologic food system treats crops grown by the farmer not as food, but as raw material to be manipulated and manufactured into numerous products. From the manufacturing point of view, a basic raw material should be as simple as possible, its properties should be standardized, and its behavior in various manufacturing processes should be predictable. Finally, the raw material should be versatile and capable of being modified and combined with other raw materials in endless ways.

Field crops such as wheat, corn, and soybeans, the mainstay of technologic agriculture, do not qualify as crude raw materials. Grain kernels and soybeans are highly complex biologic structures comprised of many types and sizes of molecules, arranged in precise substructures. Whole wheat, for example, does not fit the technologist's view of a versatile raw material: What kinds of products can be manufactured from it? Wheat can be ground and used to make bread and breadlike products, but this is about the limit of its versatility. Whole grain is already a highly complex mixture of substances, and its subsequent processing is limited by the properties of the mixture. However, if one were to start with the individual components of the grain, these constraints would vanish. The technology to accomplish this feat is available, but before the new technology becomes a reality, a shift in images must occur: The image of grain, soybeans, etc., as foodstuffs must be transformed into the image of these crops as crude raw materials that need to be broken down into their component parts before being processed into food. Wheat flour has certainly been partially refined for a long time, but contemporary refining is now being redefined in molecular terms (27).

We are still in the initial period of this image shift. Food technologists employ the old terminology of the nineteenth-century chemists and classify the grain in parts: carbohydrates (starch, sugar), protein, and fat (oil), plus small quantities of accessory factors. Nineteenth-century chemical analysis said little about the structure of the grain or seeds and nothing about the internal relationships of the components, an ignorance that suits the approach of contemporary food technology. The grain or seeds are viewed as little capsules containing a mixture of carbohydrate, protein, and fats. Bran and the accessory factors (minerals, vitamins, and unidentified entities), small in quantitiy, can be ignored; in fact, they are discarded as quickly as possible in the initial refining process. If they are deemed necessary in the final product, it is more convenient to synthesize them in sterile chemical plants and add them at a later stage.

PROCESSING BASIC FOOD ELEMENTS

Extruded soybean protein

The protein of soybeans is unique compared to that of corn or wheat, for its amino acid composition comes much closer to the composition of human protein than does that of the grains. Moreover, soybeans consist of about 40 percent protein (20 percent oil, 30 percent carbohydrate), so food technologists consider soybeans a prime source of protein. The protein exists in the form of tiny spheres surrounded by a membrane. The membrane is composed of phospholipids; lecithin is a phospholipid. This microstructure has to be shattered to refine the protein. The seeds are ground and the oil extracted with the petroleum solvent hexane. . . . The defatted flour contains protein and carbohydrate, which consists of about 50 percent protein by weight. This flour is used as an ingredient in protein-enriched bread, diet foods, cereals, infant foods, and baked goods. The flour can be further refined by treating it with alcohol or dilute acid to remove part of the carbohydrate, a process which increases the protein content to about 70 percent (33).

Soy protein is a globular-shaped protein, as opposed to the long, stringy wheat-protein molecules. For this reason it cannot be used to form a leavened dough. It does have its own peculiar properties, however, which make it very desirable to the food engineer. It dissolves readily in alkali but is insoluble in acids, and this property enables it to be "spun" into threads. The alkaline solution of the soy protein is forced through fine orifices directly into dilute acid. The protein precipitates in the form of fine threads, a process identical to that by which synthetic fabrics such as nylon are spun. The spun protein threads are tied together in bundles and passed through a solution that cements them together, then through succeeding solutions that add flavoring and coloring materials. The spun protein has an affinity for artificial flavor and dyes; it retains juices and has a meatlike texture. Thus, the bundles can be produced and cut into desired shapes, then cooked or smoked to simulate many familiar products, including beef and bacon. The product is officially labeled "textured protein" (21).

Chemically modified starch

Starchy foods such as bread, potatoes, and rice have long been used to fill the stomach with bulk. The human digestive system was mechanically designed to handle bulky materials, and a bulky diet helps to eliminate hunger pangs. (Bulk is defined as a high volume/calorie ratio. Carbohydrates have a low number of calories per unit weight to begin with. In addition, carbohydrates in the form of starches form gels which retain a lot of fluid.) Food technologists strive for bulk in their products, achieving it in various ways. The carbohydrate in corn (cornstarch) can be separated out and used as a filler in many cooked products, but chemical technology carries this basic raw material further. The starch is hydrolyzed with enzymes or with acid under carefully controlled conditions to give a variety of products low in reducing sugars (dextrose). Cornstarch, obtained directly from the corn without additional processing, has limited uses because of its high viscosity, starchy flavor, and high sugar content.

Many fabricated foods need a tasteless, soluble, nonsweet, easily digestible carbohydrate. The hydrolyzed starches, called "low D.E." (dextrose equivalency), give fabricated food such properties. These starch hydrolysates can be used, for example, to make fillings such as peanut butter for cracker sandwiches, pizzas, and toaster "pop-up" products, as well as imitation cheese and sour cream. They can also be used to carry flavor ingredients in protein products and in snack foods (25).

This particular process is only the start in transforming cornstarch into a technologic raw material. Natural starch consists of two carbohydrate components, an amylose fraction, composed of a long linear chain of polymerized glucose units, and an amylopectin fraction, a highly branched treelike glucose polymer. The glucose molecule is the basic building block of many carbohydrates. Nature arranges and combines glucose with other molecules in a variety of ways to form products such as starch and cellulose

362

Part V

(humans cannot digest cellulose). In all these products the glucose is arranged in repeating units. The chemist says the glucose units are polymerized and calls all such molecules polysaccharides; the nutritionist calls those molecules that are edible carbohydrates.

Starches high in amylose possess certain desirable properties: They form films that bar the passage of oxygen and fat, and they bind other materials into stable extruded shapes. The oxygen-proof films can be made strong enough to use as packaging materials, which means that the package can be eaten along with the contents, thus reducing the waste problem. In another application, this type of cornstarch can be pregelatinized and used in textured pastes. It imparts a pulpy texture to tomato paste and applesauce. The plant geneticist has aided in the production of this class of starches by breeding a special variety of corn that contains 70 percent amylose starch (14).

Waxy starch

The other class of starch, called waxy starch, consists of only the branched-chain polymer, amylopectin. Both waxy and ordinary starch swell in water and develop highly viscous solutions or gels. However, if the linear polymer (amylose) is present, the starch solution (on cooling) sets into an irreversible precipitate. This particular problem is overcome if the manufacturer uses only the waxy starch in applications where a thickener is needed. The waxy type of starch has been produced on a commercial scale since 1940. After solving the problem of irreversible pastes by eliminating the linear-chain fraction, the manufacturers ran into other difficulties. Modern food manufacturing involves heating and mechanical manipulations. The waxy starch gels are unstable and break down, particularly when subjected to the mechanical shear of high-powered mixers.

Chemical technology came to the rescue: the starch is treated with phosphorous oxychloride (8), a process that ties single chains of starch molecules together with phosphorus bonds. A whole new set of properties is thus created. The starch molecules become less fragile and more resistant to breakdown by mechanical shear, heat, freezing-thawing, and acid conditions. The modified starches find their way into pie fillings, creamed butter sauces, cheese sauces, gravies, and baby food (16).

Starched baby food

Chemically modified starches have been a boon to the commercial baby food industry for about 20 years. Puréed baby food made from natural starch separates into a liquid and solid phase on standing; moreover, according to the baby food manufacturers, the starch cell dehydrates into a granule that resists digestion inside the baby. This whole process is accelerated at refrigerator temperatures. Chemically modified starch solves all these problems. The baby food can be stored for long periods at room temperature or at refrigerator temperature (the lower temperature helps retain the potency of heat-labile vitamins) (32).

Although phosphorus is a natural constituent of many foods, the phosphate-starch molecular configuration created by the food technologists is a completely unnatural relationship. Questions have been raised over the safety of this material. A survey reported by the Subcommittee on Safety and Suitability of Monosodium Glutamate and Other Substances in Baby Foods of the Food Protection Committee, Food and Nutrition Board, National Academy of Sciences–National Research Council, states that infants between one and fourteen months of age consume about 2.3 percent of their daily calories in the form of chemically modified starch. One infant surveyed derived 16 percent of its calories from this substance (8).

The subcommittee's evaluation of the propriety of using chemically modified starch focused on the question of digestibility. Experimental evidence showed that the modified starch and natural starch are equally digestible (8). Such experiments ignored what else was happening in the infant digestive tract. Digestion and efficient absorption of nutrients depend a great deal on the mix of things in the digestive system. In other words, the investigation did not study the effect of chemically modified starch on other food components of the stomach. The Joint FAO/WHO Expert Committee on Food Additives (1970), meeting in Rome in 1969, reported that apart from the information on digestibility, short- and long-term studies on health hazards of modified starch are not available (10, 11).

On the other hand, over 25 billion jars of baby food have been consumed (32). Have any of the customers complained?

CHEMICAL INDUSTRY DIVERSIFIES INTO FOOD

The chemical industry experienced extremely rapid growth from World War II until about 1970. Much of the growth occurred as chemically produced products began to replace more traditional ones. Synthetic fibers, synthetic paint products, plastic containers, building materials, and chemical pesticides became the fast-growing segments of the industry. The rate of growth slackened as these segments of the industry began to mature, much to the chagrin of the industry, although optimism remains in their writings. If one goes through the last few years of the authoritative trade journal *Chemical and Engineering News*, one is struck by the fact that the main concern in every issue is growth of this or that segment of the industry, if not this year then next.

A general tapering off of the growth curve occurred in the latter part of the 1960s. Patrick McCurdy, editor of the journal, sees the slackening in the rate of growth as a time of reorganizing (23); he and his senior editor, D. M. Kiefer, see the industry changing from one that makes chemical raw materials to one that identifies with the ultimate consumer products. They note that the strength of the industry has been its aggressive diversification into any opportunity, wherever it may lead (17, 23).

Earl V. Anderson, another senior editor of *Chemical and Engineering News*, in an article entitled "The New Priorities," heralds food as a new opportunity for chemists and chemical engineers (2). The chemical modification of protein and starch I have described, though an example of chemical thinking and technique applied to food, represents quite unsophisticated chemical technology. When the full force of creative chemistry is applied to Nature's molecules, the types of food products capable of being machined to precise specifications will be unlimited.

The change in image, the biggest and most important breakthrough, has already occurred. It is no longer a case of accepting the molecules in corn or soybeans the way Nature designed them; now the molecules just become starting materials for endless chemical manipulation and transformation.

The hidden technology

The transformed image of field crops has not had any direct impact on the public. They are unaware of the change in image, and food technologists, recognizing the intrinsic conservatism in public taste, have shaped the products fabricated from their new building blocks into familiar forms. Chemically transformed soy protein, "textured protein," finds its way into products such as hamburger, bacon, beef, and milk products. Chemically treated starches stiffen pie fillings, puddings, gravies, stews, etc.—all in familiar-looking forms.

The full potential of chemical transformation of natural polymers such as starch and protein will not be realized until the public fully accepts, in their own right, the new forms possible from these fabricated products. Acceptance will probably not be long in coming, however, because patterns of public taste are rapidly shifting.

I will first consider some of the more overt ways in which public taste is molded.

TEXTURED TASTE

The objective of food technologists is to create marketable taste sensations. Much of their activity is empirical; in other words, the technologist modifies existing formulas and processes according to his own experience and intuition to obtain new products that he believes will provide acceptable taste sensations and are feasible to fabricate. If the rather vague conception of what constitutes a pleasurable taste sensation could be rendered in mathematical formulas, the task of the food technologist would be rendered more precise and it would be much easier to write the specifications of the raw materials. What constitutes a pleasurable taste sensation? To answer this question, technologists start by trying to dissect the sensations of eating.

Rheology is that branch of physics that deals with the deformation and flow of materials. Physicists classify the characteristics involved in this process as elasticity, plasticity, and viscosity, and they have developed elaborate mathematical formulas to define these properties. Food engineers, who consider food in the same terms as a piece of steel, study the same properties in food products with the idea of reducing taste and texture to a set of mathematical formulas (9). If the science of physics can provide nuclear power and atomic blasts, surely it can provide the mathematical definition of eating a piece of bread. Once they have acquired these formulas, technologists feel that they will be able to synthesize food products with predictable mouth feel and taste sensation.

Dr. J. N. Yeatman of the Division of Food Technology, Food and Drug Administration, states that sensory preception of texture depends on the deformation of food resulting from the application of pressure and/or on roughness, smoothness, or stickiness, properties estimated by sense of touch. Dr. Yeatman feels that all of these qualities should be measurable, but concedes that at the present time, in spite of progress in physical measurement, humans still perceive qualities that cannot be expressed in mathematical terms (34).

Dr. P. Sherman of the Food Science Department, Queen Elizabeth College, London, hopes that a detailed study of food structure and its interrelationships with textural properties will indicate how the latter can be modified and, furthermore, how new textural concepts can be created with fabricated foods. Once this is done, he considers the possibilities as endless (30).

Food engineers in this field appear to agree with the nineteenth-century physicist Lord William Thomson Kelvin that when you can assign numerical values to what you are speaking about, you know something about it. One should be able to relate the physical properties of food to the psychological event of eating the food, according to Dr. C. T. Morrow of the Department of Agricultural Engineering, Pennsylvania State University. He feels that it will be possible to develop the technique of psychophysical analogues, a mathematical model that explains the relationship between psychological and physical measurement (24). In other words, one would be able to predict the psychological sensations of eating just by measuring the physical parameters of the food.

Flavor

Mouth feel and the noise food makes when it is chewed comprise only two of the psychological sensations of eating. Flavor also plays a major role, and it has been defined as a sensation embracing aspects of taste and smell as well as texture. For most foods, however, the aromatic properties probably exert the greatest influence over what we regard as flavor. The aromatic components of food are volatile and frequently occur in vanishingly small concentrations. Chemists have long tried to analyze the flavor-producing components of natural foods, but only recently has chemical technology advanced sufficiently to detect trace quantities of odor-producing substances. Gas chromatography and mass spectroscopy are two highly sophisticated techniques that permit the separation and analysis of the minutest amounts of material. Over the past 15 years, chemists have compiled an impressive list of volatile constituents of dozens of natural foods. However, according to Dr. W. G. Jennings of the Department of Food Science and Technology, University of California at Davis, even with all this information it is rarely possible to construct meaningful criteria for flavor quality control, and many critical natural flavors resist duplication (15).

A place still exists for human senses, and in spite of the advances in techniques of chemical analysis, food experts still formulate new flavor sensations by trial and error. The classic flavorist mentally breaks down a flavor into various nuances and then tries to stimulate each nuance with the materials available, blending them to achieve a final effect. Occasionally, the flavorist and the analytical chemist combine their expertise. The chemist puts a complex flavor into his gas chromatograph and detects the components by running the effluent past the flavorist's nose (3).

Mechanical approximation of natural taste

Although food technology still relies heavily on human senses for guidance in formulating its products, the trend is clearly in the direction of minimizing the role of the senses by replacing it with precisely defined physical parameters. In attempting to transform their activity from an art to a science, food technologists, however, look backward to the nineteenth century—to concepts that were developed to understand a physical world. The nineteenth-century physical approach was to analyze a system, fragment it into as many bits as practical, quantitate the bits, and then use this information to resynthesize the system. Food technologists believe that the analytic concepts of nineteenth-century physics and chemistry can be applied to the subtleties and complexities of natural foodstuffs. It is highly improbable that scientists will ever be successful in duplicating natural tastes and textures, although their approximations may appear to come close.

The approximations will satisfy the food engineers, however, because they will be approximations synthesized according to scientific procedures. Moreover, all else in the system including the ultimate consumers will have to conform to what the food engineers synthesize. The raw materials used will be specified in terms of these limited physical criteria. Farmers will grow crops, and primary processors will process the basic molecules according to these criteria. At the receiving end of the system, the public will be conditioned to accept food which the technology produces according to its new scientific criteria.

Cultural conditioning of taste

An individual's acceptance of taste sensations is highly conditioned by his culture. Some cultures enjoy beetles, grubs, fresh blood, and partially digested contents of animal stomachs. All these items are highly nutritious but abhorrent to the Western mind. This fact merely stresses the effect of culture on what is acceptable as food and, moreover, stresses the visual appearance of food and the knowledge of its origin in important ingredients of the total taste experience. As René Dubos points out, the value of an article of food is determined not by the content of protein, carbohydrates, etc., but by its symbolic value—as it appeals to the appetite, the emotions, the soul (5).

The public's acceptance of engineered food products will have to be conditioned by their total cultural milieu; nevertheless, the technologic food environment itself does significantly affect public taste. It is not just a matter of the public accepting the pressures of a hyperactive food industry. Rapid two-way interaction between the public and the food industry creates a powerful resonance—each part affecting the other. One example of how this resonance operates is through rapid product change.

Product resonance

New food products rarely last more than two years, but each succeeding product represents a slight variation over the preceding one. The public is not aware of any major change in taste, texture, or appearance from one product to the next, but over successive product switches the change can become substantial. According to E. H. Fallon, former executive Vice President of Agway Inc., Syracuse, N.Y., about 7,500 new food products are introduced every year (7). Most of these new products fail quickly; consumers inform the food industry what is acceptable at any given moment.

Rapid product change and enormous product variety—the average supermarket stocks as many as 10,000 items (22)—coupled with mass distribution, become a medium for mass resonance between public and food industry. The speed-up in communication accelerates the evolution of the entire food service system.

A FEEBLE NUTRITON SCIENCE

Palatability separated from nutrition

Most practicing food technologists have very little nutritional background, and also little appreciate the impact of their efforts not only on the nutritional value of foods but also on the nutritional well-being of consumers.—G. F. Stewart, Professor of Food Protection and Toxicology, University of California at Davis (31).

Arthur Odell of General Mills is quoted as saying: "You can't sell nutrition. . . . Hell, all people want is Coke and potato chips" (18).

Food technologists are rapidly improving their skills and professional knowledge, secure in the feeling that their efforts are highly appreciated by the companies and agencies for whom they work. Technologists and scientists, as much as businessmen, like to feel that they are part of an expanding activity and that there are no limits as to what can be accomplished. These technologists and producers view the rapidly evolving food manufacturing industry as a highly stimulating place in which to work. But what of the nutritionists? They seem to be ignored. The objective of the food industry is to develop palatable products that sell well; nutritional factors, in their opinion, contribute nothing to palatability, so they are ignored.

In fact, the editor of *Food Technology,* the journal of the Institute of Food Technologists, had to justify his recent decision to insert items on nutrition in the journal normally devoted to product development, packaging, government regulations (31). However, the reason that nutrition science makes little input into food technology lies more with nutrition science than with food technology. If the technologists responsible for developing and promoting new taste sensations receive little training in nutrition, the the science of nutrition itself must be faulted.

Nutrition science fails to understand

The hearings today have shown the great difficulty in getting data that reasonable men can agree on in the field of food and diet and nutrition—we certainly have a great need for a certain body of basic research to get a fundamental basis from which we can proceed. —Senator Charles H. Percy (12).

The task of science is to understand and explain phenomena; we would expect the science of nutrition to try to understand and explain the nutrition of the contemporary food service environment. Instead, their concept of nutrition stems from nineteenth-century studies that classify foodstuffs as proteins, fats, carbohydrates, and accessory factors. To nutritionists, protein is protein, whether in the form of a piece of beefsteak or in the highly processed form of a synthetic bacon bit. Food technologists already know about proteins, carbohydrates, etc. They can look up the food values in their bible: *Composition of Foods,* Agriculture Handbook Number 8, 1963, provided by the U.S. Department of Agriculture (see table below). They do not need nutrition scientists to give them this information. They would prefer that nutrition science work out some new principles to guide them in their work. But since this is not happening, food technologists seek guidance from other scientific disciplines, for example, from the science of physics, thereby further promoting mechanization of the organic.

Nutrition science, by retaining outdated notions of nutrition, has failed to develop any new knowledge about the effects of modern food technology on human health and well-being. It provides no insight into what constitutes nutrition in the latter part of the twentieth century.... In this analysis of contemporary food technology we see the effects of having a science called nutrition that cannot explain what is happening and can provide no guidelines for a technology that engulfs all in its environment, carrying everyone in some undefined direction.

Nutrition science denies the existence of change

I have referred to both food technologists and nutrition scientists as looking backward to concepts that developed in the nineteenth century. I would like to enlarge on this point and also distinguish between technology and science. The practice of food technology is contemporary, but the principles on which it operates are those of the past and, moreover, they are mostly economic. It espouses increasing production, increasing mechanization of

The Known Nutrients According to Contemporary Nutrition Science

Proteins*	
Carbohydrates*	
Fats*	
Vitamins:	Minerals:
A*	Calcium*
D	Phosphorus*
E (tocopherols)	Iron*
K	Iodine
C (ascorbic acid)*	Fluorine
B₁ (thiamine)*	Potassium*
B₂ (riboflavin)*	Sulfur
Niacin*	Sodium*
B₆ (pyridoxine)	Chlorine
Pantothenic acid	Magnesium
Biotin	Manganese
B₁₂ (cobalamin)	Copper
Folic acid group	Cobalt
Choline	Zinc
Inositol	Chromium
Paraaminobenzoic acid	Molybdenum
	Selenium

*Nutrients listed by US Department of Agriculture. Composition of Foods, Agriculture Handbook No. 8. Washington, D.C., Consumer and Food Economics and Research Division, Agricultural Research Service, 1963.

the organic, increasing organization and centralization, and increasing standardization.

In working toward these goals, food technologists, except in the grossest sense, do not understand what they are doing to food. The food processor, for example, consciously extracts protein from soybeans because nineteenth-century science tells him this procedure will extract a class of molecules called proteins. In fact, a much more complex and subtle process is occurring to the foodstuff, of which he has only the barest grasp. No scientific theory or knowledge explains what is happening to the food value of the soybean. Nutrition science does not investigate these questions, nor does it know how to investigate them. By thinking of nutrition as a simple classification of a few categories of molecules, it denies the existence of such questions.

Although nutrition scientists complain that they are not part of the action and that food technology pays little heed to their advice on the nutritional value of food, food technology can easily incorporate classic nutrition into its methodology, if it so chooses. The FDA now requires full disclosure of the "food value" of manufactured food on the label. Food value, however, is tabulated according to the nineteenth-century classification of food values (see table). Food technology can easily furnish this information, but the regulation will have little effect on the way food is processed or marketed. Moreover, it serves as an effective screen behind which the methodology of food fabrication develops unimpeded either by scientific or by public scrutiny.

Man's redundant senses

When food technologists began to separate nutrition from palatability, they also undermined the ability of the human senses to assess the quality of the food. Texture, color, odor, taste, and feel of natural food are all human guides, not only to the nutritional value of food but also to its safety. At one time, one could use one's own senses to determine accurately the freshness of food, but man's senses no longer guide him in his choice of food items.

Food has been one of man's most direct contacts with his natural environment, and sensory exploration of his food supply every day was obligatory for survival. Now his senses have become redundant, and this deep psychological experience has vanished—replaced by a promise of a taste experience, certified by the label. As long as man is willing to trust an organization and not his own perceptions, this increasing psychological dependence on a technologic food system may be acceptable. But what is the effect of diminishing, even eliminating, the need for man to explore his environment and protect himself through his own senses?

Nutrition science and food service

The failure of nutrition science to influence the course of food technology is illustrated by what is happening in the food service field. (I have been using the expression "food service environment" to describe the total system of growing, manufacturing, merchandising, and eating food. In this section I use the term of the industry to describe the processing and selling of food through commercial eateries.)

A North American, on the average, consumes one meal in four away from home. The amount of food consumed away from home is increasing. In 1972 two experts predicted that by 1975 "we will look on institutional feeding as a natural outgrowth of our way to life, of increased population, of increased urbanization and of increased modernization" (1). At one time food was prepared and cooked on the premises of the restaurant or cafeteria, but now the trend is to do all of the preparation and most of the cooking in centralized factories. G. E. Livingston and his colleagues of Food Science Associates, Inc., review what is known about the effects of food service handling on nutritional value; not surprisingly, little is known (20). The effects on the nutritive value of preparing food on an ever-increasing scale are not studied and can only be surmised.

For example, one aspect of nutrition in which effects are easily measured is the accessory factors (vitamins and minerals). Many vitamins are destroyed by heating, and essential minerals leak into the cooking water. For this reason, careful cooks heat their vegetables for a minimum length of time in a minimum amount of water. But when food preparation is scaled up and chefs must thaw out 50-pound cartons of meat and cook vegetables in 300-gallon kettles, the time required to thaw or heat up the large mass increases considerably.

In centralized cooking, the raw materials arrive at the factory already frozen or canned. They are then made up, cooked, and divided into individual servings to be frozen and transported to the institution where they will be served. The individual servings are thawed and heated in a microwave oven to provide a freshly cooked dish. But during this process, what happens to the vitamins?

Chicken pot pie and the disappearing vitamin

Dr. P. A. Lachance and collaborators at the Department of Food Science at Rutgers University, concerned at the loss of nutrients in reheated convenience foods, decided to check commercially frozen chicken pot pies. They chose vitamin C as the indicator of nutrient level. First of all, they could not find any vitamin C in the pot pie even though it was full of vegetables. They then added a known amount of vitamin C to the thawed-out pie, refroze it, and after two days heated it to serving temperature. On reanalysis, they determined that about 25 percent of the vitamin had disappeared (19). This anecdote illustrates a deeper question for which nutrition science provides no information—the effects of combinations of ingredients (as, for example, in meat pies, stews) on the vitamin and mineral content of prepared food. The U.S. Department of Agriculture Handbook Number 8, *Composition of Foods* (table), treats each foodstuff individually and does not allow for significant losses of nutrients under conditions of commercial cooking. Dr. Lachance and his coworkers conclude that this handbook, the bible of dieticians and food professionals, does not provide accurate nutritional information for the eater.

Thus we find that even in the one area of nutrition for which analytic tools and established methodology are readily available, nutrition science does not provide any guidance. Is it any wonder that this science is not prepared to study the more profound effects of technologic processing on the nutritional qualities of food?

Dry-cleaned french fries

Centralized processing of food presents its own set of technical problems, and in the absence of any nutritional guidance, these problems are cast within the criteria of technologic food processing. Solutions appropriate to these criteria follow.

The French fried potato is the mainstay of restaurant, cafeteria, and many home meals.* One problem with frozen French fries sold for home consumption is that oven-baking of the fries gives a product inferior in texture

---

*In a survey of high-school cafeterias in the Hamilton [Ontario] area, we found that the typical teenage lunch consisted of one or two dishes of French fries, slathered with ketchup and eaten with pop or a chocolate drink. The principal of one of the schools admitted that it was an unbalanced diet, but the catering service pushed these items because they made more of a profit.

and flavor to the product prepared by frying. To solve this problem, the U.S. Department of Agriculture's Western Regional Research Laboratory, Agricultural Research Service, Berkeley, California, has engineered a solution. Fresh potatoes are cut into chip size and immersed in a bath of difluorodichloromethane (Freon 12) at about −21°F (this fluid used as a refrigerant is also a close relative of dry cleaning solvents; it is approved for food use by the FDA). The frozen chips are leached in warm water (125°F) for 15 minutes to remove sugars and other soluble constituents, and then are partially fried in oil, frozen for storage, and transported to supermarkets. According to the USDA technologists, the product is superior in overall quality to any other commercially prepared samples for home use and provides benefits to both processor and consumer (26).

Some toxicologic testing has been done on difluorodichloromethane, although the results are confusing. In one study, rats, guinea pigs, rabbits, monkeys, and dogs were exposed continuously for 90 days to 810 parts per million in the air without noticeable signs of toxicity, even though, according to the report, some of the experimental animals died (4).

Such experiments, like most experiments in toxicology, were done using healthy animals exposed to only this one agent. On the basis of this type of experiment, the FDA proclaims the refrigerant safe for human consumption. They ignore the possibility of interactions with other contaminants in the diet. We know of one example of this interaction. Piperonyl butoxide, a commonly used pesticide synergist, acts synergistically with Freon. (There is widespread domestic and industrial use of sprays containing piperonyl butoxide and a Freon propellant.) This combination caused the death of 50 percent of the newborn mice tested in one experiment, and a significant number developed liver tumors (6).

TOTALLY SYNTHETIC FOOD

Rubber, textiles, drugs, and dyes are all synthesized by means of chemical technology, but in every case the synthetic technology got its start because of a shortage of the natural product. Will totally synthetic food be the next in line? It is not [my] purpose . . . to predict the future; it is difficult enough to understand the present. But it is not a prediction to introduce the idea of totally synthetic foods, because the technology for manufacturing such foods already exists. Fat was synthesized from petroleum as long ago as 1884, and during both World Wars was manufactured on a commercial scale (29).

Proteins can be synthesized by a fermentation technology, a technique widely used to synthesize antibiotics, hormones, and amino acids. Strains of microbes (yeasts, bacteria), grown on a large scale in fermentation vessels, can be selected to produce the desired product (in this case, the protein of their own bodies). The Mobile Oil Company, for example, has found a microbe that lives on petroleum products and fixes nitrogen from the air. Petroleum contains carbon, hydrogen, and sulfur, but no nitrogen. For a microorganism to grow, a source of nitrogen must be found so that the microorganisms can make protein, nucleic acids, and other nitrogenous constituents. A process using this organism produces large quantities of protein, and already the commercially produced material is being fed to animals (13). Scientists and technologists who write articles about these developments, and note a world food shortage in the near future, confidently predict that synthetic food prepared by chemical and fermentation technology will be the next stage of our technologic diet.

Denial of alternatives

Technologists have always assumed that because something was feasible it should be done. But before the technology of fermenting protein is introduced on a commercial scale, it would make some sense to assess its effects. Once a technology has been introduced and woven into the fabric of the culture, it is too late to withdraw if it does not seem to be working out. Napoleon's dictum that an army travels on its stomach extends to the whole of society. The systems that provide and distribute food underpin the whole societal system, and once society has adapted itself to processing and distributing food in a certain manner, it is difficult to back away from that technology.

Large urban conglomerates can exist only because of the intensive agricultural and food technology currently practiced. Our urban life style becomes so dependent on each succeeding generation of technology that the only direction possible, according to the technologists, is to increase even more the technical sophistication. So powerful is this feeling that food technologists deny the existence of any alternatives. They often hold up the organic farming movement as an example of an archaic activity that could never possibly feed the masses. Such statements, however, merely expose the narrowness of their own thinking patterns and, more seriously, their refusal to consider social and cultural values.

So enamored are food technologists of the possibility of factory-produced synthetic food that the National Aeronautic and Space Agency (NASA) has organized a systems approach to speed up perfection of the technology. The systems approach embraces scientists and technologists from several disciplines, even the social sciences. But there seems to exist no room for reflective assessment of the place of this technology in society. NASA, according to Dr. John Billingham, has already decided that the chemical synthesis of food "offers the most promise as an ultimate solution" to the problem of food synthesis for space flight and lunar bases (28).

Cows and pigs to the zoo?

Reduced to its basic elements, man's food supply consists of carbon, nitrogen, hydrogen, and oxygen. The object in any food process, whether natural or synthetic, is to convert these elements into the complex organic molecules required by man. The latter two elements, derived from water, are universally available; it is the first two that must be supplied. In totally synthetic food, fossil fuel serves as the source of carbon, and nitrogen comes from the air; energy to effect the synthesis comes from burning additional fossil fuel. In field crops, carbon is derived from the carbon dioxide of the air and nitrogen from fertilizer or air. The sun provides the energy, although an enormous amount of fossil fuel energy goes into the cultivation and harvesting of field crops.

The way our society is organized it will be a matter of economics that will decide whether man-synthesized material becomes competitive with field crops as the basic source of raw material for food production. There is no plan for biologic factors in the economic system. In fact, the economic system does its best to eliminate biologic variables. Crops are subject to the vagaries of weather, whereas factory-produced raw materials are not. The constant theme of food processors is to minimize the direct participation of Nature at every stage. Millers and bakers for a very long time have strived to produce uniform products as part of their attempt to control natural variables and to further the goal of mechanization. Humans as one of the biologic variables are no more immune to these onrushing economic forces than cows or pigs.

Simplification of the man-controlled ecosystem

The continual drive of technology to subjugate natural processes goes beyond producing food molecules consistently and reproducibly. It endeavors to simplify the ecologic system, a simplification that emerges as a central theme in technologic agriculture. Synthetic food, in one stroke, effects a major simplification: It wipes out a whole tropical level of the ecologic system. To explain further, man's food chain goes from plants→animals→man. Synthetic food eliminates animals as a source of nourishment. Soy bean protein can be produced at about one-half the cost of meat. The effects of eliminating animals as a source of food will reduce man's immediate ecological cycle to plant→man, heightening the instability of his ecosystem.

Current decision-making mechanisms do not allow for reflection on this event, nor do they encourage the study of its far-reaching effects. In the opinion of established agriculture, it is better not to know. Even the relatively straightforward choice of soybean "meat" versus beefsteak has been reduced to a consideration of the quality of protein based on the traditional method of evaluating protein—distribution of amino acids. The two proteins have a similar distribution; thus the question of choice is simplified to cost.

However, nutrition science has not investigated the matter further; nothing is known about other qualities of real meat that may be significant to good health and well-being. At least beefsteak is a whole food, whereas soybean meat is a set of extracted molecules divorced from its original context in the soybean. The effects of such a divorce have not been studied, and nutrition scientists seem convinced that the fabricated soybean protein is nutritionally no different from beef protein.

References

1   Altschul AM, Hornstein I: Food in changing world (excerpts from a paper presented at American Chemical Society meeting). Food Eng 44(5) Part 1:78–79, 1972

2   Anderson EV: The new priorities. Chem Eng News 49(10): 19–22, 1971

3   Broderick JJ: Fruit flavor research. Food Technol 26(11):37, 48, 1972

4   Clayton JW: Fluorocarbon toxicity and biological action, Toxicity of Anesthetics. Edited by BR Fink. Baltimore, Williams & Wilkins, 1968, pp 77–104

5   Dubos R: So Human an Animal. New York, Scribner 1968

6   Epstein SS, Joshi S, Andrea J, Clapp P, Falk H, Mantel N: Synergistic toxicity and carcinogenicity of "Freons" and piperonyl butoxide. Nature (Lond) 214:526–528, 1967

7   Fallon EH: Future of co-op food marketing. Feedstuffs June 4, 1973, p 10

8   Filer LJ: Modified food starches for use in infant foods. Nutr Rev 29:55–59, 1971

9   Finney EE: Elementary concepts of rheology relevant to food texture studies. Food Technol 26(2):68–77, 1972

378

Part V

10   Food and Agriculture Organization. Toxicological evaluation of some antimicrobials, an-
     tioxidants, emulsifiers, stabilizers, flour-treatment agents, acids and bases. FAO Nutritional
     Meetings Report Series 40A,B,C, 1967

11   Food and Agriculture Organization. Toxicological evaluation of some food colours, emul-
     sifiers, stabilizers, anti-caking agents and certain other substances. FAO Nutritional Meet-
     ings Report Series 46A, 1970

12   Hearings Before the Select Committee on Nutrition and Human Needs of the United
     States Senate. Part 6, April 16, 1973

13   Howard J: New proteins: Animal, vegetable, mineral. New Sci 49:438–439, 1971

14   Hullinger CH, Van Patten E, Freck JA: Food applications of high amylose starches. Food
     Technol 27(3):22–24, 1973

15   Jennings WG: The changing field of flavor chemistry. Food Technol 26(11):25–34, 1972

16   Katzbeck W: Phosphate cross-bonded waxy corn starches solve many food application
     problems. Food Technol 26(3):32–33, 1972

17   Kiefer DM: Chemicals 1992: 20 years of industrial change. Chem Eng News 50(28):6–11,
     1972

18   Kotz N: Let Them Eat Promises. Englewood Cliffs, NJ, Prentice-Hall, 1969

19   Lachance PA, Ranadive AS, Matas J: Effects of reheating convenience foods. Food
     Technol 27(1):36–38, 1973

20   Livingston GE, Ang CYW, Chang CM: Effects of food service handling. Food Technol
     27(1):28–34, 1973.

21   Lockmiller, NR: What are textured protein products? Food Technol 26(5):56–58, 1972

22   Margolius S: The Great American Food Hoax. New York, Walker, 1971

23   McCurdy P: The demise of the chemical industry (editorial). Chem Eng News 50(28):1,
     1972

24   Morrow CT: Psycho-physical analogues. Food Technol 26(5):92–98, 1972

25   Murray DG, Ziemba JV: New starch hydrolysates spur product development. Food Eng
     44(5):88–90, 1972

26   Nonaka M. Weaver ML: Texturing process improves quality of baked French fried
     potatoes. Food Technol 27(3):50–55, 1973

27   Pomeranz Y, Finney KF, Hoseney RC: Molecular approach to breadmaking. Science
     167:944–949, 1970

28   Program aims at chemical synthesis of food. Chem Eng News 50(8):19, 1972

29   Pyke M: A taste of things to come, New Sci 48:512–514, 1970

30   Sherman P: Structure and textural properties of foods. Food Technol 26(3):69–79, 1972

31   Stewart GF: Nutrition and the food technologist. Food Technol 18(10):9, 1964

32   Stewart RA: The use of modified food starch in baby foods. Corn Annu pp 19–20, 1971

33   Wolf WJ: What is soy protein? Food Technol 26(5):44–45, 1972

34   Yeatman JN: Physiological aspects of texture perception including mastication. Food
     Technol 26(4):141–147, 1972

| 35 | Professors on the Take

BENJAMIN ROSENTHAL, MICHAEL JACOBSON,
and MARCY BOHM

Benjamin Rosenthal is a Democratic Representative from New
York, Michael Jacobson and Marcy Bohm are associated with
the Center for Science in the Public Interest, Washington, D.C.
Jacobson, a biochemist, is the author of *Eater's Digest* and
Nutrition Scoreboard.

Reprinted from *The Progressive*, November 1976, pp. 42–47.
Copyright © 1976 by Benjamin Rosenthal, Michael Jacobson,
and Marcy Bohm. Reprinted with permission.

"Whose bread I eat, his song I sing," was former
Senator Sam Ervin's down-home way of describing the biases that can develop when money changes hands. Ervin was talking about politicians, but
the observation applies equally to professors. The turgid prose of the University of Wisconsin's pamphlet *Faculty Rights and Responsibilities* solemnly
defines the independence of a scholar:

> In serving a free society the scholar must himself be free. Only thus can he seek
> the truth, develop wisdom, and contribute to society those expressions of the
> intellect that ennoble mankind. The security of the scholar protects him not only
> against those who would enslave the mind but also against anxieties which divert
> him from his role as scholar and teacher.

Despite such ringing platitudes and noble aims, many professors are on
the take, according to our extensive survey.

Heightened consumer awareness in recent years has led press and public
alike to rely on the academic community for objective analyses of controversial consumer problems. Unfortunately, many professors have developed
extensive ties with the same industries of which they are asked to be objective analysts. Such ties take many forms, from providing one-shot advice to
accepting long-term research grants, from representing companies at Congressional hearings to maintaining consultant relationships and even serving
on trade association committees and boards of directors. Biases can also
develop indirectly—through fraternization with industrial executives at conventions and scientific meetings, conducting seminars at corporate head-
quarters, or pursuing industry contacts to help graduate students obtain jobs.

The fields of nutrition and food science are typical. The songs many nutrition professors sing indicate that the bread they eat is baked by Ralston-Purina, Quaker Oats, Gerber, Pillsbury, General Foods, or other corporate giants.

The quality of the American diet has been the subject of many Congressional hearings, documentaries, and exposés. Americans worry about mounting evidence that our foods contribute to such widespread health problems as diabetes, tooth decay, obesity, allergies, heart disease, constipation, and bowel cancer. In fact, one nutrition expert from the University of California estimated that diet-related illnesses cost consumers $30 billion a year.

The high-fat, high-sugar, low-fiber content of the American diet has been identified as a major factor in hundreds of thousands of deaths annually. The chemical additives which saturate our foods have often been found dangerous. For example, the pesticides 2, 4, 5-T (birth defects), DDT, aldrin, and dieldrin (cancer) have all been banned from food crops. Cobalt, used to stabilize beer foam, was finally banned in 1965 after killing dozens of heavy beer drinkers. Violet No. 1 food dye (cancer), DEPC (cancer), and some uses of sodium nitrite (cancer) have also been banned in the past decade.

Despite the compelling need for experts who can subject the food industry to critical examination, the nutrition and food science communities have fallen under the $200-billion industry's influence. At the most prominent universities, eminent nutritionists have traded their independence for the food industry's favors. Our recent survey of nutrition and food science departments reveals that eminent nutritionists have abandoned their professional independence to curry the favor of the food magnates.

Harvard University's Department of Nutrition, one of the most prestigious, is riddled with corporate influence. One need go no further than the front door for the first indication—a wall plaque thanking General Foods for funding the research facilities. From there, one can proceed to the annual *Treasurer's Financial Report to the Board of Overseers of Harvard College.* The 1973 report (the 1971, 1972, and 1974 reports are similar) lists as donors to the Department of Nutrition the Amstar (sugar) Corporation, Beatrice Foods, Carnation Company, Coca-Cola, Continental Can Company, Gerber Products, International Sugar Research Foundation, Kellogg Company, Kraftco (cheese), Oscar Mayer and Co., Miles Laboratories, Monsanto, Nutrition Foundation, the Sugar Association, and more than a dozen other food industry giants, plus a smattering of drug companies. The food industry provided about $2 million [to the department] from 1971 to 1974.

Dr. Fredrick Stare, who has conducted respected studies on heart disease, has been chairman of the nutrition department at Harvard since it was founded in 1942. If a chairman—particularly one who has served for more than three decades—can be presumed to influence his department's philosophy, Stare's influence certainly encourages good will toward corporations. Harvard's working relationship with industry has been a sound financial investment for Stare and the department, judging from the plethora of corporate grants it has received. Stare has been on the board of directors of Continental Can Company, a major food packaging firm, for twelve years. He has, moreover, testified in recent years at Congressional and Food and Drug Administration (FDA) hearings on behalf of Kellogg, Nabisco, Carnation Milk, the Cereal Institute, the Sugar Association, and the Pharmaceutical Manufacturers Association.

Although Stare's widely syndicated newspaper column notes his Harvard affiliation, it makes no mention of his food industry connections. His columns and articles in defense of sugar and food additives have neglected to disclose his intimate ties to the sugar and chemical industries. *Women's Wear Daily*, for example, interviewed Stare, who declared that "most people could healthily double their sugar intake daily." His advice contradicts one of the few widely accepted nutritional principles—that Americans eat far too much sugar. In a recent column, Stare tried to dismiss the food-additive controversy: "Is there any reason for concern about food chemicals? . . . The answer is no."

Stare has refused to disclose to us the companies which currently employ him. When asked whether his corporate ties cast a shadow on his pronouncements, he maintained, "I really honestly feel I have not reduced my credibility." In the three years after Stare told a Congressional hearing on the nutritional value of cereals that "breakfast cereals are good foods," the Harvard School of Public Health received about $200,000 from Kellogg, Nabisco, and their related corporate foundations.

Yet Fredrick Stare is not the most prominent member of the Harvard nutrition department; that honor has belonged to Jean Mayer (who was recently named president of Tufts University). Mayer has repeatedly voiced his concern over food industry advertising and the quality of the American diet. He has assisted consumer advocacy groups as well as the Senate Select

Committee on Nutrition and Human Needs, which deserves credit for alerting the public to nutrition problems. Nevertheless, Mayer, like Stare, has lent his prestige to food and chemical companies.

For the past five years Dr. Mayer has been on the board of directors of Monsanto, which manufactures food flavorings, preservatives (such as sodium benzoate and sorbic acid), pesticides, fertilizer, and other food industry chemicals. Since 1972 he has also served on the board of directors of Miles Laboratories, which makes food flavorings and other additives, imitation meat substitutes, and even synthetic fruit bits. Mayer has a syndicated nutrition column comparable to Stare's. The column, like Stare's, notes the Harvard affiliation and neglects the corporate ties.

Even the University of Wisconsin, which declares that "the scholar must himself be free," is ensnared in a web of corporate connections. The University's Food Research Institute received $635,390 in 1975 from dozens of food, packaging, and drug companies and trade associations. Among the benefactors were Kellogg ($20,000), McDonald's ($20,000), Nestle ($20,000), Campbell ($20,000), Kraftco ($20,000), General Mills ($10,000), and the Institute of Shortening and Edible Oils ($60,000). The basic annual membership fee seems to be $20,000, and the funds support research projects at the Institute as well as at several other departments in the university.

The Director of the Food Research Institute is Dr. E. M. Foster, who, in responding to our survey, noted his membership in Consumers Union (i.e., he subscribes to the magazine *Consumer Reports*) but neglected to mention his membership on the board of directors of the Stange Corporation since 1972. Stange is a leading manufacturer of flavorings, colorings, spices, and other food ingredients.

Foster's scorn of consumer advocates is consonant with industry's; he believes that consumer advocates "hold the uncompromising view that industry and the regulatory agencies are in league to rip off the consumer, and they are determined to change matters through restrictive legislation. The chief tools of these self-styled consumer advocates, and they use them well, are exaggeration and facts taken out of context. . . ."

Foster, recently named to a U.S. Department of Agriculture advisory committee (as the sole university representative), has charged that consumer activists "have complicated and confused the decision-making process," which has long been dominated by corporate giants.

One of Foster's colleagues is Dr. Alfred E. Harper, chairman of [Wisconsin's] Department of Nutritional Sciences, to which the Food Research Institute also funnels grants. Harper heads a National Academy of Sciences (NAS) committee which meets every five years to determine "recommended dietary allowances" of vitamins, minerals, and protein. He has supplemented his income by consulting for G. D. Searle Company (which produces drugs and some food additives) for up to $10,000 per year, Procter and Gamble (the giant soap and detergent manufacturer that also produces Folger's coffee, Pringles, and Jif peanut butter), McGaw Laboratories, Abbott Laboratories, General Mills, and Pillsbury. Harper had held a faculty chair sponsored by General Foods at MIT, and when he moved to Wisconsin, the $50,000 support went along with him. Harper acknowledged under oath at an FDA hearing that he receives about 20 percent of his income from consultant fees.

The public receives most of its information on food problems from newspaper reports and television and radio interviews which quote consumer advocates, industry spokesmen, and apparently unbiased professors. Yet few reporters inquire into corporate ties which might bias the judgments or philosophy of the professors they cite.

Professor Paul Kifer, head of the Department of Food Science and Technology at Oregon State University, is referred to in one article as "a top food expert." Kifer assured the readers: "Don't worry about food additives. There has never been a single proven case of humans being hurt from eating normal quantities of food containing additives." Even if we leave aside the many persons who are severely allergic to food additives (one young boy who was sensitive to peanuts died a few years ago after eating ice cream that contained a little peanut butter), Kifer's statement is highly misleading.

The concern is not so much that additives will kill on the spot, but that they contribute to cancer and other problems which show up only after many years. It is impossible to link a particular death to a food additive consumed long before. That people should indeed worry about food additives is suggested by the FDA's ban on at least twenty-five apparently safe food additives over the last six decades. A number of pesticides (such as DDT) and other "incidental" additives also have been banned. The Kifer article failed to mention that he was a "food expert" at Ralston-Purina, a major agribusiness and grain conglomerate, for almost sixteen years before he moved to Oregon State. He now receives an annual honorarium from

Ralston-Purina and serves on an advisory board of the U.S. Brewers Association.

Professor Fergus Clydesdale of the Nutrition and Food Science Department at the University of Massachusetts is a frequent public defender of the food industry. At a convention of vending industry executives, Clydesdale declared, "There are no such things as junk foods, scientifically they don't exist. . . . There is nothing wrong with any product you people sell, nothing." In an article entitled "Nutrition Experts Cite Information Foul," Clydesdale wrote: "In order to supply wholesome, high quality food in today's over-populated, urbanized world, nearly all foods must be processed and preserved." Clydesdale has defended the use of sodium nitrite as a preservative in baby food—a practice which not even baby-food producers defend.

Clydesdale consults for the Carnation Co. and the National Automatic Merchandising Association, the vending industry trade association. The vending machines which are overpopulating the world preclude nutritious choices, since coffee and soda pop account for 60 per cent of all vended food, with candy, gum, and other non-nutritious items constituting another 20 per cent. Clydesdale's résumé also notes: "Informal counseling to several major food industries, as well as major [artificial] color equipment manufactures. Work in close cooperation with several food industries who are currently funding research in the color and chemical area."

Professor Theodore Labuza of the University of Minnesota's Department of Nutrition and Food Science has said: "Let's face it, the food industry has to make a profit, otherwise it will not be able to keep providing us with food." In order to help the companies, Labuza has sold his services to General Mills, Searle Biochemics (a drug company), Pillsbury, Hunt-Wesson, and Quaker Oats.

Both Clydesdale and Labuza were reluctant to disclose their current outside affiliations to us. Instead, each referred us to university administrators. Inquiries to the university department heads met with equal evasiveness. Professor Elwood Caldwell, head of the University of Minnesota's Department of Nutrition and Food Science, remarked, "All continuing consulting or retainer agreements at this university must be disclosed to and approved by its central officers and are public information obtainable from the University." Requests to University President C. Peter Magrath and others, however, proved fruitless. (Caldwell worked for nineteen years for Quaker Oats Company before forsaking his position as director of research.)

Professor R. V. Lechowich, head of the Department of Food Science and Technology at Virginia Polytechnic Institute, was another department head who refused to disclose his corporate connections, stating, "Since control of conflicts of interest are exercised, the request for names of firms and consulting fees are not pertinent to the question." Professor Bernard Schweigert, chairman of the Department of Food Science and Technology at the University of California at Davis, also refused to disclose any information. He is, however, known to serve on the board of directors of Universal Foods, a manufacturer of specialty products and a leading importer of gourmet and fancy processed foods. What Lechowich, Schweigert, and other corporate consultants realize is that secret review of conflicts of interest is tantamount to no review at all. Bringing the industry-academy nexus into the open would be the most reliable way of discouraging corporate co-optation.

Rivaling direct payments to professors as a source of bias are research grants funneled through the departments. Although industry spends far more on advertising than on academic research, it does dispense millions of dollars in grants to hundreds of professors. Food and chemical companies donate research funds to professors directly, as well as through their conduit, the Nutrition Foundation. Because government is the largest supporter of university research, industry support usually amounts to only a fraction of a department's budget.

Nevertheless, industrial grants are often substantial, and they become more crucial to some departments as the Federal Government reduces its science budget. The University of Massachusetts Department of Nutrition and Food Science, for example, receives more than one-third of its research funds from industry. The Department of Pediatrics at the University of Iowa, a major research center for infant nutrition, receives about 20 per cent of its research support from companies, including Gerber and infant formula manufacturers. The Harvard School of Public Health's Department of Nutrition receives a substantial percentage of its budget from industry, but declines to disclose the exact amount.

Any grant will induce a certain amount of gratitude on the recipient's part and discourage him from being a major critic of the donor—particularly if there is a chance for a second grant. Predictably, industry-financed studies generally support the industry's interests.

Harvard's reputation was invoked in defense of breakfast cereals in 1974, when two researchers at the School of Dental Medicine published a paper purporting to show that presweetened cereals do not contribute to tooth decay. Later that year, when consumer groups criticized high-sugar break-fast cereals in a petition filed with the FDA, the Cereal Institute (a trade association) praised the Harvard study in a press release headed "Scientific Studies Prove Cereals Don't Cause Cavities, Are Vital in Nation's Diet." Not unexpectedly, the Cereal Institute hid the fact that the Kellogg Company helped finance the study. The study, moreover, was designed in such a way that tooth decay caused by sugar-coated cereals never could be detected. So unreliable was the study that other dental specialists, including Dr. Herschel Horowitz of the National Institute of Dental Research, wrote to the *Journal of the American Dental Association,* where the Harvard-Kellogg study was published, to attack it.

The shaping of public policy by professors who have ties with industry goes far beyond teaching and interviews. Many professors of nutrition, food science, and toxicology have been appointed to public or private commit-tees that advise the Government and issue public statements that receive wide publicity.

The Office of Maternal and Child Health in the Department of Health, Education, and Welfare is the only Government agency concerned with in-fant nutrition. The Office publishes a few poorly distributed pamphlets on infant care and feeding. Its influence on infant feeding patterns is negligible compared to the role of baby food and formula manufacturers. The three baby food companies (Gerber, Heinz, Beech-Nut) and three formula com-panies (Ross, Mead-Johnson, Abbott) sponsor full-page ads in magazines read by new mothers, send salesmen to visit doctors, offer free formula to hospitals and new mothers, and place free promotional materials in government-funded clinics. The comparative impact of government and in-dustry efforts can be judged by noting that only 25 per cent of American babies are breast-fed for more than a week, and that supermarkets stock dozens of high-sugar baby foods (some providing up to 44 percent of their calories by added sugar).

The Office of Maternal and Child Health's scientific adviser is Dr. Samuel Fomon, a widely respected expert on infant nutrition. It is possible that some of Fomon's lack of zeal in getting HEW to inform women about breast-feeding and to exercise greater control over the composition of baby foods is attributable to the grants and consulting fees which he and his laboratory at the University of Iowa receive from Gerber, Mead-Johnson, Wyeth, Nestle, Ross Laboratories, and CPC International (Mazola margarine, Skippy peanut butter).

The Food and Nutrition Board is one of the most influential advisory committees. It issues authoritative reports on nutrition and food safety under the imprimatur of the National Academy of Sciences–National Research Council (NAS-NRC), a quasi-governmental agency established by Congress. According to Ralph Nader, "The Academy can be considered the preeminent forum through which individual scientists, acting as responsible citizens and rendering their best professional judgments, can have a significant impact on major technological events."

As a key adviser to the Federal Government, one would expect the Academy to avoid potential conflicts of interest by limiting participation of individuals with corporate ties. However, the composition of the Food Protection Committee of the Board indicates that potential conflicts of interest are of little concern to it. Several members serve simultaneously as professors and corporate consultants or directors. Various other members of the NAS-NRC food committees work for food and chemical companies full-time.

In the late 1960s, MSG (monosodium glutamate), a common flavoring, was alleged to cause severe burning sensations and other painful symptoms and was later shown to cause brain damage in young mice. The FDA contracted with the Academy to investigate the evidence. Yet the special seven-member committee appointed by the Food Protection Committee to study MSG had close ties to industry. The chairman of the MSG committee, Iowa Pediatrics Professor Lloyd Filer, admitted that members of his research team had recently received grants from International Minerals and Chemicals Corporation (IMC), the major producer of MSG (it makes Accent), and Gerber Products Company, which had used MSG in baby foods until public pressure forced it to stop. About 20 per cent of Filer's research funds come from industrial sources.

Filer currently consults for a variety of companies and received more than $17,000 between 1970 and 1974 for his services. He declines to disclose the names of the companies for which he consults. Filer, in addition, had been the medical director of Ross Laboratories, an infant formula manufacturer, for twelve years. Two other committee members also had done research for interested parties: Lloyd Hazelton, founder of the Hazelton laboratory, had been hired by IMC to conduct MSG studies. George Owen, professor of pediatrics at the Children's Hospital in Columbus, Ohio, published an unrelated study supported entirely by Gerber.

Phillip Boffey, author of an exposé of the political and corporate pres-

388

Part V

sures which undermine the Academy's objectivity (*Brain Bank of America*), has described the Academy's response to the partisanship of these committee members: "Filer defends these relationships by pointing out that the Committee needed knowledgeable experts and that there are few proficient food scientists who have not, at one time or other, received research support from the food industry. However, even the Academy's own staff later acknowledged that Filer should probably not have been asked to serve as chairman of the panel, though it defended Filer's probity and saw no reason why he should not serve as a member of the Committee." Filer was subsequently selected to chair the Food and Nutrition Board, a position he held until 1975.

The final report on MSG, quoting both Filer's and Hazelton's research, concluded that MSG was safe. But the committee did note, "The risk associated with using MSG in foods for infants is extremely small. The committee cannot find, however, that the usage confers any benefit to the child, and therefore recommends that MSG not be added to foods specifically designated for infants."

Senator Charles Percy, Illinois Republican, expressed concern about Dr. Hazelton's conflict of interest after the doctor testified on behalf of the Grocery Manufacturers of America, the food industry's major lobbying group. Percy commented, "He is judge and jury. Regardless of his objectivity and his competence, it appears there is a conflict of interest. . . . It is very hard to justify having people serve on a panel who have been in the employment of the very companies that are making products that they are called forth to judge."

Members of NAS-NRC committees and consultants are asked to submit a routine statement listing potential sources of bias. Yet the Academy has no criteria for deciding whether a conflict of interest actually exists. The statements are never made public; the public is simply asked to place its faith in a nebulous and ineffective process.

Individuals who work with such organizations as NAS on government contract jobs become, in effect, public employes. Their affiliations must be carefully scrutinized to assure unimpaired judgments. These individuals should be willing to disclose such information as professional consultantships when public policy is involved. Such a sacrifice does not seem to be an undue infringement of privacy where the decision rendered affects millions of lives.

The Politics and Economics of Food

In sharp contrast to the pervasive and multifarious links between professors and industry, professorial associations with consumer groups are rare. Of the eighteen professors responding to our survey who noted any association with consumer groups, half of the links consisted of token involvement, such as subscribing to *Consumer Reports* or belonging to Common Cause. Receiving *Consumer Reports* entails rather less influence than serving on a corporate board of directors or receiving a $15,000 industrial grant.

While a great many professors work closely with industry, only a small minority of professors has shown a deep commitment to working with citizens' groups. Samuel Epstein, for instance, a pharmacology professor at Case Western Reserve University, has long worked with citizens' groups and Congressional committees on problems related to food additives and environmental pollutants. Joan Gussow, chairperson of the Nutrition Education Department at Columbia Teachers College, has been especially critical of junk-food advertising aimed at young children and has worked closely with Action for Children's Television. Frances Larkin, head of the University of Michigan's nutrition department, helped students form the Food Action Coalition and organize the nation's most active Food Day activity in 1975. Nutrition professor Eleanor Williams of the University of Maryland has worked with both student and citizen activists.

The professorial practice of maintaining ties with industry is an old one which is certain to continue. It provides important information and support to companies while supplementing professors' salaries. At the same time, it impinges on professors' commitment to their students and their allegiance to professional objectivity.

Some professors who moonlight for industry, such as Stare and Clydesdale, defend industry and attack consumer activists so vehemently that they have become known as food-industry apologists. It is difficult to know the extent to which their philosophies have been molded by industrial grants and honoraria. But an even more serious consequence than creating a professional advocate is the gag-effect of company money. Intimate working relationships between professors and executives inevitably lead to friendships, sympathy, and reluctance to alienate future sources of grants or job possibilities for oneself or one's students. Pediatric nutritionists, for example, have been singularly uncritical and close-mouthed about high-sugar baby food desserts and the switch from breast-feeding to canned formula. One probable reason for this silence is the grants and supplies given by baby food and formula manufacturers to researchers in the field. Developing ties to industry causes one to overlook problems, rationalize faults, and defend policies.

As long as collaboration with industry continues to be viewed by the academic community as ethical and respectable, it is important that the public know about potential sources of bias. When professors are in a position to influence public policy, by speaking to the press or sitting on advisory committees, this information is vital. In such matters, respect for individual privacy must yield to society's right to know. When interviewing professors about matters that may affect a corporation or industry, reporters should routinely inquire into that professor's industrial ties.

A more active and formal policy is appropriate for government advisory committees. When the members of a committee are announced, corporate ties should also be listed. A less suitable policy would be disclosure of how many professors have ties with which companies, naming the businesses but not the members. This approach would provide the public with necessary information regarding conflicts of interest while completely respecting the privacy of the professors.

Dr. Dean Abrahamson, professor of public affairs at the University of Minnesota, has offered his own prescription to discourage conflicts of interest: "At a minimum I think that a listing of each faculty member's outside activities—whether recurring or not—should be maintained in the departmental office and that this file should be open to any and all that wish to look at it. It should include all outside activities, amounts of time spent, and payment received. It should also include all grants and contracts that support either that faculty member, staff and students. . . .

The Center for Law and Economic Studies, based at the Columbia University Law School, is one of the few academic institutions to adopt such a guideline. The Center's statement of policy stipulates: "Participants in the Center's research studies are required to disclose their past, present, or anticipated consultant or other relationships, whether or not compensated, with special interest groups, labor unions, corporate entities, and other institutions which may have positions on particular issues of concern to the Center in its work. They must also disclose any significant financial interests which may bear upon these issues."

New mechanisms are needed to ensure industrial research support without impairing the professor's objectivity. One alternative is establishment of a non-profit public-interest group to "launder" contributions before they reach the university. Industry would contribute money to a central pool;

professors would apply for grants, as they do to the Government. Funds would be dispensed by a panel composed of scientists without industry ties, consumer leaders, and a few industry representatives. The group would use a small part of the pool to develop priorities and criteria for giving grants.

Tight connections between the academic community and industry bode ill for responsible corporate practices, a safe food supply, and vigorous investigations. Industry has impressive resources with which to communicate its opinions to the public, particularly through publications and advertising. Society needs the academic community's help in offsetting this powerful advantage. Professors should examine current practices with a critical eye, cooperating with citizens' groups and speaking out publicly when problems come to light. The rewards for this, of course, are psychological rather than financial. But for the sake of healthy debates and healthy bodies, we can only hope that some food science professors will choose this recipe for action.

|36| Another View of "Professors on the Take"

RONALD M. DEUTSCH

Ronald M. Deutsch is an author, lecturer, and educator, particularly in the field of nutrition. Nutrition fads and fallacies are his special interest, and two of his books—*The Nuts among the Berries* and *The Family Guide to Better Food and Better Health*—became best sellers. Among his recent books are *Realities of Nutrition* and (with the National Nutrition Consortium) *Nutrition Labeling*.

From *The New Nuts among the Berries,* by Ronald M. Deutsch (Palo Alto, Calif.: Bull Publishing Co., 1977). Copyright 1977 Bull Publishing Co. Reprinted by permission.

. . . In 1976, the *Washington Star* reported: "Food scientists are accused of becoming advocates for industry practices or deliberately keeping mum on controversial issues. . . ."

The story concerned a report issued jointly by Rep. Ben Rosenthal (Dem. N.Y.) and the Center for Science in the Public Interest. The tone of the report was bitter. Consider the title, *Feeding at the Company Trough,* and such conclusions as: "Many professors are, quite frankly, on the take. . . ."

The report centered on the truths that the food industry gives some money to universities for research, and that some companies ask nutritionists for advice and pay them for their time. None of this was very revealing.

Virtually every nutrition department in the world has some industry grant support. The report chose 17 professorial examples. And they have some common characteristics. They either (1) declined to give their names and support to Food Day and other CSPI activities, (2) withdrew their names and support or (3) challenged one or more principles of consumerist attacks, such as the amount of water in baby food or the need for organic farming.

Dr. Jean Mayer, for example, is listed because of an association with Monsanto, "which manufactures food flavorings, preservatives . . . pesticides, fertilizer and other food industry chemicals." Yet in 1972, Dr. Mayer wrote the introduction to Jacobson's own book on food additives. In this, Mayer renewed the call for a review of the GRAS (Generally Recognized As Safe) list of additives.*

Dr. Fredrick Stare of Harvard was cited for statements that sugar is not dangerous and that food chemicals are not immediate sources of peril. He also "has refused to disclose to the authors of this report the companies which currently employ him."

Actually, Dr. Stare does not accept fees from industry. Even royalties for his books and columns are all signed over to Harvard.

Dr. E. M. Foster of the U. of Wisconsin's Food Research Institute is singled out. Why? "He believes that consumer advocates 'hold the uncompromising view that industry and the regulatory agencies are in league to rip off the consumer. . . . The chief tools of these self-styled consumer advocates . . . are exaggeration and facts taken out of context. . . .' "

Professor Paul Kifer of Oregon State is also chosen. Why? Because he has said that "there has never been a single proven case of humans being hurt from eating normal quantities of food containing additives." The authors of the report refute this. . . .

---

*Incidentally, the White House Conference on Nutrition, which Dr. Mayer chaired, strongly urged this review. And to clarify his own position, the author wrote one of those demands for a GRAS review into the report.

Dr. Fergus Clydesdale of the U. of Massachusetts is accused of "moonlighting." The report says that his prejudice is revealed in his statement, "In order to supply wholesome, high-quality food in today's over-populated, urbanized world, nearly all foods must be processed and preserved."

Dr. Theodore Labuza of the U. of Minnesota is indicted for his statement: "Let's face it, the food industry has to make a profit, otherwise it will not be able to keep providing us with food."

And the report concludes: "In sharp contrast to the pervasive and multifarious links between professors and industry, professional associations with consumer groups are rare. . . . Professors should examine current practices with a critical eye, cooperating with citizens' groups."

The author refrains from conclusions.

So, curiously, do the lines continue to be drawn.

But such lines are not always apparent. And both the public and its officials tend to regard consumer organizations as sources of truth without prejudice. In 1976, the Nader-sponsored Public Citizen Forum invited presidential candidates to speak. One of them who did had earlier said, "I would like to be known as the foremost protector of consumers." He reaffirmed this statement and laid out some specifics for reaching the goal, among them the needed strengthening of regulatory agencies, to which, he said, "I will appoint consumer or citizen advocates. . . . One of the goals that I have for my own appointees is that they would be acceptable to Ralph Nader."

The candidate's name was Jimmy Carter.

Through such avenues and through such people of good intention have some of the oldest errors about food and health acquired astonishing force in our own time. Thus has the need to clarify truth and fiction in nutrition acquired new urgency. . . .

Part VI
What Can Be Done?

There is no authoritative
body of comment on food.
Like all the deeper personal
problems of life, you must
face it alone.

—FRANK MOORE COLBY

Introduction to

Part VI

Eating, contrary to the general rule, is not something that practice makes perfect. In fact, for many of us, the more we practice, the worse it gets. Through ignorance or indoctrination we tend to assume that, having put about a thousand meals and countless snacks under our belt each year over the decades, we must know what we're doing. According to a recent report:

> One of the overwhelming and inescapable conclusions from all the research data we have seen is that *in the eyes of the consumers* there is no significant problem about nutrition. . . .
>
> The only recurring problem with respect to the broad area of food and health, as consumers define problems, is in the area of overweight and dieting. About 50 percent or more express concern about overweight and *claim* some form of overt activity to deal with that problem.[1]

Though confidence runs high in regard to "balancing" nutrients, the report notes, consumers actually have a poor understanding of how to achieve such balance either by the meal or by the day, and their choices are steeped in folklore. In several studies consumers were asked to describe balanced meals or menus; the question involved not the amount, but only identification of what should be consumed. Only about 50 percent came reasonably close, while 30 to 40 percent omitted one or more of the basic foods considered necessary in a menu.[2]

There are two questions that you might consider about a balanced diet—a diet furnishing sufficient calories, protein, vitamins, and minerals for your body's needs. (1) Since we are not biochemically homogeneous, and balance is a matter of degree, might your nutrition needs vary considerably from those of others? (2) Is it really necessary to eat a balanced diet *every day*? As for the "basic four" grouping, it should be remembered that it is a useful, but not definitive, guide to selecting food. There are millions of people in the world who completely eschew one of the basics, the dairy group, and enjoy good health. There are also millions who live long, healthy lives on a diet notable for simplicity rather than variety. Contrary to what is commonly believed, variety is not a guarantee of good nutrition.

One of the reasons that Americans mis-eat, falling short of the well-balanced diet that is supposedly within easy reach, is the proliferation of "fun" foods and convenience foods. These are such nutritional hybrids that the consumer is nonplused when trying to fit such products into the "basic four" categories. And even if the category is clear, how much actual nutrition is available? Consider, for instance, Pringles, which Michael Jacobson has called "the ultimate insult to the potato." How much honest potato can there be in a product the price of which involves 20 percent for the cost of the can and nearly 80 percent for the cost of processing, production, and distribution?

Is labeling the answer? Not according to one source:

> The blunderbuss approach of putting everything down in print for the hurried customer in the supermarket who may have insufficient knowledge or interest in evaluating it or time to master the terms and their relationships is likely to "turn off" a lot of people who know what they like and are not going to eat a particular food just because it carries a declaration of what the FDA regards as "good" ingredients.[3]

Modifying America's food habits promises to be a long and formidable task, often thanks to food-industry policies that are counterproductive to the efforts of nutritionists. As Joan Dye Gussow observes:

> Since eating habits are established early in life, whoever teaches a child may be the most effective nutrition educator. And who teaches today's pre-schoolers about nutrition? Television! . . . To be effective, nutrition education must enter the marketplace and hard-sell good nutrition with as much sophistication as the fun-food manufacturers. We know that a diet of ordinary foods got man into the twentieth century. We have no evidence that a diet of colas, sugar cereals, snack cakes, and mock fruit juices (even fortified) will take our children into the twenty-first century.[4]

In a 1977 report linking health and diet, the Senate Select Committee on Nutrition and Human Needs recommended reducing sugar consumption by 40 percent and salt intake by 50 to 85 percent. Also suggested was that we eat more fruit, vegetables, whole grain products, fish, and poultry and cut down on red meat, eggs, and other foods high in cholesterol or fat. Such a diet would be much like that of Americans toward the end of World War II, before the processed food industry and supermarkets began their extraordinary growth. According to the report, these changes could reduce the heart-attack rate by 25 percent, cancer deaths by 20 percent, and infant mortality by 50 percent.

The Senate Select Committee has, however, been severely criticized by numerous physicians and professional nutritionists who regard the release of its recommended "Dietary Goals" as premature and founded more on hope than on scientific fact. In hearings on responses to these dietary goals, Dr. Robert Olson, of the University of St. Louis School of Medicine, contended in his testimony:

> There is no evidence that the eating patterns of Americans constitute a critical public health problem. There is no evidence that adoption of the "Dietary Goals" will reduce health costs and maximize the quality of life. There is no evidence that the diet modifications suggested will modify the morbidity or mortality from any of the "killer diseases." There is evidence, on the other hand, that such diet modification may exacerbate malnutrition in some segments of our population.[5]

Dr. Thomas Parran, former Surgeon General of the United States, once reportedly declared that faulty nutrition is the greatest single cause of disease. While there is obviously considerable disagreement over this point among physicians, most are willing to concede that nutrition science and medical science have too much in common to remain apart. Yet physicians, for all their knowledge about health and disease, too often know as little as or less than their patients do about nutrition. According to Dr. Michael Latham of Cornell University's Graduate School of Nutrition, "Nine out of ten doctors in New York City would give wrong answers to dietary questions."[6] As Dr. Julian B. Schorr of the New York Blood Center explains it, "Often doctors are trained in nutrition by doctors who heard it from another doctor who made it up."[7]

Although Hippocrates emphasized, around 460 B.C., the universal role of nutrition in medicine, his view has been largely ignored in American medicine. Among the reasons given for this situation are that the science of nutrition, being multidisciplinary, has a "blurred image"; medical schools typically limit nutrition to the study of deficiency diseases; and nutrition is a relatively new science.[8]

According to some nutritionists and physicians, a renaissance of nutrition education in medicine and the health sciences is in the making.[9] But Dr. Esther S. Nelson, in *Selection 37,* reports that so far the programs of only about 10 percent of medical schools measure up to the need in nutrition education. She pleads for a change in this state of affairs, ending on a hesitantly hopeful note.

What about the food industry, which is not against people but which tends to see them as secondary to profits? Larry Gross asks:

> What are we to do while we wait for the food industry to undergo near-revolutionary reforms of its priorities, sense of public responsibility, and mode of overcentralized production and distribution? . . .
> . . . It is not enough to tell people what to eat; they must be able to find desirable food without inordinate effort or expense. In addition, the development of grass-roots consumerism and active alternative systems of production or marketing might well be the most effective mode of motivating the food industry in the direction of nutritional reform.[10]

In *Selection 38,* biochemist Roger J. Williams explains why the food industry must undergo "a revolutionary change in attitude"; he uses the example of "enriched" but impoverished white bread to bolster his case.[11] Williams believes that probably only an informed public opinion can force the food industry to change its attitude, arguing that "we need to realize that we need to derive *help* and *benefit,* day by day and hour by hour, from the food we eat, and that anything that does not help *contributes* to our ill health."

Clearly, Williams would not give his imprimatur to such products as Breakfast Squares, Wonder Bread, Frute Brute, Coca-Cola, and Pringles. But Harvard's Whelan and Stare contend that "these foods, like *all* foods available today, when used in moderation and in the context of a well-balanced diet, *contribute* to both our physical and psychological well being."[12]

That theirs is probably a minority opinion is brought out by *Selection 39,* in which Consumers' Research outlines the types of foods that, according to the evidence at hand, we would do well to omit from our diet. The article also points out why we should reduce our consumption of coffee and colas. (The average per capita consumption of soft drinks, many of which contain caffeine, recently almost doubled in one decade, from some 16 gallons in 1962 to roughly 30 gallons in 1972.)

Even when people do know the basic facts and principles of nutrition, they often do not behave accordingly; in fact, they seem to take a perverse delight in eating what is "not good for them." Intelligent and rational individuals frequently decline to follow that path which they believe is the reasonable one — witness, for example, the obese dietitian. A question often asked is: "How can you expect people to stick to a sensible diet when you can't even get them to stop smoking?" The answer is that no one is asking them to *stop* eating, but only to *change* their eating habits. We can use our intelligence to translate knowledge into action—to make a rational choice and to do something with that choice.

In *Selection 40,* Elizabeth Kendall ponders the psychology of our wayward eating habits, our disinclination to "have a real physiological dialogue" with our food. She concludes that we must, whatever the difficulty, forget our conditioning, take a hard look at our traditions and our needs, and realize that we have a choice.

In the last analysis, what you eat, and how much respect you have for your body, is up to you—not the nutritionist, not the food industry, not the government, not the self-proclaimed expert. As Frances Moore Lappé puts it:

A change in diet is a way of experiencing more of the *real* world, instead of living in the illusory world created by our current economic system, where our food resources are actively reduced and where food is treated as just another commodity on which to make profit—a profit on life itself. A change in diet is a way of saying simply: I have a choice. That is the first step. For how can we take responsibility for the future unless we can make choices now that take us, personally, off the destructive path that has been set for us by our forebears?[13]

References

1   Howard E. Bauman and Dudley Ruch, "Problems of Researching and Marketing Fortified Foods and Their Implications for Consumption Trends," in American Medical Association, *Nutrients in Processed Foods: Vitamins, Minerals* (Acton, Mass.: Publishing Sciences Group, 1974), p. 145.

2   Ibid.

3   "Nutritional Labeling Is Not a Guarantee of Quality!" *Consumers' Research Magazine,* January 1975, p. 2.

4   Joan Dye Gussow, "Improving the American Diet," *Journal of Home Economics* 65 (November 1973), p. 6.

5   Robert Olson, quoted in Gilda Knight, "Responses to Dietary Goals—Eggs," *Nutrition Notes* 13 (September 1977), p. 1. See also U.S., Congress, Senate, *Dietary Goals for the United States,* prepared by the Staff of the Select Committee on Nutrition and Human Needs (Washington: U.S. Government Printing Office, 1977).

6   "The Perils of Eating, American Style," *Time,* December 18, 1972, p. 75.

7   Julian B. Schorr, quoted in Richard A. Passwater, *Supernutrition* (New York: Pocket Books, 1976), p. 34.

8   See, for instance, Reva T. Frankle, "Nutrition Education for Medical Students," *Journal of The American Dietetic Association* 68 (June 1976), pp. 513–519.

9   Ibid.; and William J. Darby, "The Renaissance of Nutrition Education," *Nutrition Reviews* 35 (February 1977), pp. 33–38.

10 Larry P. Gross, "Can We Influence Behavior to Promote Good Nutrition?" *Bulletin of the New York Academy of Medicine* 47 (June 1971), p. 622.

11 For an even more negative view of the processing and "enrichment" of white bread, see William Longgood, *The Poisons in Your Food,* new rev. ed. (New York: Pyramid Books, 1969), pp. 149–162. For a surprisingly benign view, see Jean Mayer, *A Diet for Living,* Consumers Union ed. (New York: David McKay Co., 1975), pp. 28–30.

12 Elizabeth M. Whelan and Fredrick Stare, *Panic in the Pantry: Food Facts, Fads and Fallacies* (New York: Atheneum, 1975), p. 15.

13 Frances Moore Lappé, *Diet for a Small Planet,* rev. ed. (New York: Ballantine Books, 1975), p. 55.

| 37 | Nutrition Instruction in Medical Schools—1976

ESTHER S. NELSON

Esther S. Nelson is an M.D. in Vista, Calif. More than 40 years ago, at the medical and dental schools of Northwestern University and the University of Southern California, Dr. Nelson taught what was probably the first practical course in nutrition for medical students ever offered.

From *The Journal of the American Medical Association* 236 (November 29, 1976), p. 2534. Reprinted by permission of the American Medical Association. Copyright 1976, American Medical Association.

Last fall I was informed that only approximately 42 percent of our medical schools offered courses in nutrition. Having been involved in nutrition since 1916, this low figure hardly seemed possible, so a survey was undertaken to find out what the status really is.

A questionnaire was sent to the chiefs of the departments of medicine of 60 medical schools and asked these questions:

1 Do you offer instruction in nutrition?
2 How many hours of lecture? How many hours of quantitative figuring?
3 Do you have research in nutrition?

Forty-four schools responded. To question 1. seven answered "No." To question 2. thirty-four responded: two schools offer only 1 hour, eleven offer 2 to 10 hours, nine offer 11 to 19 hours, three offer 20 to 40 hours, and one has a complete department of nutrition with 13 faculty members and 20 courses leading to a BS, MA, and PhD. The remainder said that the subject was touched upon in other courses, that an elective seminar was given, that it was part of public health instruction, or that work with the dietitian was elective.

Rudiments of figuring quantitative diets are given in only seven schools. From personal communication, I understand that three schools inform students how to write a diet prescription in terms of calories and grams of carbohydrate, protein, and fat.

Twenty-seven schools are engaged in research in nutrition in areas such as mineral metabolism.

From personal experience in reaching this subject in two medical schools, I feel that anything less than 20 hours is not meaningful in providing real ability in prescribing diets.

For comparison with the teaching of human nutrition, a survey card similar to the one sent to the medical schools was sent out to departments of animal husbandry in 30 agricultural colleges and asked about animal nutrition. All responded; and *every one* teaches animal nutrition in many courses, both undergraduate and graduate; and *all* have ongoing research.

Today's general public is often well informed in many phases of nutrition, and when doctors are asked for detailed information, it is expected that it be given exactly and honestly. From this survey, much less than 42 percent of medical schools give adequate training in nutrition. Many of the courses are elective, and the number of students enrolled in those courses is unknown. It appears that only about 10 percent of the schools are measuring up to the need.

Because food is so basic to health, it is amazing that more clinical research on nutrition has not been done, not only to heal sick bodies but also to build the best possible ones in the first place. Healthy bodies are less likely to fall victims of disease than those already weakened by malnutrition.

Several of the best courses that came to light in this survey are taught by trained dietitians. This resource should be tapped more often for excellent basic knowledge. Doctors will be quick to apply this information in their practices.

Notwithstanding all the knowledge that has been uncovered and proved in the last 60 years, the surface has only been scratched in clinical research. For instance, a great deal more needs to be known about the problem of obesity, which is so prevalent that it could well be called the number one ailment of our population. The fact that so many methods of reduction by diet are constantly being offered to the public indicates that more research needs to be done. Everyone knows that starvation or limitation of food intake results in weight loss; but what foods should be limited most? Do trace minerals influence it? Do hormone changes with advancing age influence it? Why can some people eat all they want and not gain, while others have an appetite that is not sated even though calories are eaten far beyond what is needed? Does heredity influence weight? Since so many are afflicted by the miseries of being fat, I maintain much will be done for the human race if the problem of obesity is solved.

The field of nutrition is wide open, and more good can accrue to the human race from this fundamental knowledge than from any other avenue. Eventually it will come. Let it hasten.

| 38 | What the Food Industries Can Do

ROGER J. WILLIAMS

Roger J. Williams, a biochemist, was the first person to identify, isolate, and synthesize panthothenic acid. He also did pioneer work on folic acid and gave it its name. In addition to several books on organic chemistry and biochemistry, Dr. Williams have written numerous books for lay readers, including the popular *Nutrition in a Nutshell*. His most recent book, co-edited with Dwight K. Kalita, is *A Physician's Handbook on Ortho-molecular Medicine*.

From Roger J. Williams, *Nutrition against Disease: Environmental Prevention* (New York: Pitman Publishing Corporation, 1971). Copyright © 1971 by Pitman Publishing Corporation; reassigned, 1976, to Roger J. Williams. Reprinted by permission.

The food industries, though based on science, have tended to stand still (or regress) with respect to performing their essential function in society, namely, producing food of better and better nutritional quality for the consumers. Because of long-standing neglect of nutrition and the nutritional improvement of life, the food industries tend to take food quality for granted.

There is a sore need for a revolutionary change in attitude. The public, the medical profession, those who produce food by agriculture, and those who process, package, preserve, distribute, and sell foods, all need to realize that the quality of the food we eat is a problem that outranks even that of the quality of what we read in school books, newspapers, and magazines.

Scientific advances have made it possible for food to be vastly higher in quality today than it was ten, twenty, forty, or a hundred years ago; but in the food industry there has been a prevailing attitude of merely getting by the Food and Drug Administration and of waiting until some government committee prods them before trying to improve upon the food that grandma used to prepare. Even those citizens who are concerned about our food would often be content with nutrition as good as, or maybe a little better than, it was in the days of Queen Victoria.

We take it for granted that the other science-based industries will make substantial advances decade after decade. We see the development of TV and color TV, of beautifully recorded music, of transportation that can take us to the moon and back, and we take it all in stride. The textiles of today are incomparably superior to what they were when the choices were between cotton, wool, and silk; the paint industry has been completely revolutionized; our present-day lighting is a far cry from the glow produced by Edison's carbon lamp. We may swear at computers, but the industry that produces them has made unbelievable advances, and will continue to do so.

Furthermore, these advances have come from *within* the industries themselves. Can one imagine the Bell Telephone Laboratories waiting for the approval of a governmental committee before inventing the transistor? Can one imagine the textile industry sitting on its haunches for thirty years after its first production of rayon, waiting to see if vastly improved textiles might be in order? Does IBM wait for public or governmental advice as to the best ways of improving its products? If the food industries were to keep pace with the other science-based industries, they would employ experts of the highest quality who would put to shame any outsiders who might wish to tell them what to do. Where does one find outstanding experts in electronics, in textiles, in lighting, or in computer design? While academic men make their contributions, the men in the respective industries do not sit around waiting for developments to take place outside the industries.

How scientifically weak one segment of the food industry—the milling and baking industry—has been is demonstrated when one considers the story of the "enrichment" of flour and bread.

White flour and bread, though supposedly relished and in demand, has been under attack by nutrition-minded people for several decades. It is well known that white flour keeps much better than whole-wheat flour and that one reason for its better keeping quality is the fact that it will not support the life of weevils. Yet, during the milling process, the germ of the wheat grain is eliminated, and with it goes the fatty components and many of the items in the nutritional chain of life. What is left is largely starch and wheat protein; the latter, like many other vegetable proteins, is of relatively low nutritional quality.

In 1941, partially at the instigation of my older brother, R. R. Williams, now deceased, the "enrichment" of white flour and bread was instituted.[1] At that time it was decided, largely on the basis of expert help outside the industry, that thiamine, riboflavin, niacin, and iron should be added to flour and that calcium should be an optional supplement. These nutrients were added to restore, at least in part, those lost in the milling process. Many practical and technological considerations were involved in making these choices, including palatability, availability, cost, and evidence as to the probability of substantial nutritional improvement. As of the time of making these decisions, the choices were reasonable ones.

The sad part of the story is this: Since 1941, for a period of about thirty years, the milling and baking industry—lacking any substantial outside prodding—has rested quiescently on this early "enrichment." It has never made any significant attempt to improve further the nutritional quality of flour and bread.

Having become keenly aware of the situation and its importance . . . , I performed the following experiment with the technical assistance of Charles W. Bode.

Young weanling rats of four different strains, 128 in number, were placed on two bread diets. One group of sixty-four was placed on commercial enriched bread still produced essentially in accordance with the practices of about thirty years ago. A matched group of sixty-four was given the same bread which had been supplemented in accordance with more up-to-date knowledge by the addition of small amounts of minerals, other vitamins, and one amino acid, lysine.[2]

The two breads were indistinguishable in appearance, and the added nutrients at wholesale rates would cost only a fraction of a cent per loaf.

That the rats on the commercial enriched bread would not thrive was to be expected. After ninety days, about two-thirds of them were dead of malnutrition and the others were severely stunted. The rats on the improved bread did surprisingly well; most of them were alive and growing at the end of the ninety-day experiment. Their growth and development on the improved bread was on the average seven times as fast as on the commerical bread.[3]

It is my contention that the milling and baking industry should have been doing experiments like this for decades, and should have been moving consistently in the direction of better bread by whatever routes seemed most appropriate to the experts. As a science-based industry, the milling and baking industry should be expected to advance. Bread holds—or should hold—a unique position as the staff of life, a staple basic food. If the food industry is not interested in improving our daily bread, it is not to be expected that it will be much concerned about other foods.

Actually, "enriched flour" (it should, on the basis of present knowledge, be called "deficient flour") is used in the preparation of a multitude of other products such as cakes, cookies, crackers, pastries, doughnuts, biscuits, muf-

~~~~~~

RATING CEREALS

Scientific studies conducted by Consumers Union and reported in the February [1975] *Consumer Reports* have shown that Maypo 30-Second Oatmeal with Maple Flavor, Cheerios and Special "K" are "far and away the most nutritious" of all the cereals tested.

Groups of weaned rats were fed one of each kind of test cereal and nothing else. Three control groups of weaned rats were fed a standard laboratory diet, eggs only or milk only. How did the cereals compare as the only food?

Three—Maypo, Cheerios and Special "K"—did well. Twenty were of significantly lower nutritional quality than the top three. They included Sun Country Granola-Regular, Quaker 100 Percent Natural Cereal, Total, Post Grape-Nut Flakes. Twenty-one were found of sufficiently low nutritional value to be considered deficient. They included Sugar Frosted Flakes, Kellogg's Corn Flakes, Product 19, Rice Krispies and Sugar Pops.

~~~~~~

fins, waffles, pancakes, macaroni, noodles. All of these would be far better nutritionally if the flour were not needlessly so deficient.

Furthermore, the complacent acceptance of the limited "enrichment" with thiamine, riboflavin, niacin, and iron has held back the nutritional improvement of all other cereal products. When corn or rice or breakfast foods are "enriched," the same four nutrients are added, as though these constituted an exclusive "sacred quartet" and no other nutrients could be of concern. There are many other nutrients—pyridoxine, pantothenic acid, folic acid, vitamin B_{12}, vitamin A, vitamin E, magnesium, and the trace elements—that need to be thought of in any real enrichment program. Some of these are probably sorely lacking in many diets—especially when these diets include many products made from "enriched" flour. People who eat substantially more bread and related products than the average (often those with lower incomes) are liable to be badly deficient in the items that we used in our feeding experiments to supplement commercial bread.

I personally feel keen disappointment in the failure of the food industry to advance, because most of my scientific life has been devoted to exploring and increasing our knowledge about nutrition. My endeavors have resulted in the discovery, isolation, and synthesis of one key vitamin, pantothenic acid; I have named another—folic acid—and have contributed by the microbiological approach to our knowledge about many others. Yet the vast amount of information and insight into nutrition gained in the last thirty years by hundreds of investigators has netted very little in terms of improvement in the food industries. This is a disgrace.

When our experiment involving the improved bread was reported to the National Academy of Sciences in October 1970, and the story got into the newspapers, I began to get protests from the Millers' National Federation and the American Institute of Baking. Their arguments rested largely on the thesis that bread was not supposed to be eaten alone and that other foods fill in the deficiencies of bread.

While bread need not be by itself a perfect food, it is nevertheless about as basic as a food can be. If it is grossly deficient and the deficiencies can be readily and inexpensively corrected, it should be the self-imposed responsibility of the milling and baking industry to see that it is done.

The Millers' National Federation published an interview with its president, C. L. Mast, Jr., the day after my paper was given to the National Academy. Mr. Mast said, in part: "If competent nutrition authority recommends any other additions to enriched flour and bread, you may be sure that the milling-baking industry will do its utmost to meet what it considers its responsibility in providing essential nutrients in such form that they meet public acceptance."

This sounds encouraging, except that it is the milling and baking industry itself that should provide the authorities and not wait for outsiders to tell them what to do.

In the same statement, Mr. Mast said, "the Millers' National Federation and the American Bakers Association had petitioned the Food and Drug Administration, November 5, 1969, for permission to treble or quadruple the amount of iron in enrichment, and subsequently asked Food and Nutrition Board support of a proposal to increase by 50 percent the amount of thiamine, niacin, and riboflavin in the enrichment formula."

These requests, particularly the latter one, reveal a singular lack of understanding of modern nutritional principles. From the perspective of 1941, the suggestion that more thiamine, riboflavin, niacin, and iron be added may sound reasonable; but from the perspective of thirty years later, it is ridiculous to stutter like a broken record about the "sacred four." Thiamine, riboflavin, niacin, and iron are no more indispensable in the scheme of life than are pyrodixine, pantothenic acid, vitamin E, folic acid, magnesium, and the trace elements, all of which are lost to a substantial degree in the milling process.

In our rat feeding experiments, we left the iron, thiamine, riboflavin, and niacin strictly alone, and improved the bread enormously by adding minor amounts of *other* nutrients. These nutrients were either not readily available in 1941, or their importance was not fully recognized. A lot of things can happen in science in thirty years.

One bit of philosophy accepted by some of those who supported the "enrichment" program involved making the white bread as nearly equivalent as possible, nutritionally, to whole-wheat bread. I see no reason why such a philosophy should be adhered to today. Why shouldn't modern bread be vastly *better* than old-fashioned whole-wheat bread?

It is well known that wheat proteins are poorly balanced in amino acid content so far as human consumption is concerned.[4] The amount of lysine, one of the essential amino acids, is, for example, far too low; and the nutritional value of bread and the availability of the protein in it would be greatly increased if it were supplemented with lysine. Since this is an economical and completely harmless procedure,[5] I can see no argument against it. There is nothing sacred about the composition of whole wheat that should make us slavishly follow its dictates in our search for good food.

It would be out of place for me or anyone else who lays no claim to expertness in milling and baking technology to outline precisely how the industry should proceed. This is *their* business. They should greatly improve our daily bread by whatever means they can—by including the germ in the flour, supplementing with milk powder and/or soybean flour, adding vitamins, minerals, and amino acids, or whatever. Since they have already moved part way in the direction of supplementation with specific nutrients, it seems logical that they should try further moves in the same direction. Our experiment suggests one possibility, but it is only a suggestion. Every possible means should be explored. The important thing is that bread, a staple food, be improved nutritionally.

One of the weak links in the enrichment program has been lack of attention to newer knowledge about the calcium-magnesium situation. The addition of calcium to bread was placed on an optional basis. It still is; some bakers put it in, others do not. In 1941 the human requirements for magnesium were not known to be high, nor had a magnesium-deficiency disease been demonstrated in man.[6] The Food and Nutrition Board gave estimates of the magnesium needs of human beings for the first time in their 1968 edition of its publication on "Allowances."[7] For a young man, this need is set at 400 milligrams per day, about one-half of the calcium need!

If the calcium addition is made to "enriched" bread (it should be, and there should be uniformity), then by all means magnesium should be added also. Extra calcium calls for extra magnesium, since a balance needs to be maintained. Magnesium deficiency is probably widespread, and increasing the intake of magnesium is an important measure recommended for protecting against heart disease.

Trace elements need to be thought of also; many vital ones are present in whole wheat and are removed in the milling process.[8] All of these matters should be of great concern to the milling and baking industry.

A key to this entire problem lies dominantly in the area of public education. If medical scientists and the general public were aware that the nutritional environment of our body cells and tissues hinges on what we eat—every mouthful contributes—and that this environment determines the degree of health we possess, then the public would be continually complaining about the poor nutritional quality of the flour and bread, and the industry would be forced to act. When the best that the baking industry can offer an infant for a snack is a soda cracker or some other washed-out tidbit, it is time for a change.

I have dwelt upon the problem of "enriched" bread because it is such a staple food, and the neglect of it is accompanied by a disregard of the nutritive value of foods in general. Improvement of all present-day foods should be on our minds.

The canning industry has, on the whole, done a good job in preserving the better-known nutrients from destruction during the canning process. What is needed now is attention to the nutrients that are just as indispensable as thiamine, riboflavin, niacin, and iron, but that have received far less attention. Tables designed to give information about the nutritive value of foodstuffs rarely mention such items as vitamin B_6 (pyridoxine, etc.), pantothenic acid, vitamin B_{12}, and folic acid, and yet these are indispensable to life, and there is evidence that deficiencies are commonplace.

Since two of these nutrients exist in nature in various forms, the problem of knowing precisely how they are affected by canning or other food processing is not simple. Part of the burden of proof with respect to their retention should rest with the food processors, who need to be concerned about the loss of all essential nutrients.

We need to develop a different psychological attitude toward eating. Instead of reassuring ourselves by saying, "Enriched bread (or breakfast cereal) is harmless; it won't hurt me," we need to realize that we need to derive *help* and *benefit,* day by day and hour by hour, from the food we eat, and that anything that does not help *contributes* to our ill health.

We have developed something of this attitude toward our cats and dogs, who fare better at the supermarket than we do. They have fewer choices, but most of the foods offered them are compounded scientifically and are far superior nutritionally to what their owners eat. People who would not think of feeding a dog bread, doughnuts, and coffee, or waffles and syrup, eat such foods with abandon.

We (and the food industry) need to appreciate that for young children the "headstart" we may attempt to give them educationally may be more than cancelled by the "hindstart" we give them nutritionally. The brain cells of children need to be furnished an adequate nutritional environment so that brain development can take place. As it is, the brain cells of many youngsters are forced to limp along as best they can in a poor environment induced by deficient nutrition.[9] This is a most serious situation.

Who in these days can say that the environment doesn't matter? Whenever we eat "enriched" bread or any other product that is needlessly deficient, we help along the development of a poor environment. Every food we eat should contribute in a *postive way* to the development of a better environment. At present it is easy in a supermarket to pick out hundreds of items which *detract from* rather than contribute to a good cellular environment. The entire food industry should have as its aim building up better internal environments for children and adults.

Agriculture, too, needs to join in the scientific quest for better food. While it is impossible to produce, by agriculture, foods that are lacking in nutritional value, we have it in our power to grow vastly improved foods through better soil use and more intelligent fertilization.

This is a complicated field of endeavor, since soils vary considerably and require different fertilization for different plants. It may be that some plants can be improved in nutritional value far more than others by proper fertilization. But over the country we have a large number of agricultural experimental stations and regional laboratories, many of which should be directing their major energies precisely toward the unravelling of these problems. Because the whole science of nutrition (as it applies to real people) has lagged terribly, agriculture has tended to fall into the same rut as the rest of the food industry, and to be satisfied if the food it produces is about as good as our grandfathers had. Agriculture can and must move ahead in the production of better grains, better fruit, better vegetables, better melons, better meats, better eggs, better milk.

The food industry as a whole, including agriculture, needs to be increasingly concerned about the problem of contaminating the internal environment of our bodies by the free use of additives which have no nutritional value and are always capable of doing harm . . .

It is too much to expect that the internal environment of our body cells and tissues will be completely free from all contaminants. (The air we breathe, and the water we drink, is never *absolutely* pure.) But it is the food industry's responsibility, zealously to guard this internal environment, not only by putting the right things into it, but also by leaving the destructive things out.

Food technology is far too complicated to make it possible for an outsider to discuss in detail just what the various branches of the food industry should do about specific additives.[10] What we need to develop in the food industry is adherence to the motto of the future: "Better and better food." When this is followed, additives will be held to an absolute minimum. The idea that an additive is acceptable if it helps sales and does not make the customer noticeably ill must be discarded. I believe an informed public will force this change in attitude.

Indeed, it is on the power of an informed public opinion that we shall probably finally have to rely to effect most of the significant improvements in our nutritional situation. I do not underestimate the difficulty of creating an informed opinion, but in view of the tremendous interest in our macroenvironment which had developed in a few years, it is by no means unreasonable to hope that a similar interest can be stirred up with respect to our microenvironments.

Of course, the teaching of nutrition to home economics students would be vastly simpler if there were fewer vitamins, minerals, and amino acids to worry about. But we have to take nature the way we find it. If we simplify matters too much, we do violence to truth.

In a booklet *Eat to Live,*[11] put out by the Wheat Flour Institute of Chicago (1970), a deplorable full-page illustration shows a pyramid of ten children's blocks labelled "The 'Key' Nutrients." These individual blocks represent vitamin A (at the top), then two B's (thiamine and niacin) next, then beneath them C, another B (riboflavin), and D, and on the bottom row Protein, Calcium, Iron, and energy.

This is a most unfortunate picture, because what it says is fundamentally untrue. In order for our cells and tissues to have a proper environment, we need to have adequate supplies of a *team* of nutrients, and the team is as strong as its weakest member. Pyridoxine (vitamin B_6), pantothenic acid, cobalamine (vitamin B_{12}), and folic acid are absolutely essential nutrients, just as are thiamine, niacin, and riboflavin. Phosphate, magnesium, potassium, and the trace elements are just as indispensable as calcium and iron.

Abbreviated nutrition, which is adequate with respect to only some of the needed nutrients, can only lead to diminished health and early death. This kind of nutrition is easily attained; our children, with all their candy bars, potato chips, soft drinks, and "enriched" bread live with it all the time, and we adults sometimes fare little better. The kind of nutrition we crucially need, what the food industry should provide us, is *complete nutrition*—the kind that leads to abundant health.

Notes

1 Williams, R. R. *Toward the conquest of beriberi.* Cambridge, Mass.: Harvard University Press, 1966.

2 To each pound of "enriched" flour was added: pyridoxine, 2 milligrams; pantothenate, 4.5 milligrams; cobalamine, 2.2 micrograms; vitamin A, 2160 units; vitamin E, 20 milli-

grams; folic acid, 0.5 milligrams; L lysine, 0.5 milligrams; calcium, 300 milligrams; phosphate, 713 milligrams; magnesium (oxide), 150 milligrams; manganese (sulfate), 20 milligrams; copper sulfate, 4 milligrams.

As the experiment progressed, supplementation with vitamin D was also included. Under the conditions of our experiment this seemed to make no substantial difference. We look upon the particular formulation used as primarily illustrative. Undoubtedly, the nutritional value could have been increased further by adding more lysine, but under present conditions this would have increased the cost materially.

3   Williams, R. J. "Should the science-based food industry be expected to advance?" Paper presented to Natl. Acad. of Sci., Oct. 21, 1970; published as a chapter in *Orthomolecular Psychiatry,* David R. Hawkins and Linus Pauling, eds. San Francisco: Freeman [1973].

4   Horn, M. J., et al. "The distribution of amino acids in wheat and certain wheat products." *Cereal Chem.,* 33:18, 1956.

See also Orr, M. L., and Watt, B. K. *Amino acid content of foods. Home Eco. Res. Rep* No. 4, Superintendent of Documents, U.S. Government Printing Office, Washington, D.C., 1966; Csonka, F. A. "Amino acids in staple foods. I: Wheat *(Triticum vulgare)."* *Jour. Biol. Chem.,* 118:147, 1937; Albanese, A. A., ed., *Protein and amino acid nutrition.* New York: Academic, 1969, p. 18.

5   Wilcke, H. L. *Proceedings Amino Acid Conference.* MIT, Sept. 1969.

Wilcke found that the lowest-cost solution to the problem of completing the amino acid requirements in wheat protein was by adding pure lysine. Since it can now be purchased at $1.00 per pound, this was more economical than adding either animal or soy protein. For an excellent coverage of the procedure and need of fortifying wheat protein, see Altschul, A. M. "Amino acid fortification of foods." *Third Inter. Cong. Food Sci. & tech.,* SOS 70, Aug. 9–14, 1970.

6   Flink, E. B. "Magnesium deficiency syndrome in man." J.A.M.A., 160:1406, 1956; Vallee, B. L., et al. "The magnesium deficiency tetany syndrome in man." *New Eng. J. Med.,* 262:155, 1960; Tambascia, J. J. "Magnesium deficiency tetany syndrome in man." *J. Med. Soc. N.Y.,* 59:530, 1962; Shils, M. E. "Experimental human magnesium depletion: I. Clinical observations and blood chemistry alterations." *Am J. Clin. Nutr.,* 15:133, 1964.

7   *Recommended dietary allowances,* 1968. (7th rev. ed.) "A report of the Food and Nutrition Board, National Research Council." National Acad. Sci., Washington, D.C., 1968.

8   Czerniejewski, C. P., et al. "The minerals of wheat, flour and bread." *Cereal Chem.,* 41:65, 1964.

Also, in his article on the need for trace metal chromium in human nutrition, Schroeder accounts for part of the chromium deficiency in the tissues of Americans (based on a comparison with other peoples) as due to its removal in food processing, particularly in the refining of wheat. See Schroeder, H. A. "The role of chromium in mammalian nutrition." *Am J. Clin. Nutr.,* 21:230, 1968.

9   The data demonstrating this statement is extensive. One good study of this problem is found in Giok, L. T., Roxe, C. S., and Gyorgy, P. "Influence of early malnutrition on some aspects of the health of school-age children." *Am. J. Clin. Nutr.,* 20:1280, 1967.

10   Turner, J. S. (project director). *The chemical feast*. The Ralph Nader Study Group Report on Food Protection and the Food and Drug Administration. New York: Grossman, 1970.

11   *Eat to live*. Chicago, Ill.: Wheat Flour Institute, 1970.

|39| Some Constructive Ways to Improve Your Diet

CONSUMERS' RESEARCH

Consumers' Research is an independent, nonprofit scientific, technical, and educational nongovernmental public-service organization.

Reprinted from *Consumers' Research Magazine,* October 1976 (Vol. 51 of the Handbook of Buying Series), p. 62, by permission of Consumers' Research Inc. Copyright © 1976 by Consumers' Research, Inc., Washington, N.J. 07882.

The evidence at hand indicates that the consumer would do well to eliminate, so far as practicable, from his selection at the grocery store all of the following:

• Foods containing artificial colors (often labeled as "certified colors") and artificial flavors, and foods labeled as containing preservatives and other chemical additives and chemically modified substances (e.g., modified starch, hydrogenated or hardened oil).
• Steaks, so-called (made from beef "flakes" compressed to look like solid meat), and most foods made from mixes, including cakes, cookies, doughnuts, bread, etc.
• Uncooked or rare meat, or roast pork that is not fully cooked and has not reached an internal temperature of 170° at least (preferably a little higher). Bacteria or parasitic worms often present in meats and fish and not killed by the heat of broiling or baking can cause serious illness.
• Overfat meat, likely, in the case of beef, to be found in the prime and choice grades and in ground beef sold under various names, especially

hamburger (even when marked "extra lean" ground round), self-basting turkeys (wrong type of fat in the basting fluid). Lean meats, low-fat hamburger, and naturally fed poultry are available for many people willing to go to some trouble to obtain them. (Duck, inherently very fat, is best avoided.)
• Cured "meat products" and luncheon meats, so-called, especially chicken, turkey, and ham loaf, and similar products made and preserved with chemical additives and in no way comparable in flavor with the "real thing."

Coffee and Colas

There is a growing suspicion that the habitual drinking of coffee in which many millions of persons indulge many times every day has come to a point where the practice can be a distinct menace to health. The danger of harm exists not only to the large number of persons who for medical reasons should avoid coffee and caffeine-containing drinks such as Coca-Cola, Pepsi Cola and Dr. Pepper, but to the average typical American who is very likely not aware that coffee and caffeine are under suspicion as dangers to health.

Scientists have isolated in coffee a substance that contributes to hardening of the arteries, and so could tend to be a cause of heart attack. It is their view that the chlorogenic acid in coffee can interact with preservatives present in cheese, pork products, and some other foods to produce potent cancer-causing agents known as nitrosamines.

Caffeine in coffee stimulates acid secretion, and removing the caffeine in making decaffeinated instant coffee was found not to eliminate this action. Coffee has some unfavorable effects on health that cannot be accounted for on the basis of caffeine content alone, as is indicated by the fact that decaffeinated coffee has been found to affect coffee drinkers in the same unfavorable way as untreated coffee. It is known that decaffeinating coffee does not completely remove ingredients that cause undesirable effects on health and well-being.

Recent researches have shown that trichloroethylene, used in the process of decaffeinating coffee beans, is a cancer-inducing solvent. Some residues of the solvents used to extract caffeine (all are toxic) may be expected to remain in the finished product, or the solvent treatment will have caused unwholesome changes of some unknown kind in processing the coffee.

The average American consumes a

- Imitation dairy products (cheese spreads, imitation cream cheese, "coffee whiteners").*
- Potato chips, instant mashed potatoes, presweetened cereals, sherbets.
- Fried foods and all kinds of foods which have been subject to overheating

*EDITOR'S NOTE: It is often assumed that these products are high in polyunsaturates. They are not.

little over two cups a day, in the winter season, but some people, even physicians, drink as many as 10 or 15 cups a day, with effects that may be manifested as nausea, dizziness, irregular heartbeat, circulatory problems, restlessness, or instability. Coffee has been associated with heart attacks, high blood pressure, bladder cancer, and possibly birth defects. It has been shown to be associated with development of ulcers, with the risks higher in women. The xanthines in coffee may aggravate gout, and may present some hazard to the many persons on their way to becoming diabetic.

About 60% to 65% of the bottled soda consumed in the U.S. contains some caffeine; abnormalities termed "caffeinism" have been observed among young cola drinkers. . . . It would appear that few mothers are aware of the unsuitability of cola drinks, and they should not allow young children to drink coffee, tea, or any of the cola drinks. A 60-pound child drinking three colas would be taking an amount of caffeine about equivalent pharmacologically to a 175-pound man consuming 8 cups of coffee a day. Remember that caffeine is a common ingredient in drugs that people take when they want to stay awake.

. . . In one study in Utah and Idaho, data on reported problem pregnancies suggested that miscarriages, death of fetuses, and stillbirths could be associated with drinking coffee to excess. . . .

Many assume that cocoa is harmless and therefore may be given freely to children. This is not true, as a cup of cocoa may contain 50 mg of caffeine, not far below the amount in a cup of coffee and an amount that corresponds to an adult dose of caffeine as a medicine; such a dose is not at all suitable for the small body of a child. . . .

or charring, including French-fried foods of all kinds and burnt or blackened "charbroiled" steaks, hamburger, chops, chickens, etc.

• Breads made with bleached flour, or with cake flour, commonly used in fancy breadstuffs. (Bread made of the preferable unbleached flour tends to have a grayish rather than a pure white tint.)

• Foods that do not clearly specify the ingredients used, or that use initials instead of the full name for some (e.g., BHT for butylated hydroxytoluene), and any and all foods and beverages, ice cream, sherbet, puddings, cakes, soft drinks, etc., that are labeled as containing artificial color (actually coal-tar dyes), often described on labels as "certified" food color.

• Mushrooms to which a preservative has been applied (e.g., sodium bisulfite).

• Foods high in fat, starch, and sugar, including crackers, cookies, sweet cakes, sugared buns, Danish pastry, and all fancy desserts and pastries.

• Prepared and convenience foods labeled as containing hydrogenated (hardened) fat, vegetable gums, monosodium glutamate, disodium inosinate and guanylate, brominated oil, imitation butter flavor, diacetyl, propylene glycol, ethylenediamine tetraacetic acid.

Good nutrition depends far less on how many dollars we spend than upon the good sense and discrimination we use in our purchasing at food stores. A final word: *get the habit of reading food labels;* they are often so placed and in such typefaces as to make them hard to read. They will faze you at first (many are meant to), but with experience and a little study you can learn from them what not to buy for [your] health. . . .

|40| On Food— and the American Psyche

ELIZABETH KENDALL

Elizabeth Kendall, who writes mainly on the dance, recently contributed two scripts to the WNET "Dance in America" series. She is now completing a book on how modern dance emerged out of American culture over the years 1900–1931.

Reprinted from *Mademoiselle,* December 1974, pp. 40, 48, and 57, by permission. Copyright © 1974 by The Condé Nast Publications, Inc.; reassigned, 1978, to Elizabeth Kendall.

Traveling south on the train from Paris to Nimes, I found an article on dieting in *Elle,* a French women's magazine. Attracted to all diet articles, I began to read. "When someone eats," the French nutritionist writes, "she doesn't nourish just her body, but also her appetite, her heart, her memory." That is a surprising thing to hear about the subject of dieting. An American article about the same thing stresses duty; dieting becomes something unpleasant but necessary for one's "image," and advice is in the form of gimmicks, rewards, and self-conscious jokes. Jean Trémolières, this nutritionist (actually a philosopher, I think), talks about diet in the context of his own culture, with its profound respect for taste and the institution called "a meal." He notices a growing anxiety about weight among the women in France, feels it goes against their cultural roots, and warns readers they are being "brutalized" by the media's version of the ideal, ultra-skinny woman. Wishing for an ideal shape is an adolescent's disease, he says, and we are far too preoccupied by that wish. He compares a woman (or anyone) trying to learn a new system of eating to a centipede who can't remember which of his thousand feet to run away on. A person used to eat what was right for him or her through instinct; it used to be a "natural impulse to accept oneself."

That impulse is long gone in America, or at least among the women I grew up with. It is normal to find one's appearance wrong, all wrong. I began dieting, typically, around the age of 11, and then entered the dance world, which is filled with people who are hypersensitive to food. One learns a lot on the diet circuit about black moods and despair over broken resolves.

At this point I am beginning to think that the only workable approach is to calm down.

That is why the common sense of Trémolières' article was such a relief to read. He claims that dieting is not possible without real awareness of what you are doing when you eat. Enjoy taste, he says, experience food as material for your flesh, rather than as fuel or party favors. But is that possible to do, or are we traumatized about our food? Myself, I am deathly afraid of eating too much. That fear is ridiculous since I am not "fat"—and yet every woman I know is similarly afraid. So many times we say to ourselves or to each other that we have been "bad" or "virtuous"—a clue that if Puritanism is fading on some cultural fronts, it is a vital force among women dieters in this country. It's not so much that fear of damnation actually prevents us from overeating; it's rebelling against imagined restrictions that blocks our true taste. When I eat something I don't want to eat, like a piece of cake, I don't taste *it,* just its forbidden-ness. Preconceiving the food had destroyed its gut effect.

This failure to taste in depth is what links dieting to American problems about food in general. The food subject preys on the public mind nowadays. Everyone seems to be restlessly searching for a new diet, and so we have millions of new health food stores, earth bookbooks, TV interviews with vitamin experts, etc. We are acting as though we have inherited no guidelines, as though the American way of eating has been all wrong and the only thing to do is start all over again. The French moderation and tradition-sense gave me a new focus. I started wondering about what in our national culture makes us so disturbed about food.

We accuse ourselves of too much pill-taking, of ministering to ourselves without waiting to hear what our bodies are saying. We eat the same way—Alka-Seltzer on top of spaghetti. The demand is for the shallow sensations, the ones you don't have to wait for. In fact, refusal to wait might be a main cause of this awful mediocrity in our food. We never wait to really sense what happens to food below the neck. We spring up from the table—on to the next activity. Only a few of the dancers I know and some wise souls who keep company with their instincts, have a real physiological dialogue with their food.

I was watching the French this summer, who have an inherited diet and eating routine: a small breakfast on getting up, then many-coursed meals at "midi" and "soir." At those sacred hours even the autoroutes are empty of cars because French people of all ages are eating a French meal and taking their time about it. No one ever imagines tampering with the basic ingredients of the meal. Two of my French friends, unconventional in most things, were astonished when I put a piece of cheese on a cookie. The American "anything goes" approach to food is not at all the kind of exploring a French person may do with taste. To be daring in French food terms means to experiment among the tiniest mutations, watched over by one's ancestors, by the literary guardians of the French culinary tradition and by one's own finely tuned instincts.

In my American childhood there was nothing sacred about food, although we middle-class suburbans had a rough sort of system and even some essentials—hamburgers, frozen vegetables, boxed desserts. (That is still the diet in suburbs like mine. Last year I polled some high school and junior high classes in Newton, Massachusetts; almost every child liked those same foods and thought they were the right foods to eat.) But our eating habits had none of the force of a tradition, because individual whims always counted for more. If you liked pizza for breakfast, that was fine. No one's (almost no one's) taste was offended. The spirit of mixing was a large part of the way we ate. People appreciated things like outlandish sandwiches: banana, peanut and Marshmallow Fluff, a grim example which has undoubtedly been eaten many times. We have also borrowed from other cultures, so that pizza, chop suey, Polish sausage seem "American" by now and you can buy them frozen.

But food "pragmatism" causes a vast confusion when middle-class children leave the suburban refrigerators for good. Our diets go haywire. A random sampling right now of eating habits among 20- to 25-year-olds in places like Berkeley or Cambridge (those are the extremes) reveals a circus. Someone eats only raw foods, someone eats only cooked vegetables and grains, someone else eats only meat and eggs, someone eats pizza exclusively, someone eats nothing but ice cream, someone eats all grapes, someone is fasting. Nor are there any recognized meal times—meeting to eat is hard because no one's meals are synchronized with anyone else's. The whole spectrum is pure chaos.

Everyone is lamenting about how far away push-button nutrition has brought us from our biological roots, but the talk is nothing—the realization has to be experienced. Once in Nice I came across a crockery jar in a friend's cupboard—it was a special kind of local mustard with the seeds still in it—and I suddenly understood that mustard grows. It's a plant, not a yellow substance manufactured for hot dogs. The French mustard looked and tasted like part of the cycle of growing and dying things on this earth, which includes me since I ate it. That is how food must have been, once.

So we are searching for simple needs and real organic food. But the search is not sensible, because we are spending large amounts of energy trying to forget the food we were raised with. I wonder if you can do that. It is a pleasure to discover Swiss chard and sunflower seeds, but what about the fact that came out of the French article: that we eat foods as symbols while we are eating it for nourishment? It's true. I can't deny that every time I'm sick I feel like eating a certain breakfast cereal—even though another me now refuses to touch that cereal since it is made of worthless refined flour with four arbitrary vitamins pumped in. Anyone who tries to feel sentimental about familiar foods like breakfast cereals or Hostess Twinkies has to deal with a fond taste for packaged nothing.

But the package-taste is there. My first morning home from France I ate a soggy grilled corn muffin in a 23rd St. café. It tasted really good. It tasted like all the funky, worthless stuff we swallow in this country and still manage to get through the day fairly cheerfully. A taste is like an emotion—you can't pretend it doesn't exist. You can only pay more attention to it and try to figure out why it's there. It probably belongs to the stubborn nostalgia for a middle-class childhood—which after all everyone has a right to feel.

But everyone also has the right to something more essential—health. We each need to find a system of eating that works, and mine (when I find it) will be slightly different from anybody else's. Whether dieting or just trying to be healthy, we walk a thin line between two impulses. It is easy to sink back into the synthetic foods that our non-tradition has prepared us for. It is even easy to do the opposite—throw out all those familiar foods and become affected by pure ingredients and no more animal flesh. The hard thing to do is to forget the conditioning, really examine traditions and needs and listen to our bodies. The search for the right foods is very long, and harder I think for Americans than for the French, who have pride in their own nutritional history. We need to hear calm and thorough advice. We need to stop being told we are neurotic. We need more information and fewer evangelical cure-alls. We need to believe we ourselves can do the choosing.